Principles of Facial Reconstruction

A Subunit Approach to Cutaneous Repair

Third Edition

Thieme

Principles of Facial Reconstruction

A Subunit Approach to Cutaneous Repair

Third Edition

Wayne F. Larrabee Jr., MD, MSH
Clinical Professor of Facial Plastic Surgery
Department of Otolaryngology—Head and Neck Surgery
University of Washington;
Director
Larrabee Center for Facial Plastic Surgery
Seattle, Washington, USA

David A. Sherris, MD
Professor and Chairman
Department of Otolaryngology
Jacobs School of Medicine
University at Buffalo
Buffalo, New York, USA

Jeffrey C. Teixeira, MD, MBA
Assistant Professor
Department of Surgery
Uniformed Services University of the Health Sciences
Bethesda, Maryland, USA

Kate Sweeney
Medical Illustrator

501 illustrations

Thieme
New York • Stuttgart • Delhi • Rio de Janeiro

Library of Congress Cataloging-in-Publication Data
is available from the publisher.

Important note: Medicine is an ever-changing science undergoing continual development. Research and clinical experience are continually expanding our knowledge, in particular our knowledge of proper treatment and drug therapy. Insofar as this book mentions any dosage or application, readers may rest assured that the authors, editors, and publishers have made every effort to ensure that such references are in accordance with **the state of knowledge at the time of production of the book.**

Nevertheless, this does not involve, imply, or express any guarantee or responsibility on the part of the publishers in respect to any dosage instructions and forms of applications stated in the book. **Every user is requested to examine carefully** the manufacturers' leaflets accompanying each drug and to check, if necessary in consultation with a physician or specialist, whether the dosage schedules mentioned therein or the contraindications stated by the manufacturers differ from the statements made in the present book. Such examination is particularly important with drugs that are either rarely used or have been newly released on the market. Every dosage schedule or every form of application used is entirely at the user's own risk and responsibility. The authors and publishers request every user to report to the publishers any discrepancies or inaccuracies noticed. If errors in this work are found after publication, errata will be posted at www.thieme.com on the product description page.

Some of the product names, patents, and registered designs referred to in this book are in fact registered trademarks or proprietary names even though specific reference to this fact is not always made in the text. Therefore, the appearance of a name without designation as proprietary is not to be construed as a representation by the publisher that it is in the public domain.

Thieme addresses people of all gender identities equally. We encourage our authors to use gender-neutral or gender-equal expressions wherever the context allows.

Thieme Medical Publishers, Inc.
333 Seventh Avenue, 18th Floor
New York, NY 10001, USA
www.thieme.com
+1 800 782 3488, customerservice@thieme.com

Cover design: © Thieme
Cover image source: © Kate Sweeney
Typesetting by Thomson Digital, India

Printed in USA by King Printing Company, Inc. 5 4 3 2 1

ISBN 978-1-68420-106-8

Also available as an e-book:
eISBN 978-1-68420-107-5

I dedicate this third edition to my wife Amy and my son Gregory who have been always supportive of my reconstructive projects with Global Surgical Outreach.

Wayne F. Larrabee Jr., MD, MSH

I dedicate this third edition to Doris M. Jones, an inspiration throughout my life.

David A. Sherris, MD

I dedicate this to my husband, Tim, and my family for the continuous support throughout this journey.

Jeffrey C. Teixeira, MD, MBA

Contents

Preface

Our goal in this third edition of *Principles of Facial Reconstruction: A Subunit Approach to Cutaneous Repair* is to present a guide to reliable, effective techniques of facial reconstruction. We have emphasized key surgical principles in a clear, graphically consistent manner. Rather than presenting a menu of many possible techniques for each problem, we have selected one or two that have proven most effective and reliable in our hands. The defect sizes deemed appropriate for each flap are only meant as guidelines for less experienced surgeons. Obviously, this approach leads to some necessary oversimplifications, and many patients will not fit exactly into the confines of our flow diagrams. The clinical experience of the senior surgeon, as always, is required to develop a surgical plan for an individual patient. Because our readers are already accomplished surgeons, we have concentrated our efforts on which approach to select for a given facial defect and on sharing specific technical points we have found useful.

It will be noted that we have emphasized the facial aesthetic units and subunits throughout. This organizing principle is conceptually important, although its significance is greater in some units (the nose) than in others (the cheek). Certain conventions have been followed for consistency. Examples of these conventions are provided on the opposite page.

There are a number of excellent, comprehensive books available on flap repair. We have not attempted to duplicate those. We have elected to concentrate on soft tissue defects of moderate size and have therefore excluded discussions of larger flap reconstructions, including free flaps, repair of structures such as the facial nerve, and hard tissue repair.

Acknowledgments

We have involved a number of experienced and respected facial surgeons in algorithm evaluation. Although the final choices rested with the three editors, we acknowledge the great assistance provided by Drs. Peter Hilger, Holger Gassner, Ferdinand Becker, Ted Cook, Vito Quatela, J. Regan Thomas, Ritchie Younger, and John Zitelli. The illustrations and computer graphics were developed by Kate Sweeney; the quality of her efforts is self-evident. Thanks to Prakash Naorem, our editor at Thieme Medical Publishers, for his enthusiasm and interest in getting this new edition published. We also wish to express our appreciation to Dr. Amit Bhrany, J. Timothy Heffernan, Craig S. Murakami, and Bryan S. Sires for the outstanding clinical photographs they have contributed to this new edition. Finally, thanks to our contributors for their commitment to this project.

Wayne F. Larrabee Jr., MD, MSH
David A. Sherris, MD
Jeffrey C. Teixeira, MD, MBA

Illustration Key

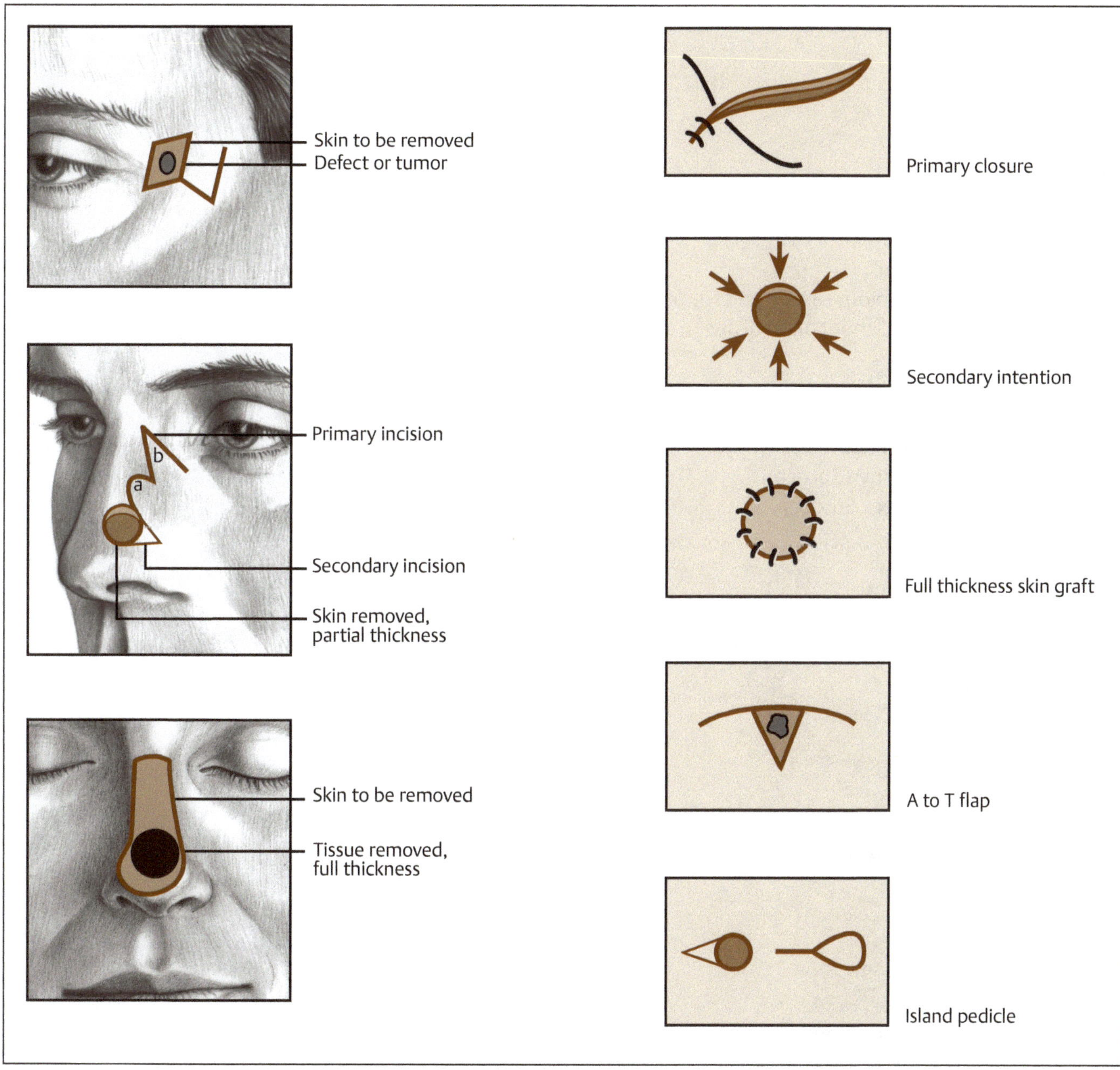

Contributors

Amit Bhrany, MD
Clinical Associate Professor
Department of Otolaryngology—Head and Neck Surgery
University of Washington School of Medicine
Seattle, Washington, USA

Kathleyn Brandstetter, MD
Facial Plastic & Reconstructive Surgeon
Department of Head & Neck Surgery
Kaiser Permanente
San Leandro Medical Center
San Leandro, California, USA

Craig Cupp, MD, EdD
Facial Plastic & Reconstructive Surgeon
Franciscan Medical Group
Gig Harbor, Washington, USA

J. Timothy Heffernan, MD
Oculoplastic Surgeon
Swedish Hospital
Seattle, Washington, USA

Wayne F. Larrabee Jr., MD, MSH
Clinical Professor of Facial Plastic Surgery
Department of Otolaryngology—Head and Neck Surgery
University of Washington;
Director
Larrabee Center for Facial Plastic Surgery
Seattle, Washington, USA

Craig S. Murakami, MD
Clinical Associate Professor
Facial Plastic Surgery
Department of Otolaryngology—Head and Neck Surgery
Virginia Mason Medical Center
Seattle, Washington, USA

David A. Sherris, MD
Professor and Chairman
Department of Otolaryngology
Jacobs School of Medicine
University at Buffalo
Buffalo, New York, USA

Bryan S. Sires, MD, PhD
Clinical Associate Professor
Allure Facial Laser Center and Medispa
Department of Ophthalmology
University of Washington
Kirkland, Washington, USA

Jeffrey C. Teixeira, MD, MBA
Assistant Professor
Department of Surgery
Uniformed Services University of the Health Sciences
Bethesda, Maryland, USA

1 Soft Tissue Biomechanics and Physiology

Summary

This chapter focuses on the biomechanical properties of the skin with respect to wound healing, importance of the aesthetic units and subunits of the face with respect to reconstruction, as well as the importance of relaxed skin tension lines with respect to design or your repair.

Keywords: biomechanics, subunits, relaxed skin tension lines, creep, wound healing, wound breaking strength

An understanding of the biomechanics of soft tissue, the vascular supply to skin flaps, the aesthetic units and subunits of the face, and the relaxed skin tension lines of the face is important in the design of an effective repair for a specific facial defect.

Skin is anisotropic and nonlinear and has time-dependent properties. Anisotropic means that the skin's mechanical properties vary with direction. Relaxed skin tension lines (RSTLs) are the lines of minimal tension of the skin; incisions parallel to them are under the least possible tension while healing (**Fig. 1.1**). Perpendicular to the RSTLs are the lines of maximal extensibility (LMEs). A fusiform excision made parallel to the RTSLs and closed in the direction of the LMEs will result in the least closing tension and the best scar.

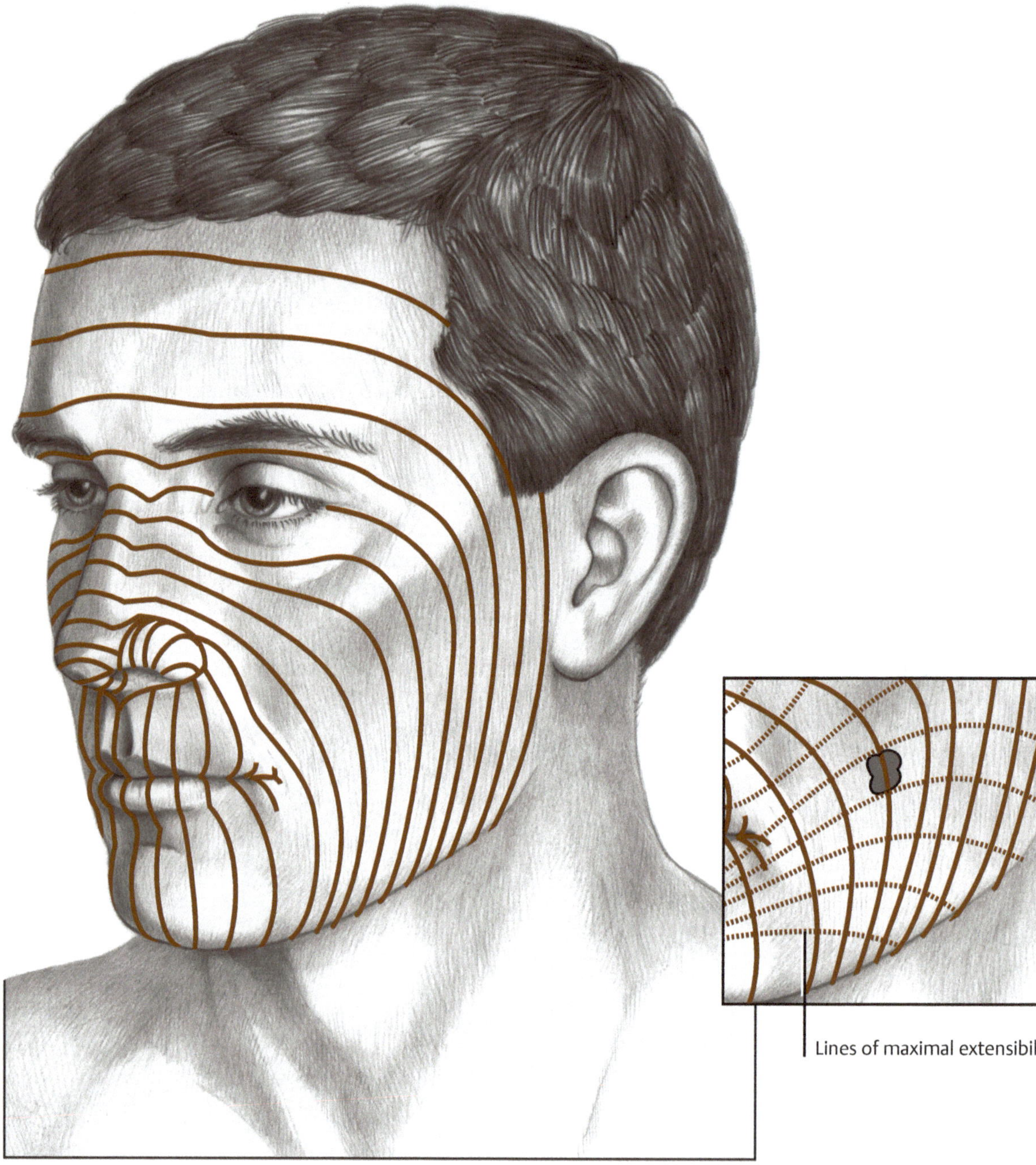

Fig. 1.1 Relaxed skin tension lines and lines of maximal extensibility.

Skin is nonlinear; as it is stretched, progressively more force is required to deform it. These changes are typically described as a stress–strain curve, where stress represents force per unit area, and strain represents the change in length divided by the original length (**Fig. 1.2**). In section I of the curve, a relatively small stress produces a large strain. This section of the curve corresponds primarily to the deformation of the delicate elastic fiber network; the loss of these fibers with age or sun exposure results in a shift of the curve to the right. In section II of the curve, a progressively larger amount of force is required to stretch the skin, which correlates with a progressive change in orientation of the collagen fibers, from relatively random orientation to one parallel to the direction of the force. In section III of the curve, a large amount of force is required to obtain any increased length. The tension required to recruit more tissue at this point in the stress–strain curve is detrimental to wound healing and should be avoided by turning to other solutions, such as skin flaps or grafts, rather than primary closure.

Skin has time-dependent properties and is not totally elastic. Repeated stretching of a section of skin results in a response change termed "hysteresis," in which the stress–strain curves are shifted to the right. Stress relaxation describes the decrease in skin tension seen over time if a segment of skin is stretched to a given length and maintained at that length. Creep describes the increase in length of skin seen over time when a given tension is applied to that segment of skin. The histologic and physiologic changes associated with creep are realignment of collagen fibers to a parallel orientation, fragmentation of elastic fibers, tissue dehydration by the displacement of fluid, and a migration of tissue in the direction of the vector of applied force. These properties are used in immediate tissue expansion. New skin is not formed in this procedure; rather, existing skin is recruited to allow moderate-sized defects to be closed with less tension.

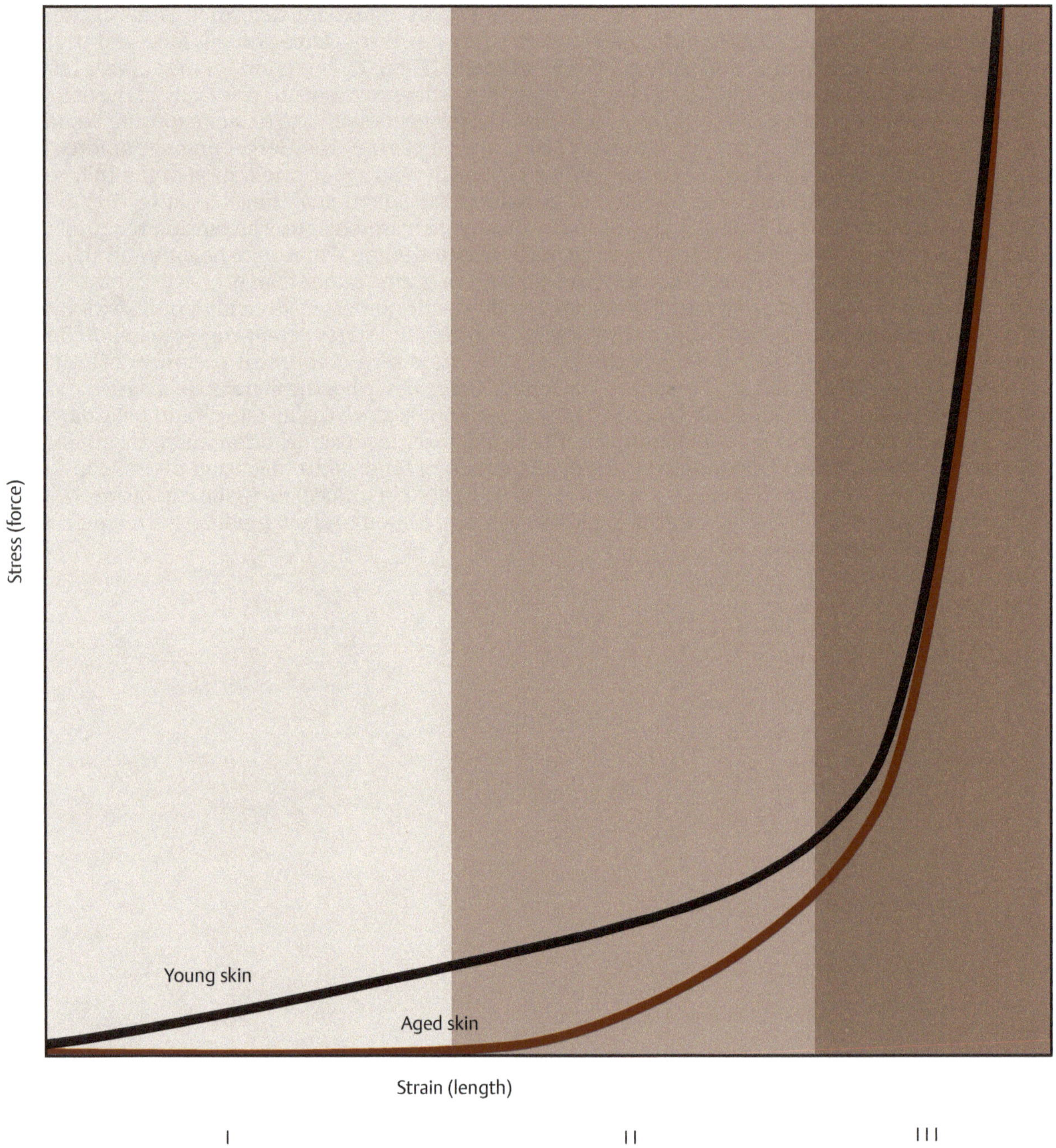

Fig. 1.2 Stress–strain curve for young and aged skin.

The abundant vascularity of the facial soft tissues allows for creative reconstructive possibilities. The subdermal plexus provides the vascular supply for the majority of the local flaps discussed in this book. Musculocutaneous and septocutaneous vessels can occasionally be incorporated in the flaps to further increase the blood flow.

Wound-closing tension is a key variable in wound healing. Excess closing tension can result in wound slough, due to decreased blood flow in flaps of borderline viability. Wounds closed under tension are more prone to hypertrophic scar formation. In addition, certain areas of the face, such as the upper lip and mandibular line, are prone to develop wide or hypertrophic scars. This propensity is probably due to underlying muscular movement, causing increased wound tension during healing. Of note, recent studies have demonstrated that when the musculature underlying an incision in the forehead is injected with botulinum toxin type A at the time of wound closure or shortly thereafter, the scar that results is of superior cosmetic appearance. This finding has been proven for the forehead in a blinded trial, and one would speculate it to be true in other incision sites where the movement of underlying musculature may cause wide or hypertrophic scars. The mechanism of effect is tempaorary paralysis of the surrounding musculature to decrease the tension on the wound during the critical first 2 to 3 months of healing. When using botulinum toxin type A, the surgeon must take care not to effect important functions adversely for the sake of a better scar. Risks must be discussed with the patient prior to using this technique of wound immobilization. Since our previous edition, further studies continue to show improvement in scar appearance with the additional use of botulinum toxin type A for facial scars to include cleft lip repair. Further studies are underway in the use of botulinum toxin type A with other scar reducing modalities such as laser therapy. At this time, botulinum toxin type A use in the prevention of hypertrophic or keloid scar is undeniable with minimal risk or adverse reactions as seen with intralesional steroid injections such as skin atrophy or telangiectesia. Finally, wound-closing tension can distort other local landmarks, such as the eyelid, ala, vermilion, and brow. These distortions are often temporary, but judicious use of flaps when primary closure results in distortion of local structures is an important concept.

Wound-breaking strength is a measure of the force necessary to separate the edges of a fresh wound and is minimal until day 7 (**Fig. 1.3**). In fact, the tensile strength of a wound never exceeds 80% of normal skin. A long-lasting absorbable or permanent subcutaneous suture closure is imperative to relieve tension over time and prevent scar widening during healing.

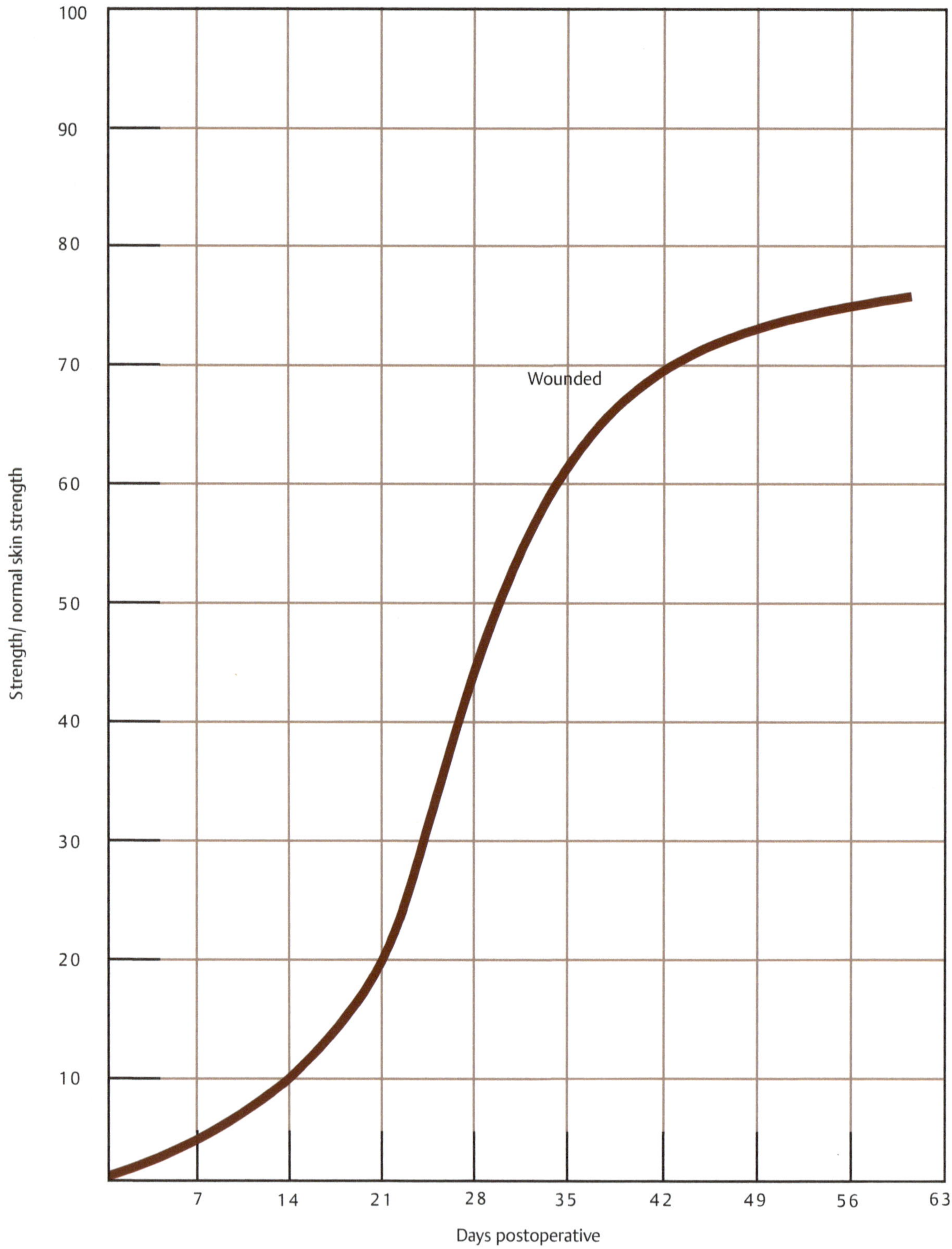

Fig. 1.3 Wound-breaking strength. Adapted with permission from Levenson SM, Geever EF, Crowley LV, Oates JF, Berard CW, Rosen H. The healing of rat skin wounds. Ann Surg 1965;161:293–308.

The face is divided into aesthetic units, which are further divided into subunits (**Fig. 1.4**). The units and subunits are based on skin thickness, color, elasticity, and underlying structural contours. Precise planning of a facial reconstructive procedure requires analysis of the size and location of a defect in relation to the entirety of the involved subunit or subunits. Incisions parallel to RSTLs, within unit or subunit borders, and in the midline of the face result in the least perceptible scars.

The following chapters represent our approach to reconstruction of the face based on aesthetic units and subunits. The aesthetic units are generally best reconstructed with tissue from the same unit. This similar tissue provides the best color, thickness, and texture match to that which has been lost. When defects are too large to reconstruct from the same aesthetic unit, tissue from surrounding units is generally recruited. Local skin flaps will generally provide the most appropriate tissue match.

Suggested Reading

Baker SR. Fundamentals of expanded tissue. Head Neck 1991;13(4):327–333

Baker SR, Swanson NA. Local flaps in facial reconstruction. St. Louis: CV Mosby; 1995

Borges AF. Elective incisions and scar revision. Boston: Little, Brown; 1973

Borges AF. Relaxed skin tension lines. Dermatol Clin 1989;7(1):169–177

Borges AF. Relaxed skin tension lines (RSTL) versus other skin lines. Plast Reconstr Surg 1984;73(1):144–150

Carrero K, Martin L, MA W, LIN HF, Yin XF, Zhou BB. Botulinum toxin type A for the treatment and prevention of hypertrophic scars and keloids: Updated Reveiw. J Cosmet Dermatol 2019; 18(1): 10-15

Dzubow LM, Zack L. The principle of cosmetic junctions as applied to reconstruction of defects following Mohs surgery. J Dermatol Surg Oncol 1990;16(4):353–355

Gonzalez-Ulloa M, Castillo A, Stevens E, Alvarez Fuertes G, Leonelli F, Ubaldo F. Preliminary study of the total restoration of the facial skin. Plast Reconstr Surg (1946) 1954;13(3):151–161

Larrabee WF Jr. Design of local skin flaps. Otolaryngol Clin North Am 1990;23(5):899–923

Levenson SM, Geever EF, Crowley LV, Oates JF III, Berard CW, Rosen H. The healing of rat skin wounds. Ann Surg 1965;161:293–308

McGregor IA. Local skin flaps in facial reconstruction. Otolaryngol Clin North Am 1982;15(1):77–98

Peacock EE. Wound repair. 3rd ed. Philadelphia: WB Saunders; 1984

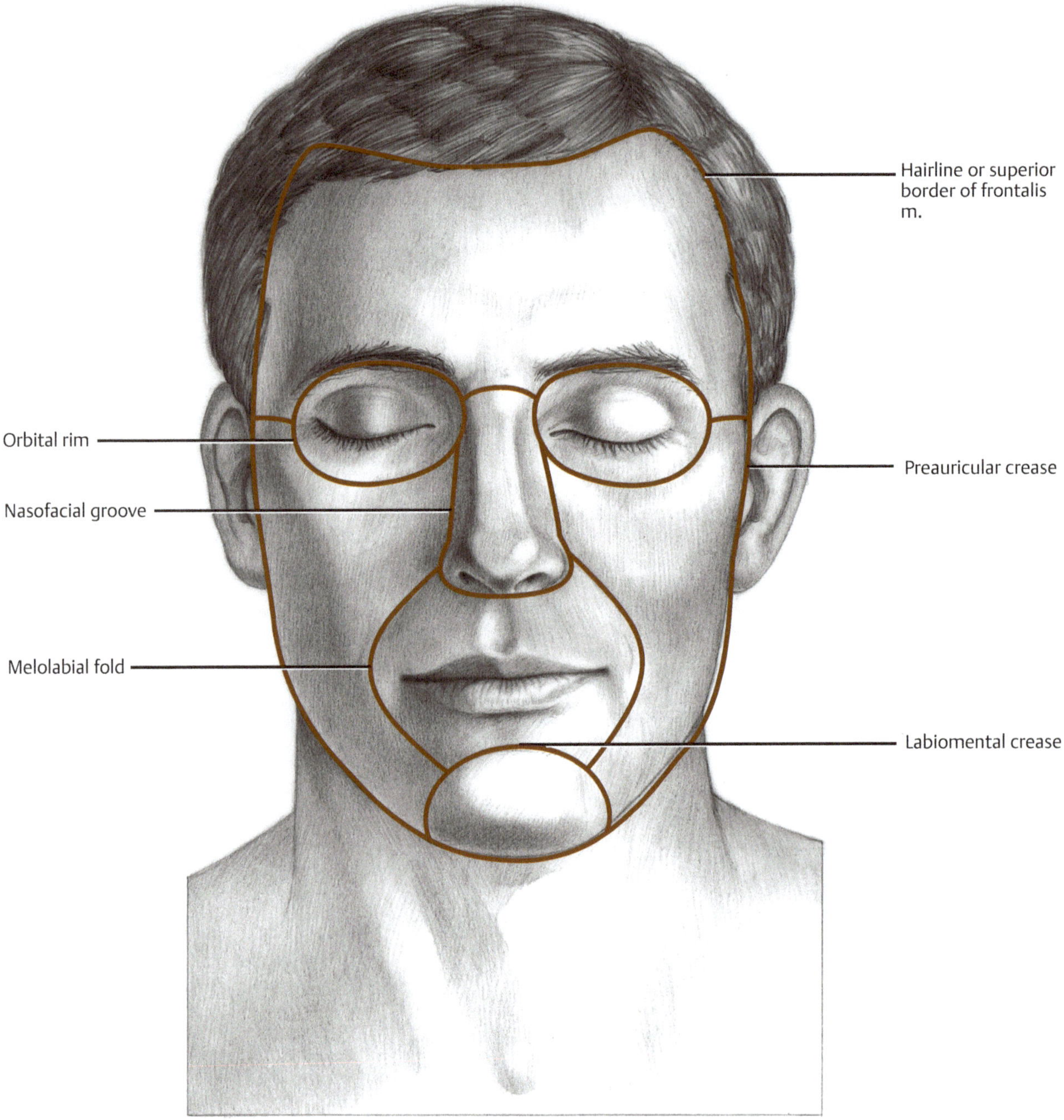

Fig. 1.4 Aesthetic units of the face.

2 Fundamental Techniques

Summary

This chapter reviews such techniques employed in facial reconstruction covering wound closure and care, defect shape, healing by secondary intention, skin and composite grafts, various flaps (advancement, rotation, rhombic, bilobed, and note), Z-plasty, and dermabrasion.

Keywords: skin graft, composite graft, wound closure, secondary intention, advancement flap, rotation flap, rhombic flap, Z-plasty, bilobed flap

♦ Wound Closure

Proper wound closure starts with the initial incision. Incisions should be perpendicular to the skin, except in areas like the scalp, where they are beveled to prevent hair follicle damage (**Fig. 2.1**). Consult Sherris and Kern's *Essential Surgical Skills* (see Suggested Reading) for an in-depth evaluation and hands-on pointers on wound closure techniques. That book especially is useful to the younger student of surgery and will work as an adjunct to the contents of this book. Pearls of wound closure and handling are mentioned in the pages that follow.

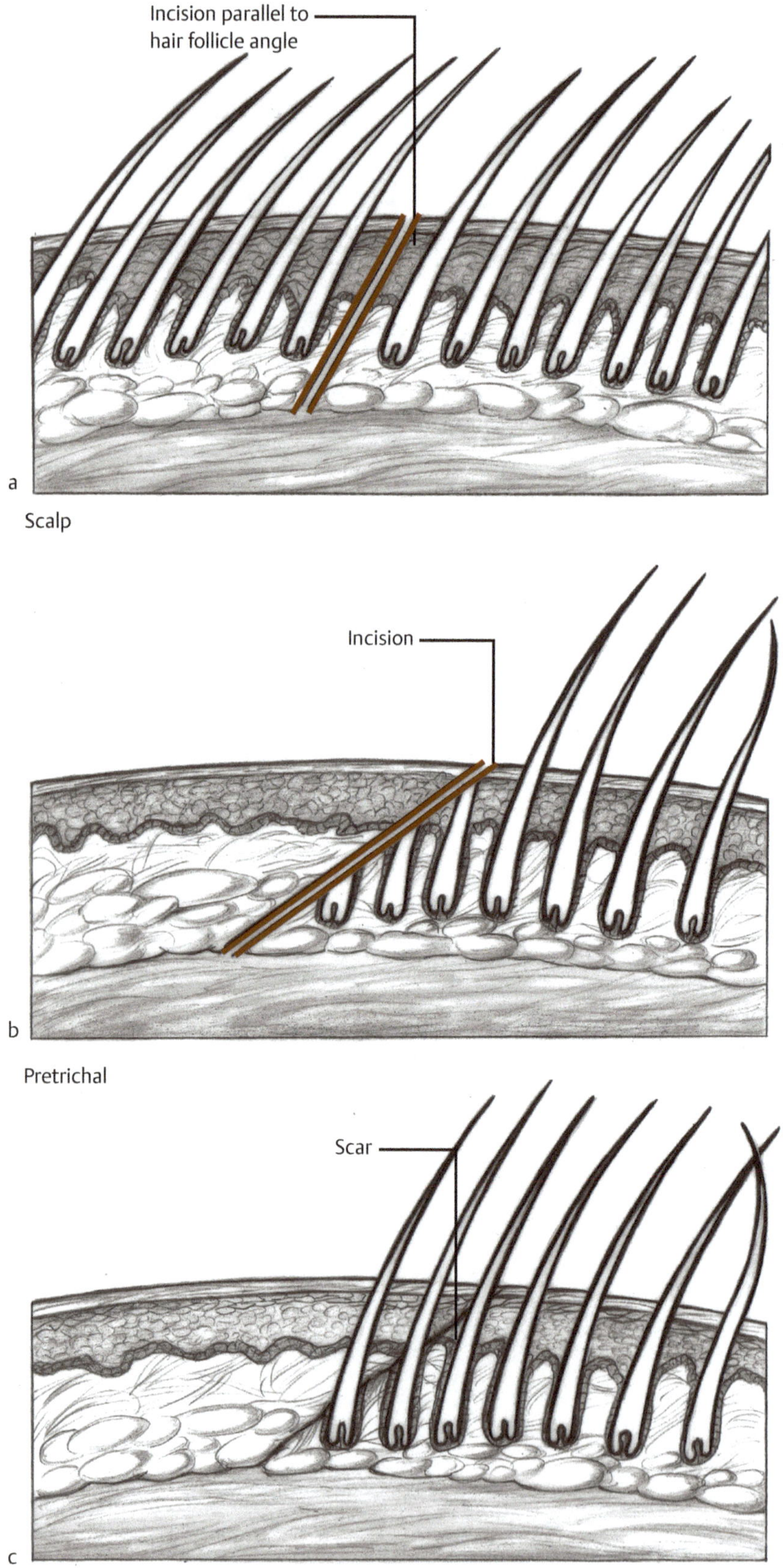

Fig. 2.1 Incisions (**a**) within the hair and (**b**) the hairline and (**c**) growth of hair through the scar.

The deep layers of the flap are closed with absorbable suture at the dermal and/or subcutaneous level (**Fig. 2.2**). The deep closure decreases wound-closing tension, decreases dead space in the wound, and aids in eversion at the skin edge. The skin edge is closed with 5–0 to 7–0 nonabsorbable suture, initiated with the needle perpendicular to the skin. Staples can be used in closure of the hair-bearing scalp after galeal closure.

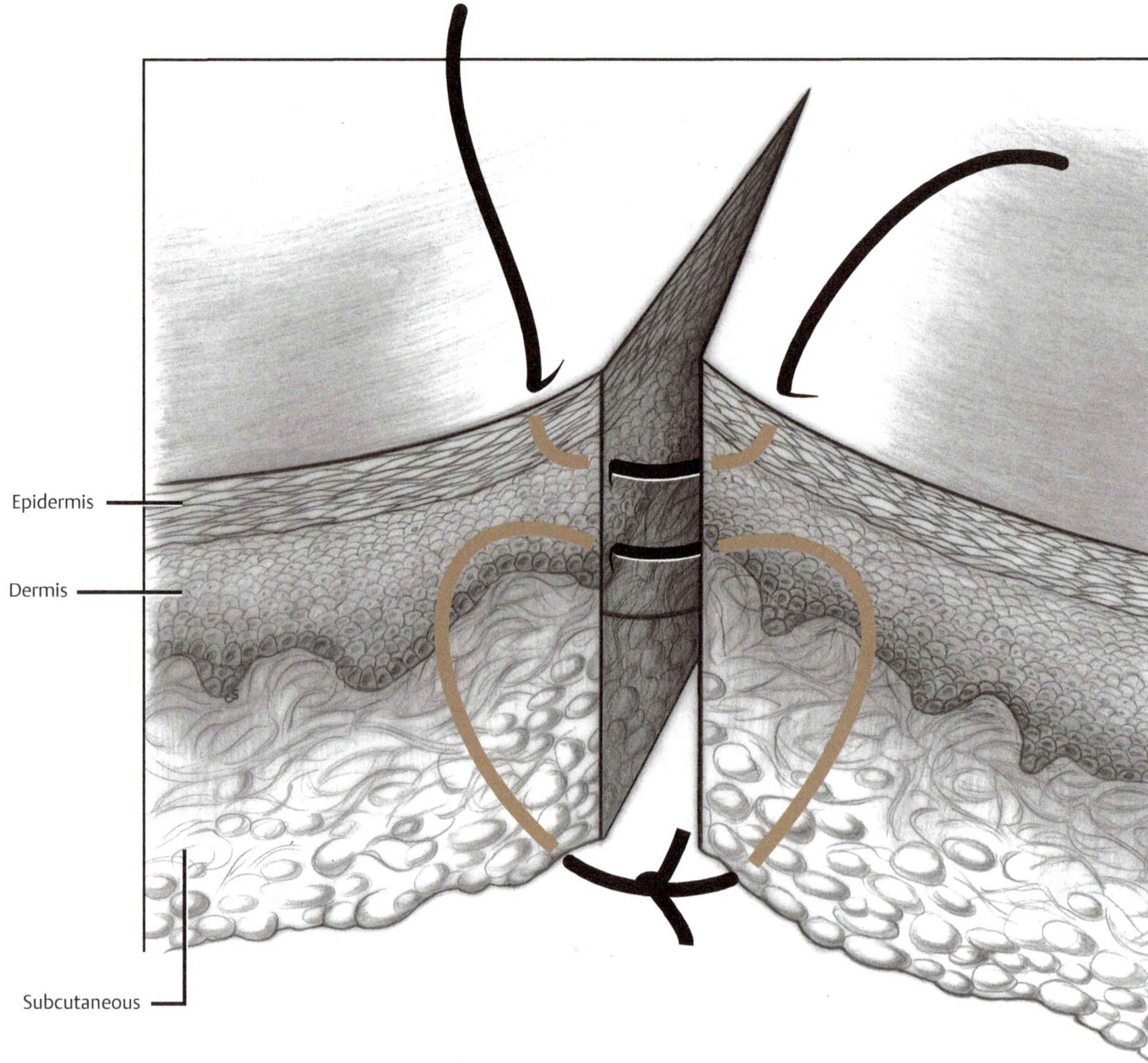

Fig. 2.2 Suture placement.

Standing cone or "dog-ear" deformities commonly occur during flap inset and skin closure (**Fig. 2.3**). A Burow triangle must be excised to treat these deformities. The simplest method is to hold the cone under slight upward tension and make the first skin cut from the base of the redundant tissue to the apex of the wound, approximately paralleling the relaxed skin tension lines (RSTLs). The excess tissue of the other side is then overlapped and excised.

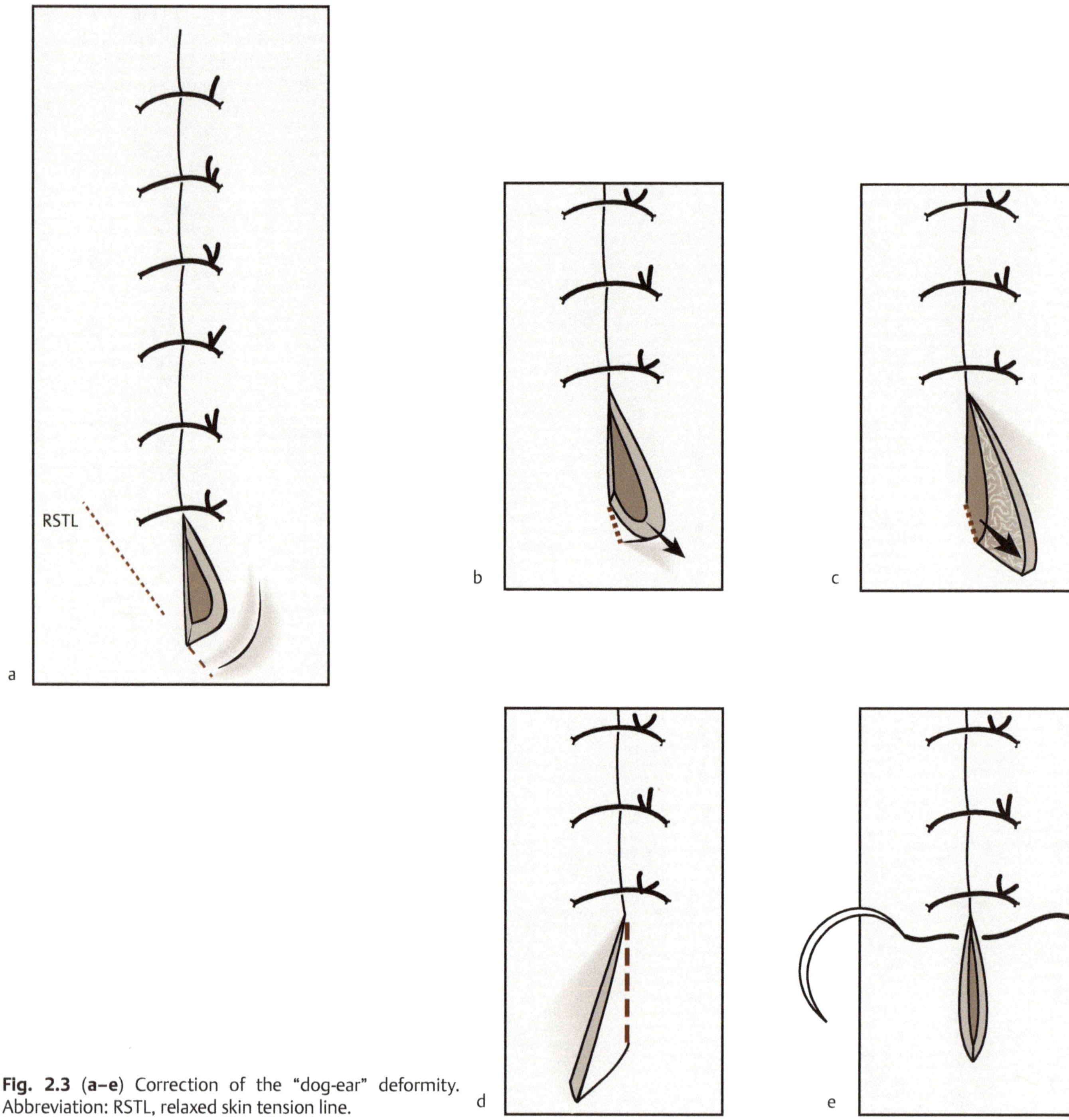

Fig. 2.3 (**a–e**) Correction of the "dog-ear" deformity. Abbreviation: RSTL, relaxed skin tension line.

♦ Wound Care

The suture line is typically coated with antibiotic ointment and covered with a nonadhesive gauze. Slight pressure can be obtained by taping the wound with paper or elastic tape.

Nasal wounds are treated with a rhinoplasty dressing to prevent hematoma formation and to aid in redraping of the skin–soft tissue envelope. The rhinoplasty dressing we employ is a paper tape attached with Mastisol, then cloth tape, and finally covered with an Aquaplast cast. The advantage of this dressing is that the cast is pliable at application and can be easily detached with minimal soft tissue envelope disruption by pouring Detachol directly onto the dressing.

Wound dressing can be removed in 24 to 48 hours, though nasal casts are usually removed at the time of suture removal. After dressing removal, the suture line is cleaned with hydrogen peroxide and coated with an antibiotic ointment three times per day.

Skin sutures of the face can typically be removed at day 4 to 6. Sutures of the eyelid skin can be removed at day 3 to 5, and sutures of the hair-bearing scalp at day 7 to 10. Wounds are sometimes reinforced with Mastisol and Steri-Strips for an additional week after suture removal. If the wound is under significant tension, then sutures should be left in longer, with the understanding that the likelihood of suture marks is increased.

If there is concern for hypertrophic scarring or keloid formation, then silicone gel sheeting is applied to the wound either immediately or after suture removal. Patients are instructed to use the sheeting as long as possible each day and definitely at night for 2 to 3 months. Patients are monitored in the postoperative period, and triamcinolone is injected into the scar at 4- to 6-week intervals to help prevent these untoward events.

♦ Defect Shape

Most cutaneous defects resulting from Mohs chemosurgery are approximately circular in shape. The technique of Mohs excision also results in saucerized defects with beveled edges. The descriptions of flap designs that follow are based on a variety of defect shapes, including triangular, equilateral parallelogram, and circular. Many times the best flap design available for a given defect corresponds to a different shape than the original defect. One commonly has to remove some normal tissue and convert the defect into a larger, though more appropriately shaped, defect for proper flap closure. Flap design and drawing on the patient with a marking pen should be completed prior to removal of any normal tissue that results in a larger defect. Generally, the flaps are transferred to close the donor site, and only then is the normal tissue excised. Even if the defect shape is appropriate for the planned flap, a 1- to 2-mm edge of the wound is usually excised in a perpendicular fashion for better wound closure.

♦ Healing by Secondary Intention

Defects in concave regions of the face heal favorably by secondary intention (**Fig. 2.4**). These areas include concave surfaces of the ear and nose, the temporal forehead, the glabellar region, the medial canthal subunit, the perialar/melolabial fold, and the philtral subunit of the lip. Large defects may be partially closed with local tissue advancement or "purse-string" sutures to decrease the area of the defect, thereby decreasing healing time. In areas with exposed cartilage, such as the auricle, small stab incisions or dermal punch excisions can be performed to allow granulation tissue from the opposite side of the cartilage and thus speed healing.

Healing by secondary intention requires wound care for weeks to months. The patient must be well informed and willing to accept the abnormal appearance during the healing phase. The wound is coated with antibiotic ointment and covered with a nonadherent dressing. The dressing is changed twice daily and the wound cleaned with hydrogen peroxide.

If healing by secondary intention results in an unfavorable outcome or causes distortion of local anatomical landmarks, revision surgery may then be performed. The process can be interrupted at any time and the defect repaired with a skin graft or local flap. In these cases, wound contracture will usually result in a defect that is smaller, shallower, and more easily repaired than the original.

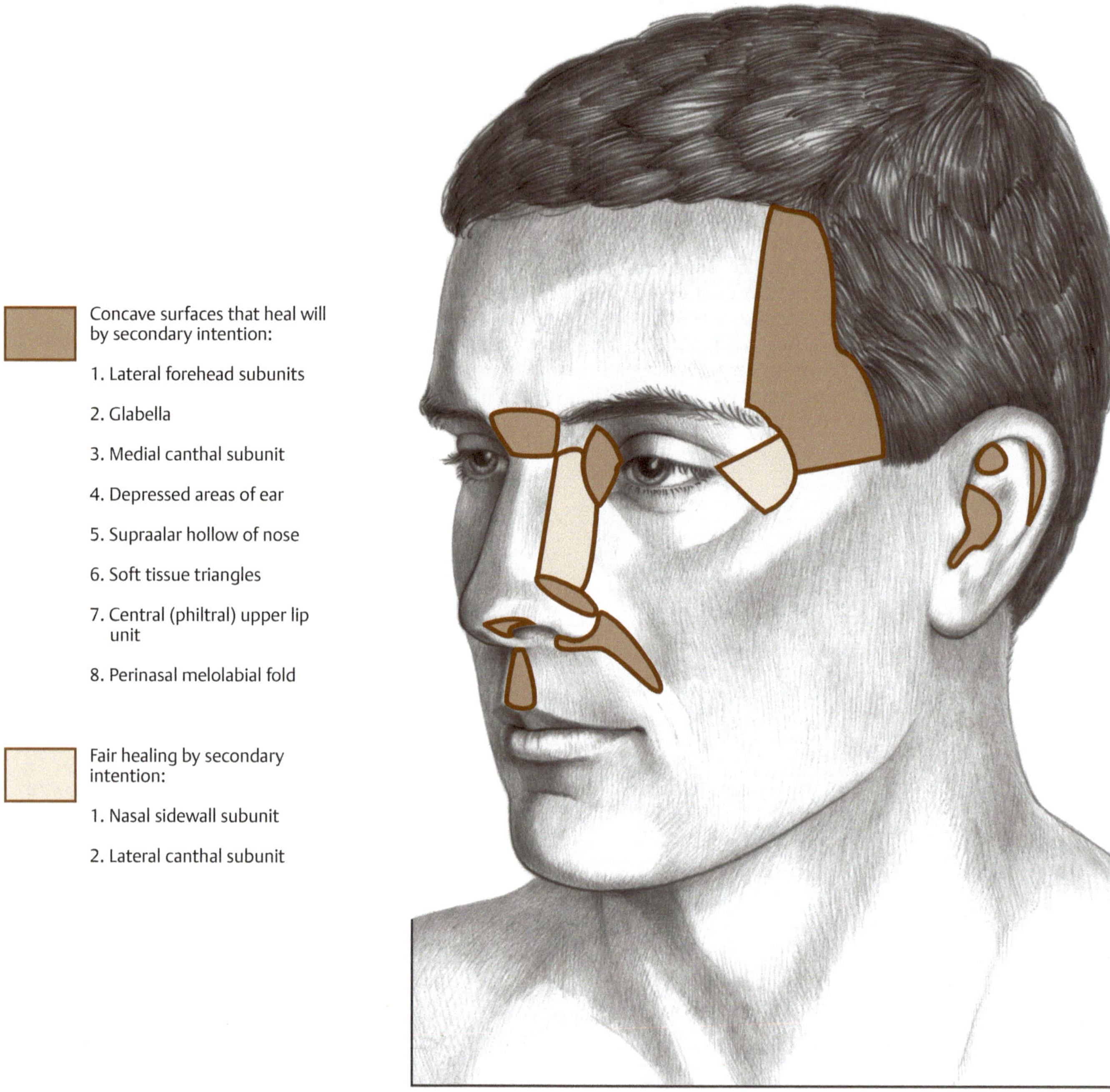

Fig. 2.4 Areas appropriate for healing by secondary intention.

♦ Skin Grafts

Split-thickness skin grafts (STSGs) are rarely used in facial reconstruction. They are generally harvested from the thigh or buttocks. A power-driven dermatome set at a thickness of 0.015 to 0.016 inch provides an adequate STSG. After harvesting the graft, the donor site is covered with a porous dressing. The graft is "pie crusted" to prevent seroma or hematoma formation.

Full-thickness skin grafts (FTSGs) are used for smaller defects (1–5 cm) and are usually harvested from head and neck sites. Color, thickness, and texture of the defect region are assessed to determine the most appropriate donor site. FTSGs are commonly harvested from the upper eyelids, the preauricular region, the postauricular region, the melolabial crease, and the supraclavicular region. When using upper eyelid skin, a blepharoplasty on the opposite eye is sometimes necessary to maintain symmetry; occasionally skin from both upper lids may be necessary for a given defect. Using a template from the defect, the proposed FTSG is marked and excised with minimal underlying subcutaneous tissue. The donor site defect is closed primarily with standing cone excised as needed.

The optimal defect bed for either an STSG or an FTSG is vascular and does not contain bare bone or cartilage. The best tissue for the bed is muscle or granulation tissue, though grafts also take well on subcutaneous tissue, perichondrium, or periosteum. If a defect contains cranial bone devoid of periosteal coverage, a local pericranial flap can be raised and used as a bed. Alternatively, drilling the bone down to the diploic space can create a vascular bed. Exposed cartilage can be treated with multiple stab incisions or dermal punch excisions to allow granulation tissue growth from the deep surface and to create a vascularized bed for grafting. A temporoparietal fascia flap can also be used to cover large areas of exposed bone or cartilage.

The FTSG is pie crusted with multiple stab incisions prior to placement. The skin graft should be further fixed to the wound bed with several placating sutures, as well as a tension-free closure at the wound edge. Once the skin graft has been sutured into place along the graft–defect margin, the site is bolstered for 3 to 5 days to prevent shearing of the graft bed surface. Cotton saturated with antibiotic ointment, nonadherent gauze (Telfa), and foam are commonly used bolster materials. Bolster sutures should be placed a few millimeters distal to the graft–defect interface to prevent cratering of the wound margins. If a seroma is noted at bolster removal, it is drained with stab incisions. Antibiotic ointment is placed on the site until healing is completed.

♦ Composite Grafts

Composite grafts used in local facial reconstruction usually contain skin and cartilage. The most common donor site is the ear, whereas the most common recipient sites are the nasal alar rim and columella. Composite grafts up to 1.5 cm in diameter may be used, though the risk of necrosis increases dramatically as size increases. Composites of 1 cm or less are preferred. Survival is enhanced in grafts that have contact with the donor bed on more than just the margins. For example, a graft in which only the alar margin is through and through and in which the remainder of the defect is skin only, will generally survive quite well, even with a partial-thickness area greater than 1.5 cm^2. A tongue-in-groove placement, with the composite graft cartilage sandwiched between donor site skin and mucosa, will stabilize the graft and enhance survival.

No bolster is applied after the graft is inset. The graft is kept cool for 2 or 3 days postoperatively with iced saline. A short course of oral steroids is given perioperatively, and the graft is kept moist with antibiotic ointment during healing. Initially, these grafts appear pale, and over the first few days they become quite blue. Occasionally, epidermolysis and superficial skin slough occur in the first week. The graft then appears to become more pink over the ensuing weeks. These grafts should rarely, if ever, be used in patients who smoke, in radiated fields, or in other patients with any impaired vascular supply.

♦ Advancement Flap

An advancement flap is the simplest to design and in its most basic form involves advancing the edges of a fusiform excision together. Tension is at the wound edge and perpendicular to the incision line. Rectangular advancement flaps are used primarily in the forehead, but occasionally elsewhere (**Fig. 2.5**). They can be used in either a unilateral or a bilateral fashion, depending on the location of the excess tissue to be advanced. The length of each flap is generally about twice the width, although the excellent blood supply of the face will generally permit longer flaps if needed. The primary tension is at the closure of the donor site, perpendicular to the incision. When advanced, the flap width decreases slightly; therefore, the width is normally designed slightly wider than the defect size. The disparity in flap side length (shorter) and donor side length (longer) can be adjusted at closure by a combination of the principle of "halving" and Burow triangle excision, as needed. The Burow excision can be placed at one or more sites to be camouflaged in the RSTLs or at a natural anatomical boundary.

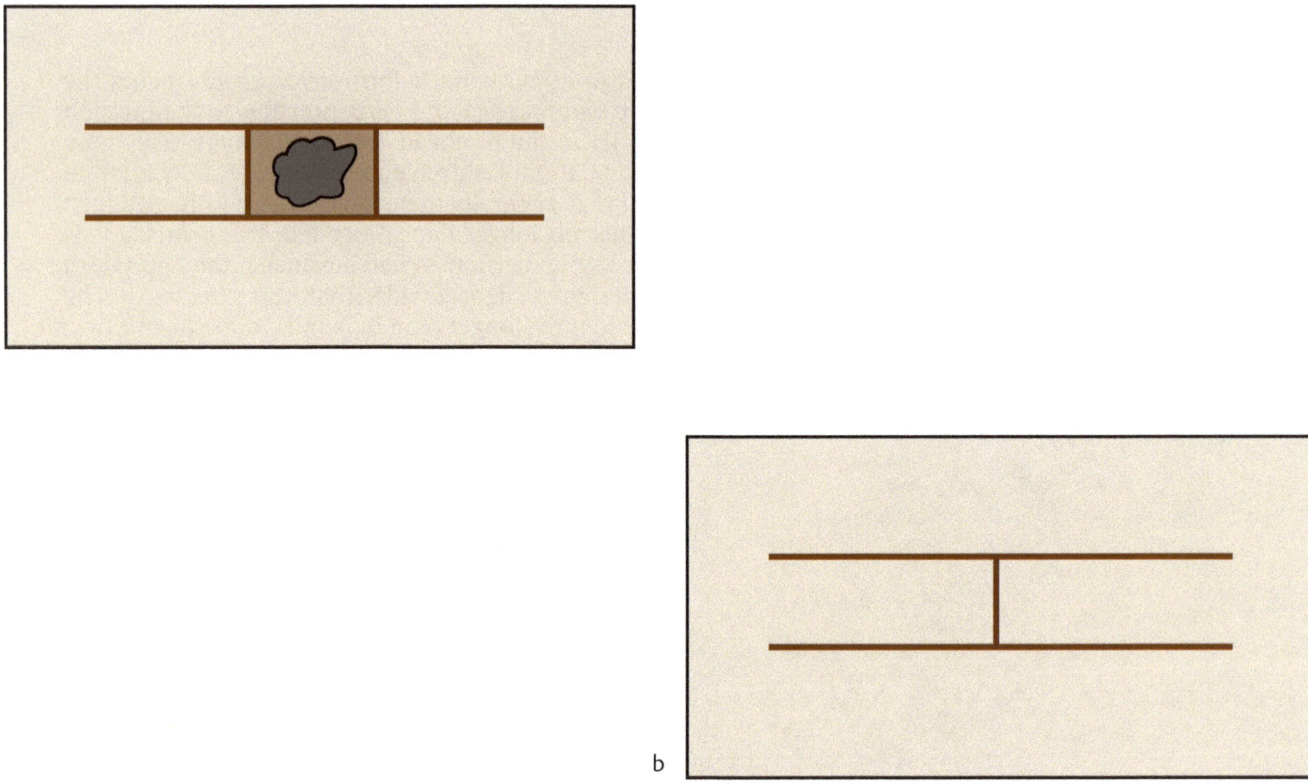

Fig. 2.5 (**a, b**) Rectangular advancement flap.

♦ Rotation Flap

The rotation flap is best applied to a triangular defect. Round or oval defects will need to be converted to a more triangular shape to allow closure without a standing cone formation. The flap is designed off one of the peaks of the triangle (**Fig. 2.6**). The incision line runs parallel to the RSTLs or within the border of aesthetic units/subunits. The principle of halving and the use of Burow triangles must be applied to close the longer defect side and the shorter flap side. Burow triangles should not be excised prior to advancing and insetting the flap, as precise prediction of the amount of redundant tissue is difficult. Burow triangles can be excised, as needed, at any point along the larger side and do not need to be excised at the base.

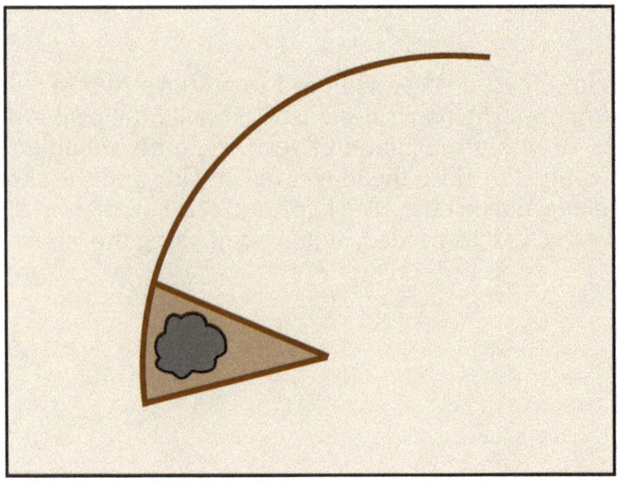

a

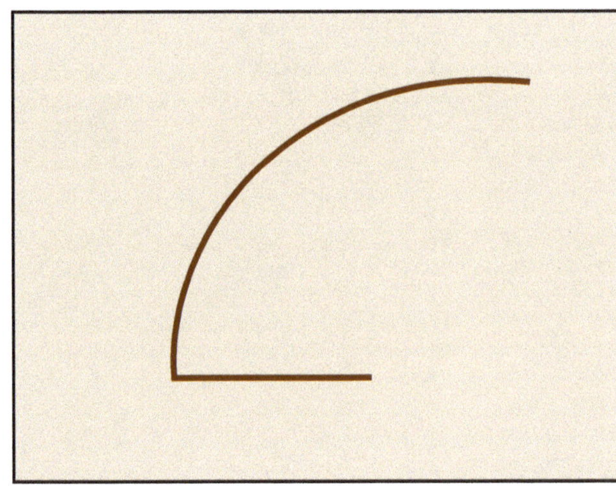

b

Fig. 2.6 (**a, b**) Rotation flap.

♦ Rhombic Flap

The rhombic or Limberg flap is an equilateral parallelogram flap designed to fill a defect of the same size and shape (**Fig. 2.7**). The classic rhombic flap is designed with two 60-degree angles and two 120-degree angles. All sides of the defect and the flap are the same length. The first limb of the flap is drawn as an extension of a line connecting the 120-degree angles. All sides of the defect and the flap are the same length. The second limb is drawn at a 60-degree angle to the end of the first limb and parallel to one of the adjacent sides of the rhombic defect. The point of maximal tension is at the closure of the donor site. The donor site closure should approximate the RSTLs and thus be perpendicular to the lines of maximal extensibility. The point of maximal tension should be approximated first with a subcutaneous suture.

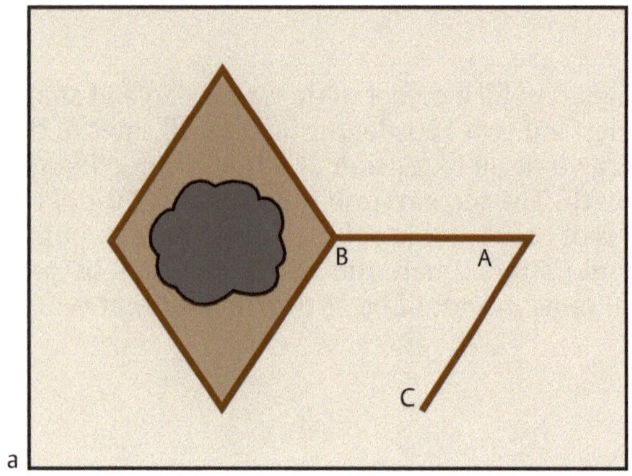

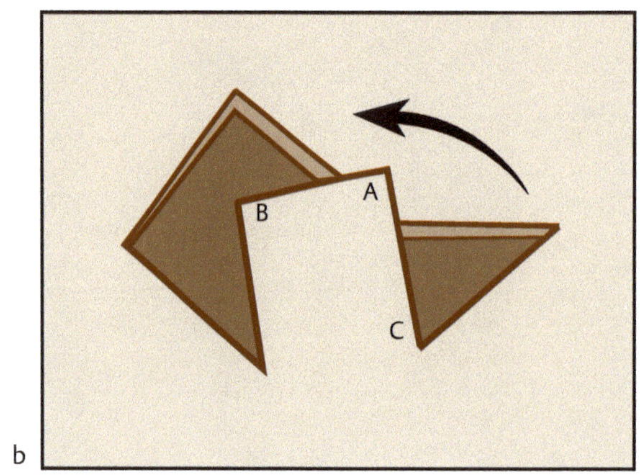

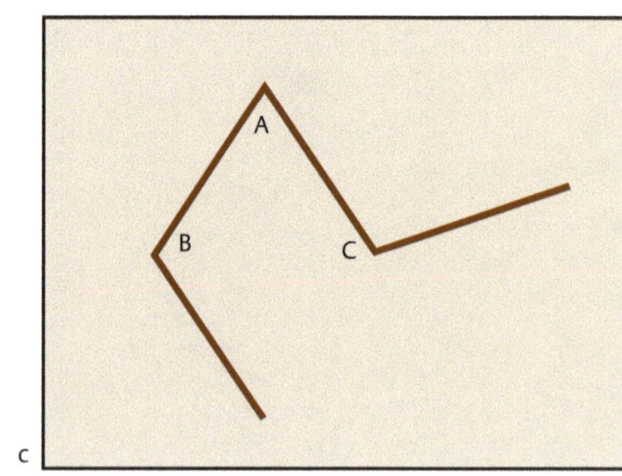

Fig. 2.7 (**a–c**) Rhombic flap.

♦ Bilobed Flap

The classic bilobed flap comprises of two flaps at 90 degrees to one another, with total flap rotation of 180 degrees (**Fig. 2.8a**). Depending on local anatomical landmarks, the angle between the flaps can be decreased to 45 to 50 degrees, with total flap rotation of 90 to 100 degrees (**Fig. 2.8b**). The lesser rotation results in both decreased standing cone formation and wound tension. The variability in angle also allows the design of the flap closures in RSTLs and at aesthetic unit/subunit boundaries.

The first flap, drawn adjacent to the defect, is designed the same size or slightly smaller than the defect, and the second flap is designed 25 to 50% smaller than the first flap. The second flap is designed and incised with the Burow triangle at the peak of the flap to both facilitate donor site closure and provide extra tissue to place in the primary flap donor site. The first donor site is closed with the second flap, plus a V to Y advancement at the distal donor site, as necessary. The second donor site is closed primarily. Area ratios of the flaps can be varied, depending on where excess tissue is present.

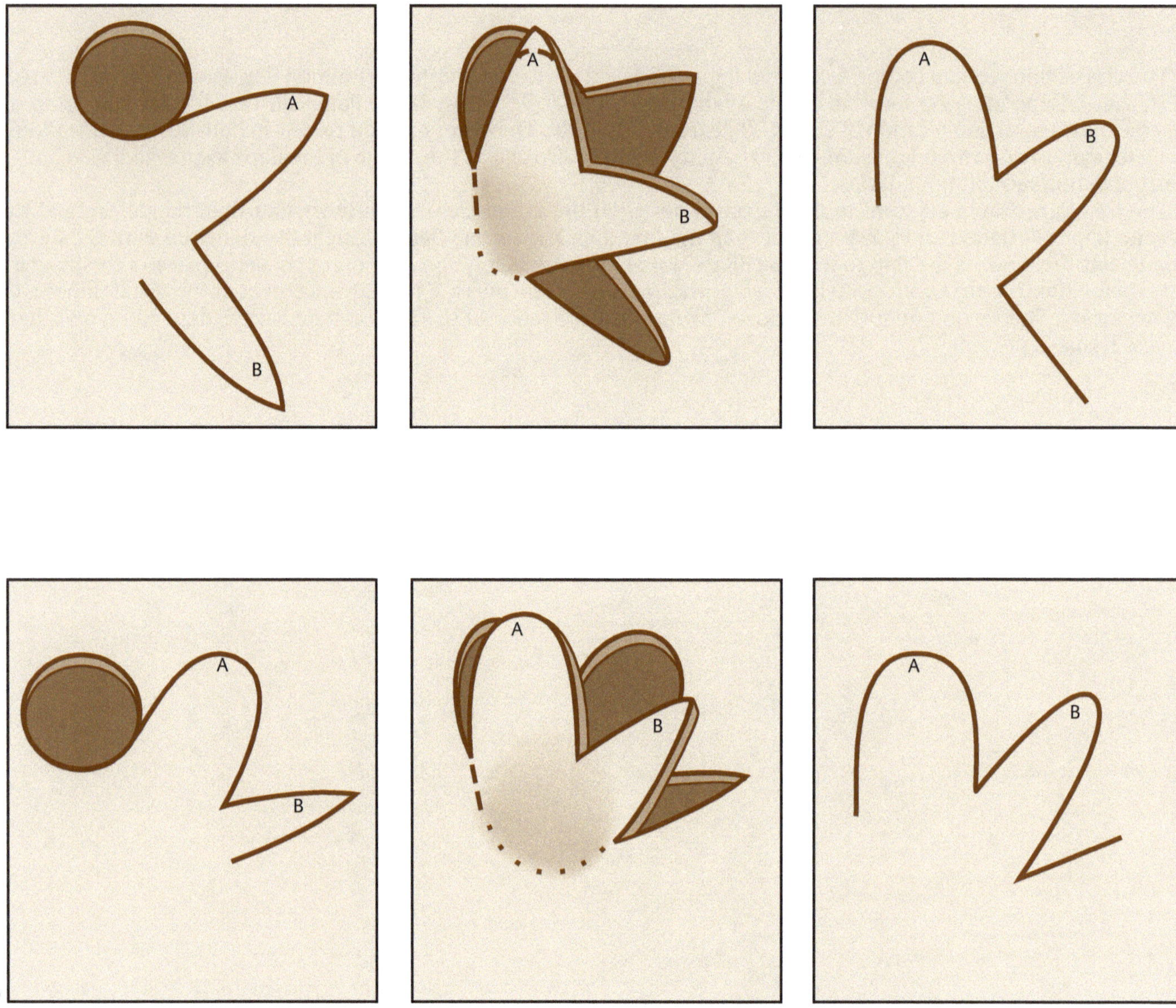

a b

Fig. 2.8 (**a**) Classic bilobed flap. (**b**) Zitelli modified bilobed flap.

♦ Note Flap

The note flap is a triangular transposition flap designed to close a circular defect (**Fig. 2.9**). A tangent is drawn off the edge of the defect, approximately parallel to the RSTL. This limb is ~1.5 times the diameter of the defect. A second limb is drawn at 50 to 60 degrees off the first limb, away from the defect. The second limb is approximately the same length as the defect diameter. The tip of the flap can be de-epithelialized or trimmed at inset. The major tension is at the closure of the triangular flap donor site. The note flap is somewhat smaller than the defect and therefore is not generally used for defects >1.5 to 2.0 cm. Flap transposition creates a small standing cone at the base of the flap, which is removed at the time of the primary procedure with a Burow triangle.

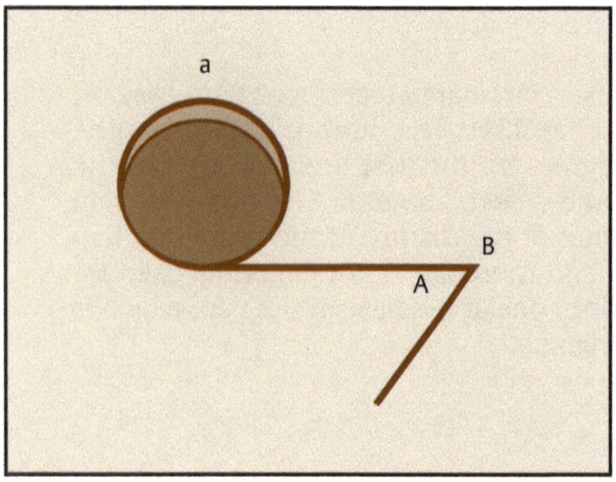

a

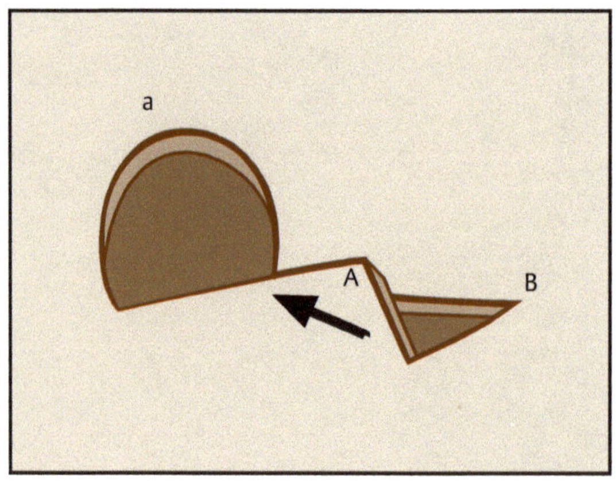

b

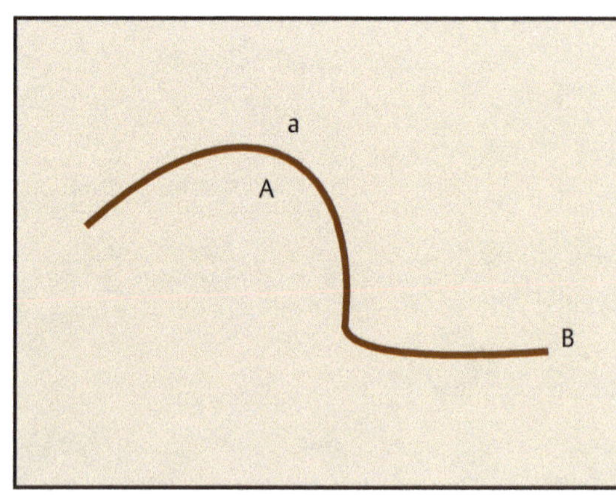

c

Fig. 2.9 (a–c) Note flap.

♦ Z-Plasty

The two main uses of Z-plasty are to lengthen a scar and to reorient a scar or landmark into a more favorable location. The classic design consists of two identical and adjacent triangular flaps transposed on one another (**Fig. 2.10**). The angle of the tip of each flap usually varies between 30 and 60 degrees. The larger the angle, the greater the length gained in the scar. The length of each of the three limbs is equal and is usually limited to 1 cm in the head and neck. Multiple running Z-plasties can be used for larger defects.

In designing a Z-plasty, first mark the RSTLs and borders of local anesthetic units/subunits. The angle of the flaps is chosen depending on whether the goal is maximum scar lengthening or repositioning of local tissue. The orientation of the central limb of the Z-plasty changes by 90 degrees, whereas the location of the lateral limbs does not change. Thus, the lateral limb location must be chosen so that the final scars will be favorably aligned in relation to the RSTLs and aesthetic unit borders. Visualizing the final result is accomplished by assuming the nonflap sites (AB and CD in **Fig. 2.10a**) stay in approximately the same position, and that the central line simply changes position from CB to AD (**Fig. 2.10b, c**). A simple rule of Z-plasty design is that the limbs of the Z-plasty can be drawn in only two ways. The design that makes the limbs of the Z-plasty most parallel to the RSTLs is the correct design choice in nearly every case.

For scar revision, the scar can be removed as an ellipse on the BC axis and reoriented at the same time with Z-plasty. Multiple Z-plasties are simply designed as a series of individual ones.

Fig. 2.10 demonstrates the effect of a Z-plasty adjacent to a defect. This adjunctive Z-plasty has been described by Borges to assist in difficult wound closures.

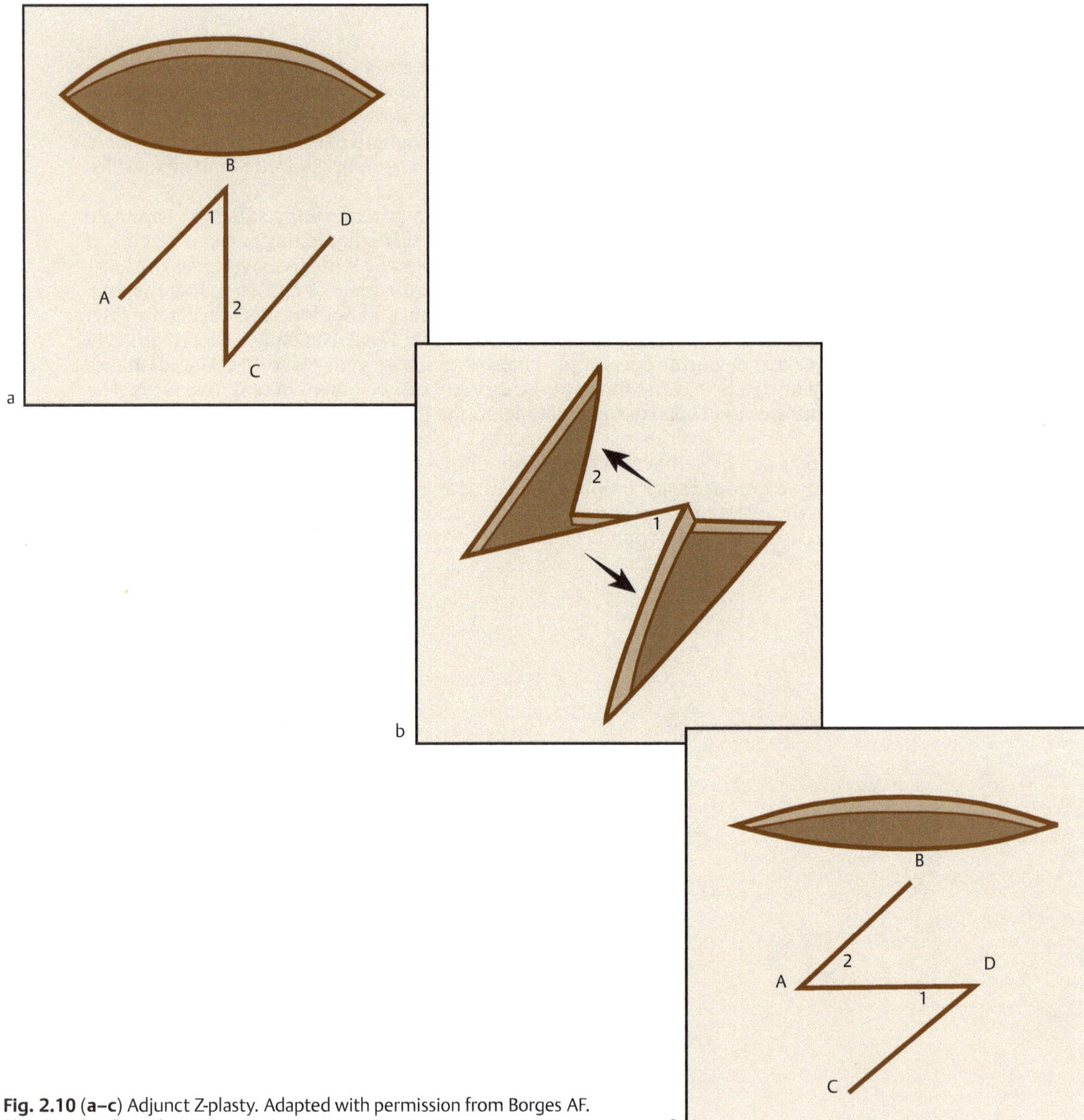

Fig. 2.10 (**a–c**) Adjunct Z-plasty. Adapted with permission from Borges AF. The rhombic flap. Plast Reconstr Surg 1981;67:458–466.

♦ Dermabrasion

Most incisions and flap reconstructions will benefit from postoperative dermabrasion. This simple technique will effectively reduce mild-to-moderate contour abnormalities and color discrepancies between donor and recipient site skin. Keloids are not appropriate for dermabrasion, as the technique may result in exacerbation of the problems.

In cases of local flaps, the incision itself should be dermabraded. In cases of regional flaps, such as a forehead flap for nasal reconstruction, the entire recipient site aesthetic unit and flap should be dermabraded. The timing of dermabrasion has been controversial. We have found optimal results with dermabrasion performed 4 to 6 weeks after surgery, but improvement can also be obtained at any later time period.

Dermabrasion is easily done in an office setting, although eye protection and surgical masks should be worn by the staff at all times, as the procedure results in aerosolization of blood and tissue. Prophylactic antiviral medications should be given prior to perioral dermabrasion. Prior to dermabrasion, the skin is cleansed, and any contour abnormalities are marked with a surgical marker. Local anesthesia is obtained with injection of local anesthetic and/or freezing with refrigerant spray. In cases where injected local anesthetic is used, the skin is pulled taut with countertraction, and dermabrasion is performed. When freezing is used, there is less need for countertraction, as the skin is dermabraded while in a temporary solid state. Refreezing of an area is avoided, as it is less effective, and tissue damage is more likely.

Both wire brushes and coarse diamond fraise attachments are effective. In either case, the depth of dermabrasion should be into the papillary dermis. Full-thickness defects beyond the dermis will create scarring and should be avoided. A good end point is when all the ink markings placed in the contour abnormalities are gone.

Care is taken to feather the edges of the dermabraded area for more subtle transition into normal skin.

After dermabrasion, the area can be covered with sponges soaked in 1% lidocaine and 1:100,000 epinephrine for both aesthetic and vasoconstrictive effects. The wound can be dressed with a polyethylene oxide gel dressing (Vigilon) or simply coated with petroleum jelly or antibiotic ointment. If an initial dressing is used, then it is removed in 24 hours. The patient is instructed to cleanse the area in a warm water shower three times a day. Antibiotic ointment or petroleum jelly is applied to the area after the shower to keep the area moist. Once all crusting has stopped, typically at 7 to 10 days after the procedure, the patient is allowed to discontinue the application of ointment and to reapply makeup to the area.

Suggested Reading

Becker FF. Facial Reconstruction with local and regional flaps. New York: Thieme-Stratton; 1985:45–54

Borges AF. The rhombic flap. Plast Reconstr Surg 1981;67(4):458–466

Fann PC, Hartman DF, Goode RL. Pharmacologic and surgical enhancement of composite graft survival. Arch Otolaryngol Head Neck Surg 1993;119(3):313–319

Gassner HG, Brissett AE, Otley CC, et al. Botulinum toxin to improve facial wound healing: a prospective, blinded, placebo-controlled study. Mayo Clin Proc 2006;81(8):1023–1028

Larrabee WF Jr. Design of local skin flaps. Otolaryngol Clin North Am 1990;23(5):899–923

Larrabee WF Jr, Sutton D. The biomechanics of advancement and rotation flaps. Laryngoscope 1981;91(5):726–734

Larrabee WF Jr, Trachy R, Sutton D, Cox K. Rhomboid flap dynamics. Arch Otolaryngol 1981;107(12):755–757

Limberg AA. Mathematical principles of local plastic procedures of the surface of the human body. Leningrad: Medgiz; 1946

Otley CC, Sherris DA. Spectrum of cartilage grafting in cutaneous reconstructive surgery. J Am Acad Dermatol 1998;39(6):982–992

Ridenour BD, Larrabee WF. Skin flap design: physiology and biodynamics. In: Meyers AD, ed. Biological Basis of Facial Plastic Surgery. New York: Thieme; 1993:72–104

Sherris DA, Gassner HG. Botulinum toxin to minimize facial scarring. Facial Plast Surg 2002;18(1):35–39

Sherris DA, Kern EB. Essential surgical skills. 2nd ed. Philadelphia: WB Saunders/Mosby; 2004

Thomas JR, Holt GR. Facial scars, revisions and camouflage. St. Louis: CV Mosby; 1989:123–136

Walike JW, Larrabee WF Jr. The 'note flap'. Arch Otolaryngol 1985;111(7):430–433

Zitelli JA. Secondary intention healing: an alternative to surgical repair. Clin Dermatol 1984;2(3):92–106

3 Scalp

Summary

This chapter focuses on the principles and anatomy that are pertinent and important with respect to reconstruction of scalp defects. Specific consideration is given to undermining and layered closure as well as the use of tissue expanders for larger defects.

Keywords: scalp, tissue expanders, rotation flap, layered closure, galea, advancement flap

The scalp is composed of five layers, recalled by the mnemonic SCALP: skin, subcutaneous fat, galea aponeurosis, loose connective tissue, and pericranium. The galea is a strong, fibrous sheet with firm connections (via the occipitalis muscle) to the nuchal ridge posteriorly and the frontalis muscle anteriorly. The tight attachments existing between the scalp, skin and the galea significantly reduce tissue mobility in the subcutaneous planes.

Undermining in the subcutaneous plane is difficult due to extreme vascularity and it risks injury to the hair follicles. Scalp flaps are easily undermined just beneath the galea, because the space is occupied by loose connective tissue with few blood vessels. Even wide undermining at this level, however, leads to disappointingly small improvements in flap tension. Subpericranial elevation is also avascular, but it yields even less tissue laxity.

Blood supply is arranged in a radial pattern from the following five arteries: supratrochlear, supraorbital, superficial temporal, postauricular, and occipital. Abundant blood supply allows for the design of numerous small random pattern flaps. Large transposition flaps should incorporate one of the previously named arteries.

Hair emerges from the scalp at an angle. The direction in which the hair is angled varies with the scalp region. Scalp incisions should be beveled parallel to the hair follicles to preserve them (see **Fig. 2.1**). In areas where hair shaft direction varies, care is needed to align the incision correctly. In the pretrichal region, incisions should be beveled opposite the direction of hair follicles to allow hair regrowth through the incision.

Scalp wounds should be closed in two layers to prevent scar widening and loss of hair. Buried 2–0 or 3–0 permanent or long-lasting absorbable sutures are placed in the galea, using care to not injure hair follicles. The skin is closed with 4–0 or 5–0 monofilament sutures or staples. When the wound is under tension, galea sutures are placed ~1 cm back from the edges to prevent tissue tearing. In addition, galea-releasing incisions parallel to the blood supply of the flap, just through the galea, and spaced 1 to 2 cm apart will further decrease wound-closing tension.

Thick and inelastic, the scalp is resistant to such standard techniques as advancement and transposition flaps. Rotation flaps are the main reconstructive technique for scalp defects. Large defects are usually treated by tissue expansion, along with rotation or advancement flaps, as dictated by the location of the defect.

The scalp should be palpated to establish the directions of greatest mobility and the flaps designed accordingly. Scalp tissues that are closed under tension tend to stretch back up 30 to 50% of the distance closed. This problem can be reduced by using galea sutures at the time of closure.

In the typical scalp, defects <3 to 5 cm in size can be closed with either unilateral or bilateral rotation flaps (**Fig. 3.1**). Bilateral flaps are usually selected to distribute closing tension over as much area as possible. Unilateral flaps are used primarily for defects adjacent to the hairline. The length of the sides of the rotation flap (or flaps) is typically four to six times the defect diameter to allow adequate rotation. One can design either a single or double rotation flap of maximal length, then cut back only partially to determine the actual length required (**Fig. 3.2**). Wide undermining in the subgaleal layer must be performed to facilitate scalp movement. Hair provides camouflage for what may seem to be inordinately long incisions for relatively small defects. The defect site is closed first. Then the long limbs are closed, using the technique of halving to distribute tension. The two limbs of the bilateral rotation flaps do not have to be equal in length, and usually are not, unless the defect is located exactly in the center of the scalp. In the situation where bilateral rotation flaps are insufficient to close a defect, one or more additional flaps may be created to convert to a "pinwheel" flap design.

Small standing cones ("dog ears") commonly form during flap closure and will usually resolve with healing. Large standing cones can be removed using the standard Burow technique. Rotation flaps used for repair after excision of benign areas (e.g., burn scars or nevi) can be designed, incised, and rotated over the lesion prior to its removal. If necessary, a partial excision can be performed and a second stage planned.

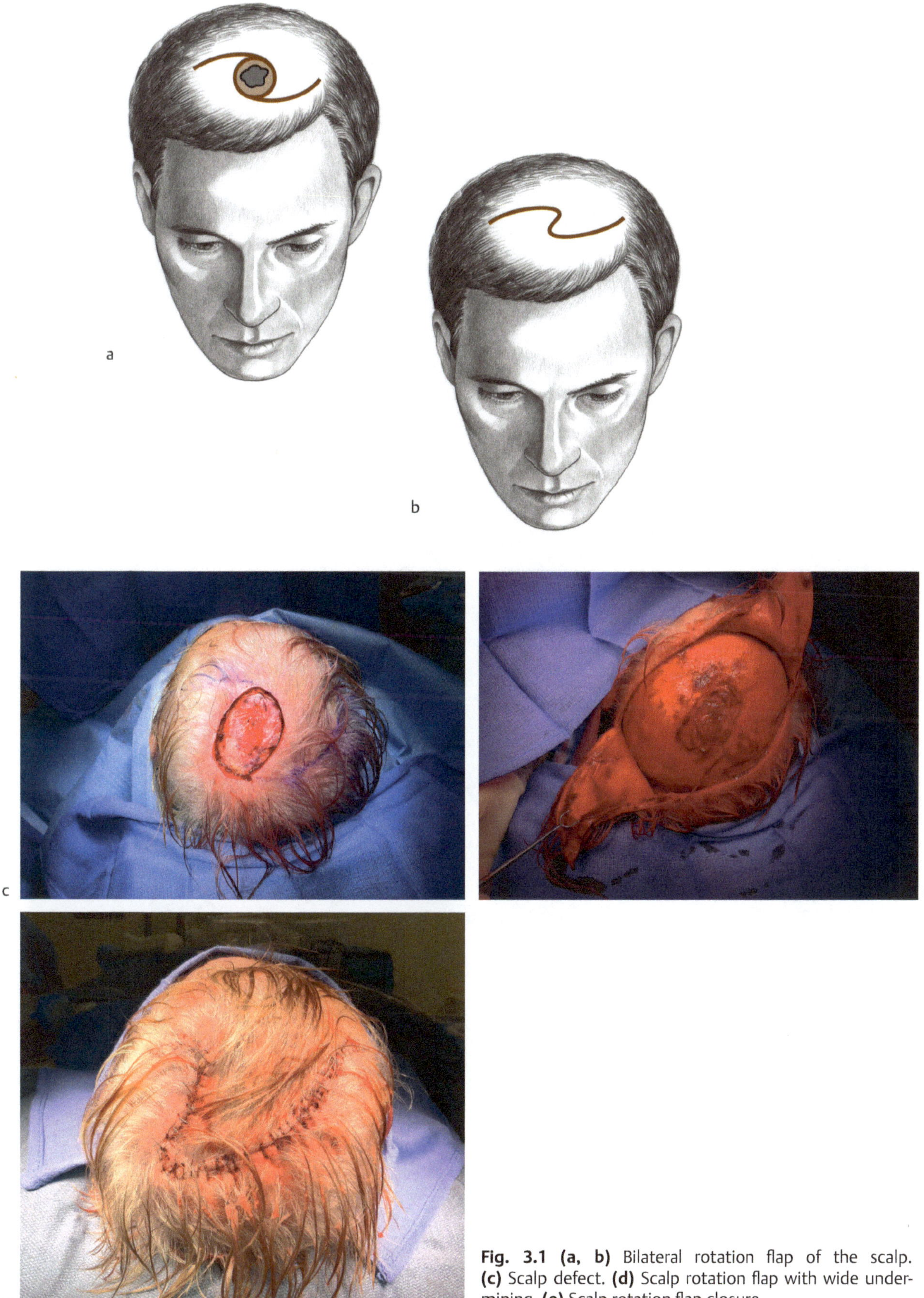

Fig. 3.1 (a, b) Bilateral rotation flap of the scalp. **(c)** Scalp defect. **(d)** Scalp rotation flap with wide undermining. **(e)** Scalp rotation flap closure.

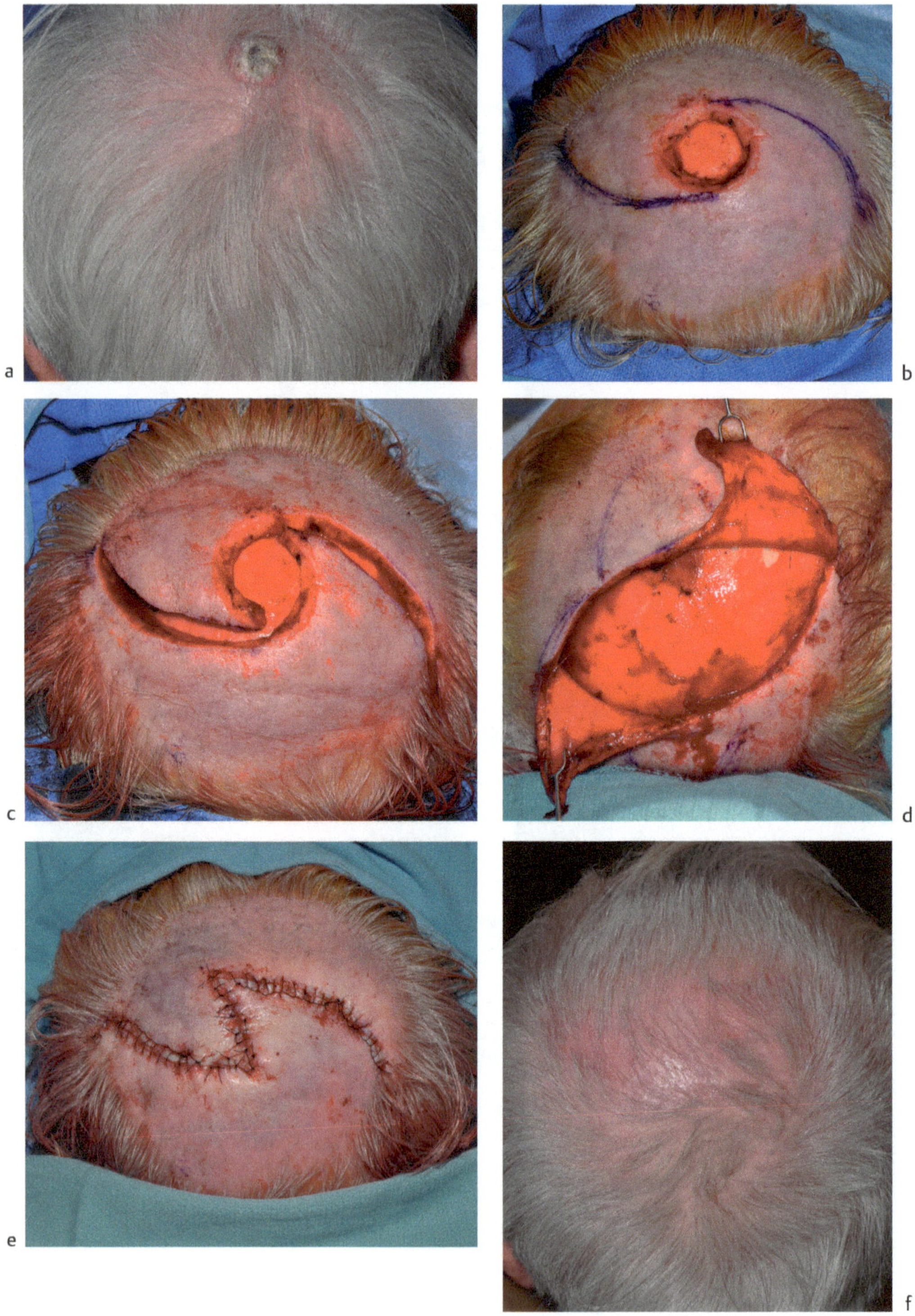

Fig. 3.2 (a) Lesion. **(b)** Defect of the scalp. **(c)** Incisions. **(d)** Bilateral rotation flap closure. **(e)** Closure. **(f)** Healed wound.

If complete closure is not possible and pericranium is present, the wound can be left to heal by secondary intention, or a skin graft can be placed to complete coverage. Split-thickness skin grafts (STSGs) can be placed directly on the pericranium or on the diploic space (after drilling to this surface) with excellent viability. Skin grafts placed on bare bone will frequently fail, resulting in an extended healing period and increased chances of osteomyelitis. Once healed, the skin graft can be serially excised, or tissue expansion can be employed to achieve complete scalp coverage.

Tissue expansion is the technique of choice for defects that cannot be closed with rotation flaps (**Fig. 3.3**). If possible, tissue expansion should be accomplished prior to removal of the primary lesion (**Fig. 3.4**).

If the lesion has been previously resected, then the defect can be allowed to heal by secondary intention or closed with an STSG until tissue expansion can be completed. In the case of a rectangular tissue expander, the expander base should be roughly 2.5 times the size of the defect to be closed. When using a round expander, the diameter of the expander should be 2.5 times the size of the defect. The expander shape should be chosen depending on what type of flap is to be used.

Although rotation flaps are most commonly used in scalp reconstruction, advancement flaps are sometimes preferred after tissue expansion because of the availability of the additional tissue. The shape and position of the tissue expander should be carefully planned to provide the appropriate amount of expanded tissue in the proper location. The preferred expander is placed between the galea and the pericranium, via the smallest incision that will accommodate it. The incision is placed at the junction of the defect and the normal skin, except in the case of the previously placed skin graft that is to be serially excised. In this case, the tissue expander is placed through an incision as far as possible from the skin graft to prevent dehiscence of the graft–skin junction. The injection portal is placed at least 6 cm from the balloon through the same incision. The skin and subcutaneous layers of the incision are closed with permanent sutures.

At the time of placement, 25 to 50 mL of saline should be placed in the expander to obliterate dead space and prevent hematoma formation. Expander inflation is started 2 weeks after the primary surgery and is executed on a weekly or twice-weekly basis. Each expansion session is continued until there is too much local discomfort to continue or until the tissue overlying the expander blanches. Saline is then withdrawn until the discomfort is tolerable or the blanching disappears. Expansion is continued until the circumference of the dome formed is two to three times that of the defect.

At the time of tissue expander removal, the initial incision is usually made at the junction of the defect and the normal skin on the side of the tissue expander. The flap is advanced into position prior to skin graft removal to ensure closure of the defect site. Further releasing incisions are made, as necessary. The capsule underlying the expanded tissue may be left in place or removed for better contour. The wound is then closed in layers.

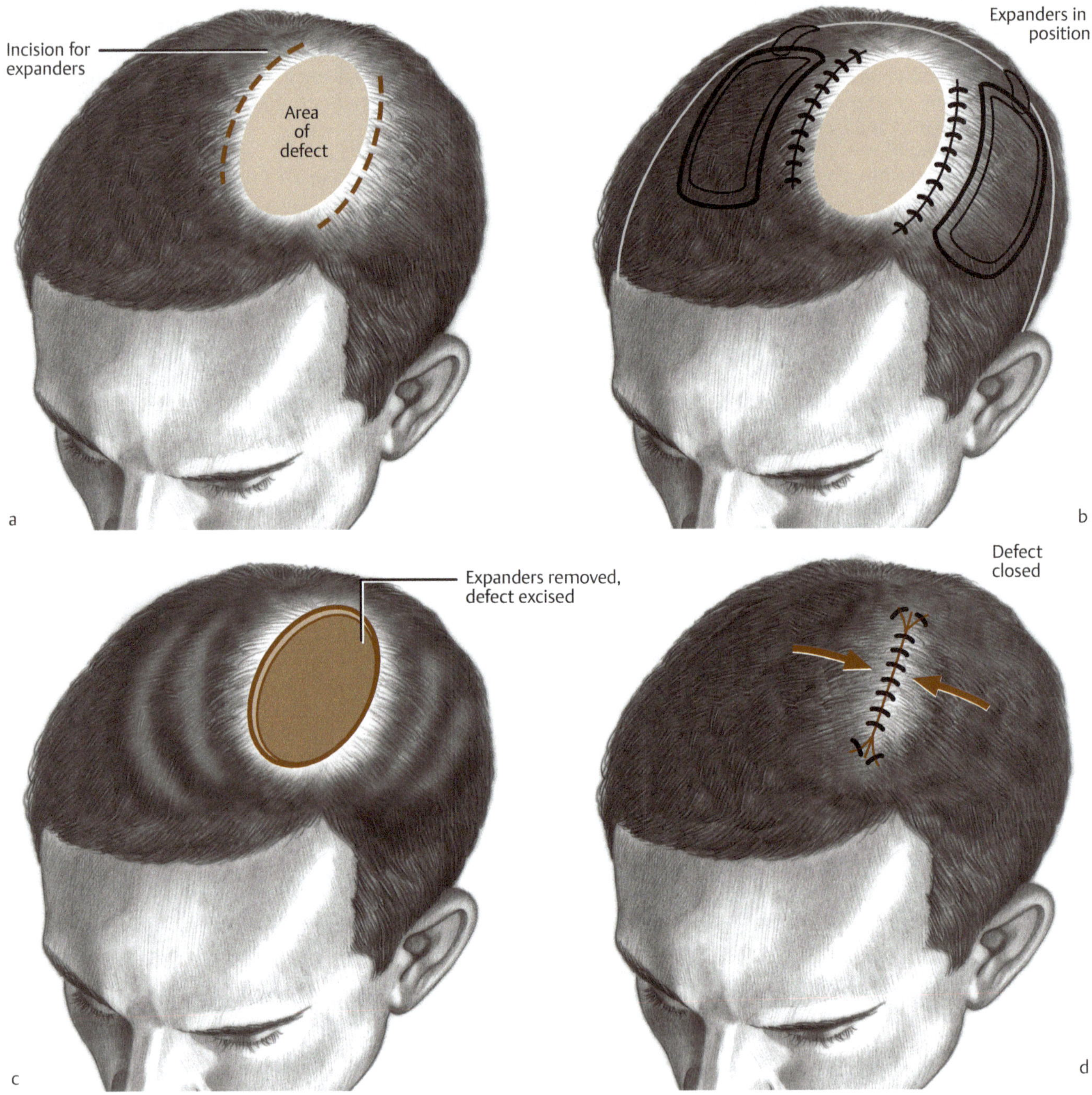

Fig. 3.3 (a–d) Tissue expansion of the scalp.

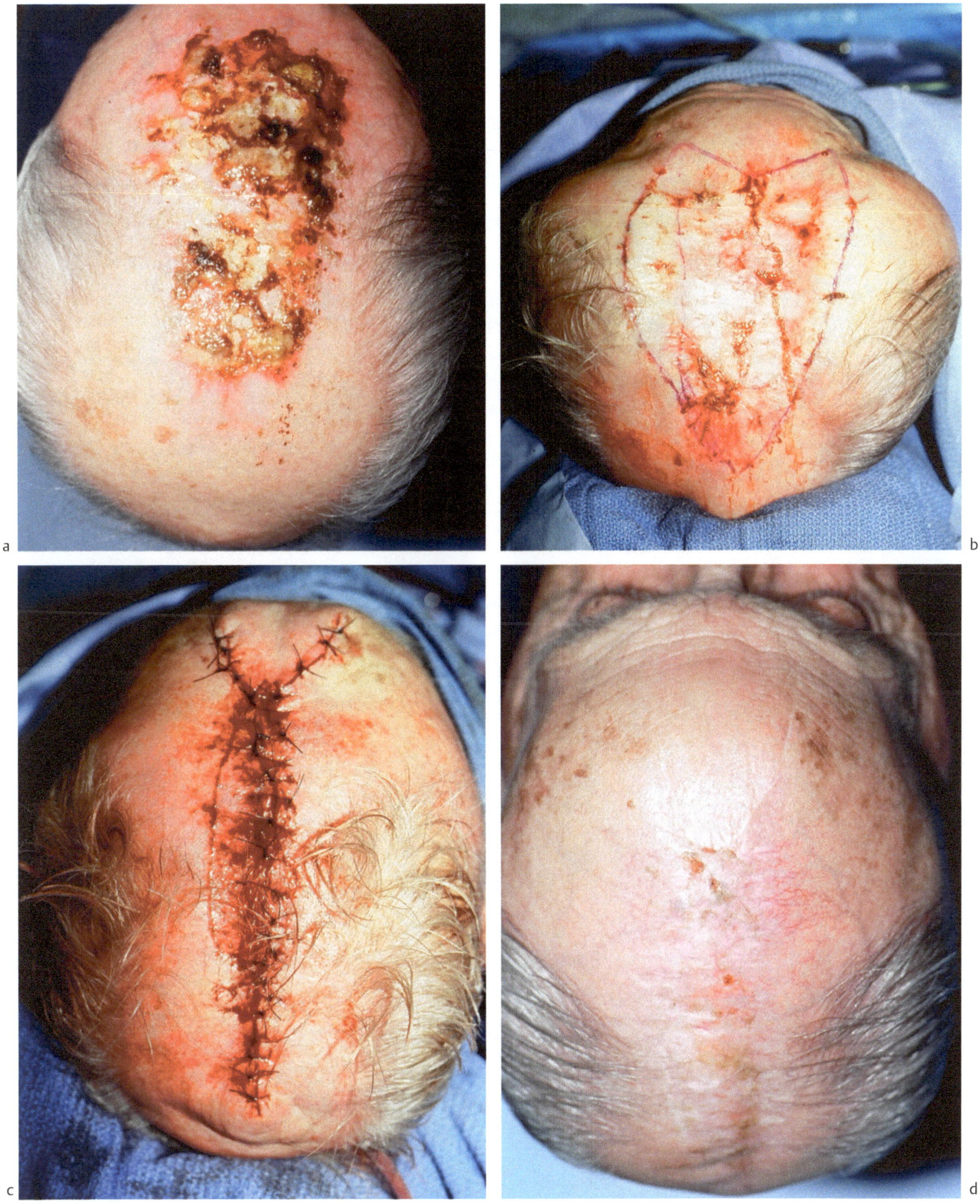

Fig. 3.4 (a) Large lesion of the scalp. **(b)** Tissue expanders in place at the time of lesion excision. **(c)** Scalp closure. **(d)** Healed wound.

Suggested Reading

Baker SR, Swanson NA. Tissue expansion of the head and neck: indications, technique, and complications. Arch Otolaryngol Head Neck Surg 1990;116(10):1147–1153

Bardach J. Scalp reconstruction using local flaps and free skin grafts. In: Local Flaps and Free Skin Grafts. St. Louis: Mosby Year Book; 1992:193–211

Jurkiewicz MJ, Hill HL. Open wounds of the scalp: an account of methods of repair. J Trauma 1981;21(9):769–778

Lesavoy MA, Dubrow TJ, Schwartz RJ, Wackym PA, Eisenhauer DM, McGuire M. Management of large scalp defects with local pedicle flaps. Plast Reconstr Surg 1993;91(5):783–790

Maves MD, Lusk RP. Tissue expansion in the treatment of giant congenital melanocytic nevi. Arch Otolaryngol Head Neck Surg 1987;113(9):987–991

Minor LB, Panje WR. Malignant neoplasms of the scalp: etiology, resection, and reconstruction. Otolaryngol Clin North Am 1993;26(2):279–293

Murakami C. Complications of local facial flaps. In: Eisele D, ed. Complications in Head and Neck Surgery. St. Louis: CV Mosby; 1993:743–755

Orticochea M. New three-flap reconstruction technique. Br J Plast Surg 1971;24(2):184–188

Tolhurst DE, Carstens MH, Greco RJ, Hurwitz DJ. The surgical anatomy of the scalp. Plast Reconstr Surg 1991;87(4):603–612, discussion 613–614

van Rappard JHA, Molenaar J, van Doorn K, Sonneveld GJ, Borghouts JMHM. Surface-area increase in tissue expansion. Plast Reconstr Surg 1988;82(5):833–839

4 Forehead

Summary

This chapter reviews the fundamental techniques and anatomy associated with forehead defects. The forehead is subdivided into several forehead subunits based on locations. We provide a "decision tree" for treatment based on these subunits with specific attention on whether there is involvement of the hairline or eyebrows.

Keywords: temporal forehead, central forehead, A-to-T Flap, rhombic flap, temple, frontalis, primary closure

The anatomical boundaries of the forehead unit are the natural hairline (in patients without alopecia), the zygomatic arch, the lower border of the eyebrows, and the nasal root (**Fig. 4.1**). The upper extent of the forehead unit in patients with alopecia can be identified as the most superior extent of the frontalis muscle. Typically, a distinct superior crease of the forehead marks this spot. The hairline and eyebrows provide camouflaged anatomical boundaries in which to hide incisions. These hair-bearing areas simultaneously limit flap designs to those that do not distort the natural hairline and eyebrow shape.

The forehead unit can be divided into five subunits. Anatomically, the central forehead is an extension of the scalp and retains many similar characteristics. Central forehead skin is thick, rather inelastic, and tightly adherent to the underlying frontalis muscle. On either side of the central forehead is the lateral forehead or temple region, which is more elastic and often acts as a reservoir of tissue for reconstruction. The frontalis muscle is not present in the temple, and the skin is loosely attached to the underlying temporalis fascia. In addition, whereas the central forehead is convex, the temple is somewhat concave. The eyebrows are subunits unto themselves with hair-bearing skin.

The relaxed skin tension lines (RSTLs) run horizontally in the central forehead, as demonstrated by the typical forehead wrinkles. Upon reaching the temporal scalp, they curve in an inferior direction.

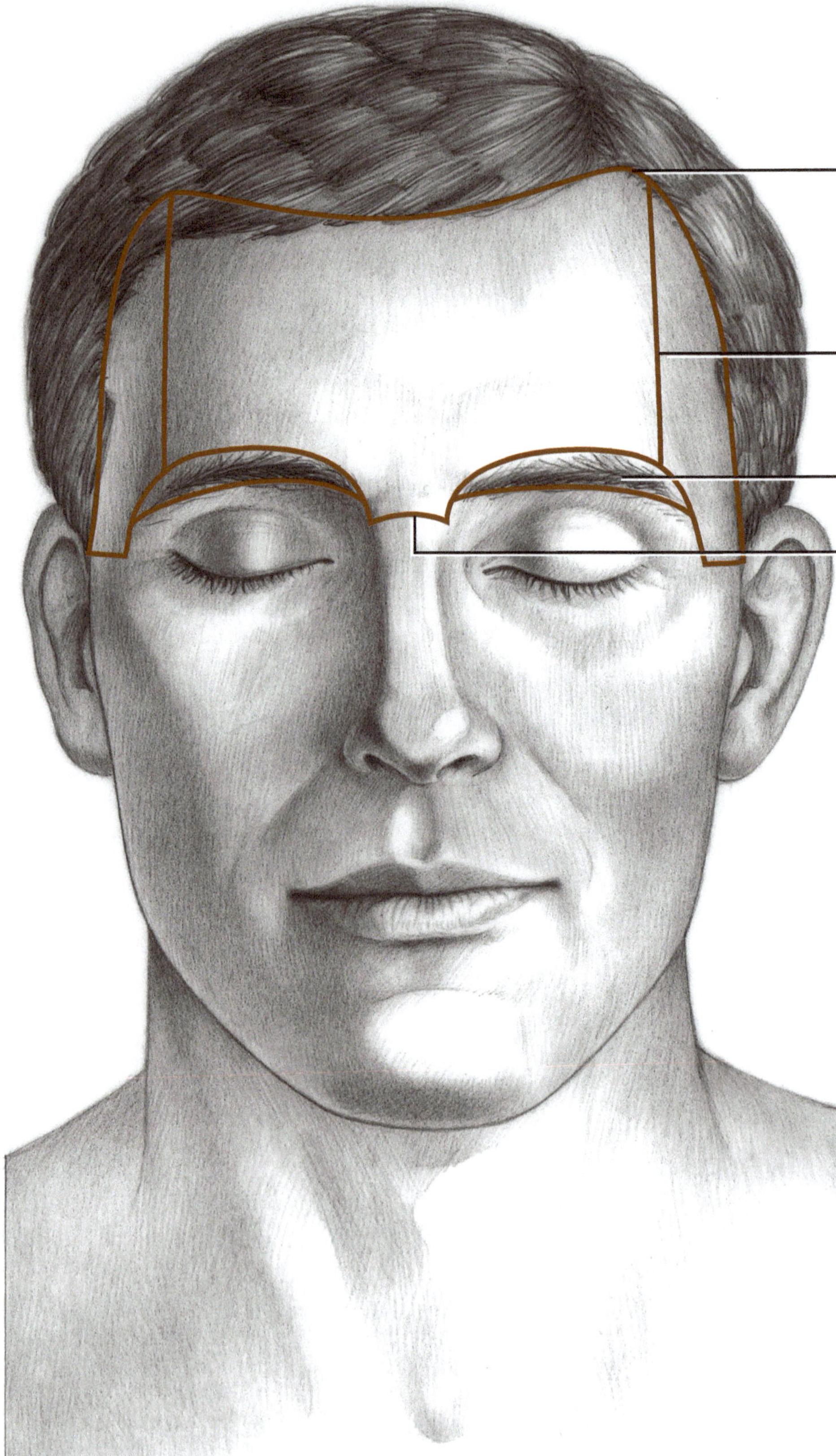

Fig. 4.1 Aesthetic subunits of the forehead.

Sensory innervation to the central forehead originates from branches of the supraorbital and supratrochlear nerves (**Fig. 4.2**). Medially, these sensory nerves branch immediately, pierce the overlying muscle fibers, and run superiorly in a superficial subcutaneous plane. More laterally, the nerves run for quite a distance under the frontalis muscle, rather than in the subcutaneous plane. If care is taken when raising flaps, these large sensory branches can be identified and preserved. The origin of the supraorbital nerve can usually be palpated at the foramina in the superior orbital rim border. The supratrochlear neurovascular bundle is usually very close to or within the glabellar creases. This landmark is especially useful when elevating paramedian forehead flaps for nasal reconstruction.

Small defects of the forehead can be closed in a fusiform manner, but a long incision is often required to avoid standing cones at either end; this is preferable to using an M-plasty, which extends outside the RSTLs and is therefore more noticeable. Fusiform repairs should be limited to locations and sizes that do not elevate the eyebrow. Vertical incisions in the central forehead between the medial extent of the brows heal exceptionally well. Midline closures take advantage of the lax tissue in the temple. The M-plasty technique can be used in the inferior extent of a vertical closure, to take advantage of the camouflaging effect of the glabellar wrinkles, and to avoid traversing into the nasal aesthetic subunit.

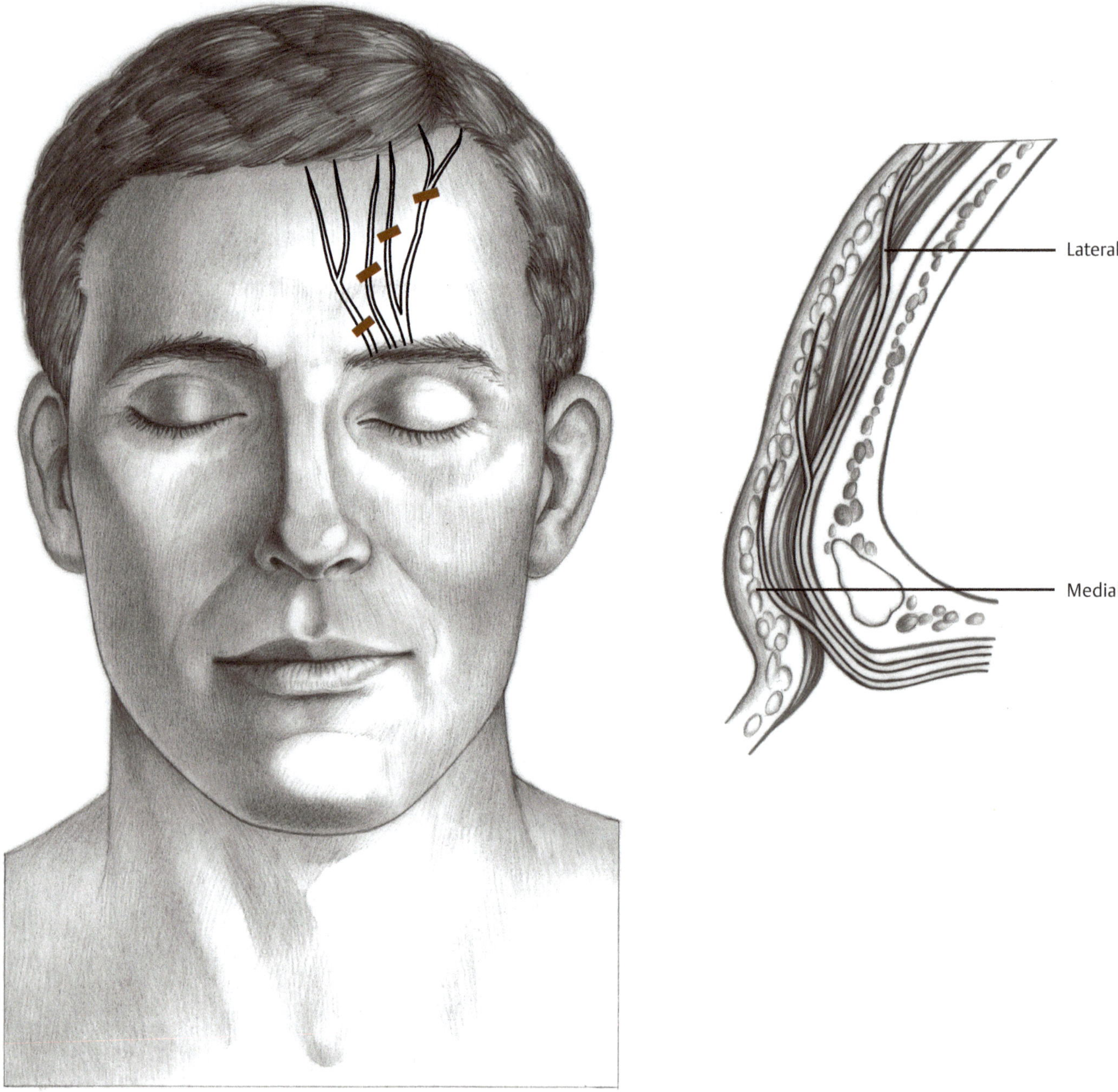

Fig. 4.2 Sensory innervation of the forehead. Adapted with permission from Fatah MF. Innervation and functional reconstruction of the forehead. Br J Plast Surg 1991;44:351–358.

Larger forehead defects are best repaired with flaps (**Fig. 4.3**). Skin grafts provide a poor match in thickness and color, and at best they should be considered a temporary measure. Central forehead defects are repaired primarily with advancement and rotation flaps using incisions placed in the RSTLs or hairline. These central forehead flaps take advantage of the more lax tissue found laterally in the temple region.

Central forehead defects should be assessed for both horizontal and vertical tissue tension. The closure with least tension is selected. The rectangular advancement flap is the repair of choice for most moderate-sized defects of the central forehead (**Fig. 4.4**). The long arms of the flap are usually placed in existing wrinkle lines. If a single advancement flap is inadequate, bilateral flaps are used. The vertical limb is placed in the midline by varying the length of the long limbs of each of the advancement flaps planned. For superficial defects with intact subcutaneous tissue, the flaps can be elevated in the subcutaneous plane, just superficial to the frontalis muscle. If the defect extends to the depths of the galea or the periosteum, then the flaps are incised to the depth of the periosteum, and a deep-layer galea closure is used. Releasing incisions in the galea may be needed to decrease wound-closing tension. Care in incising and elevating flaps may allow preservation of sensory nerve branches.

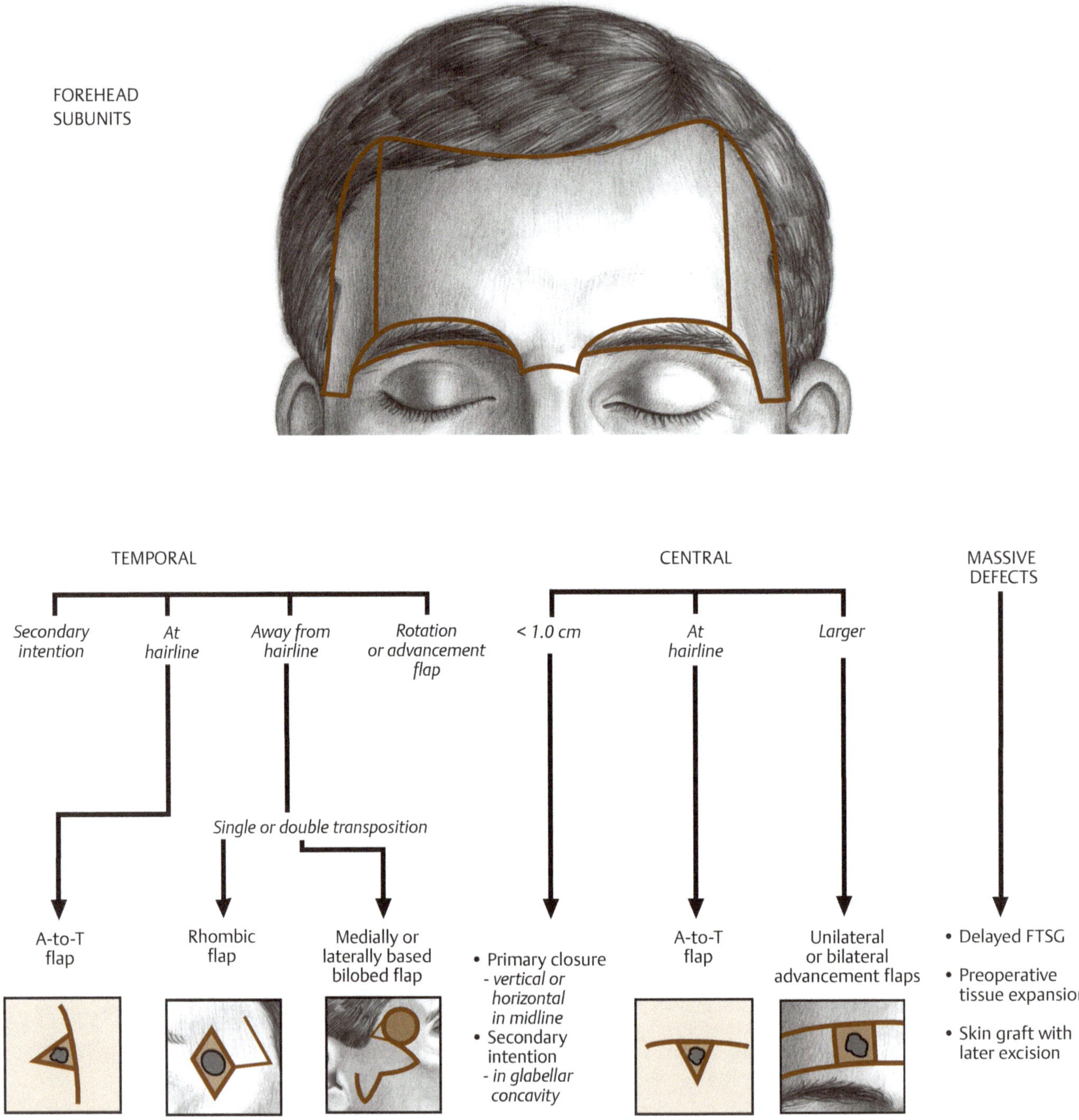

Fig. 4.3 Forehead subunits. FTSG, full-thickness skin graft.

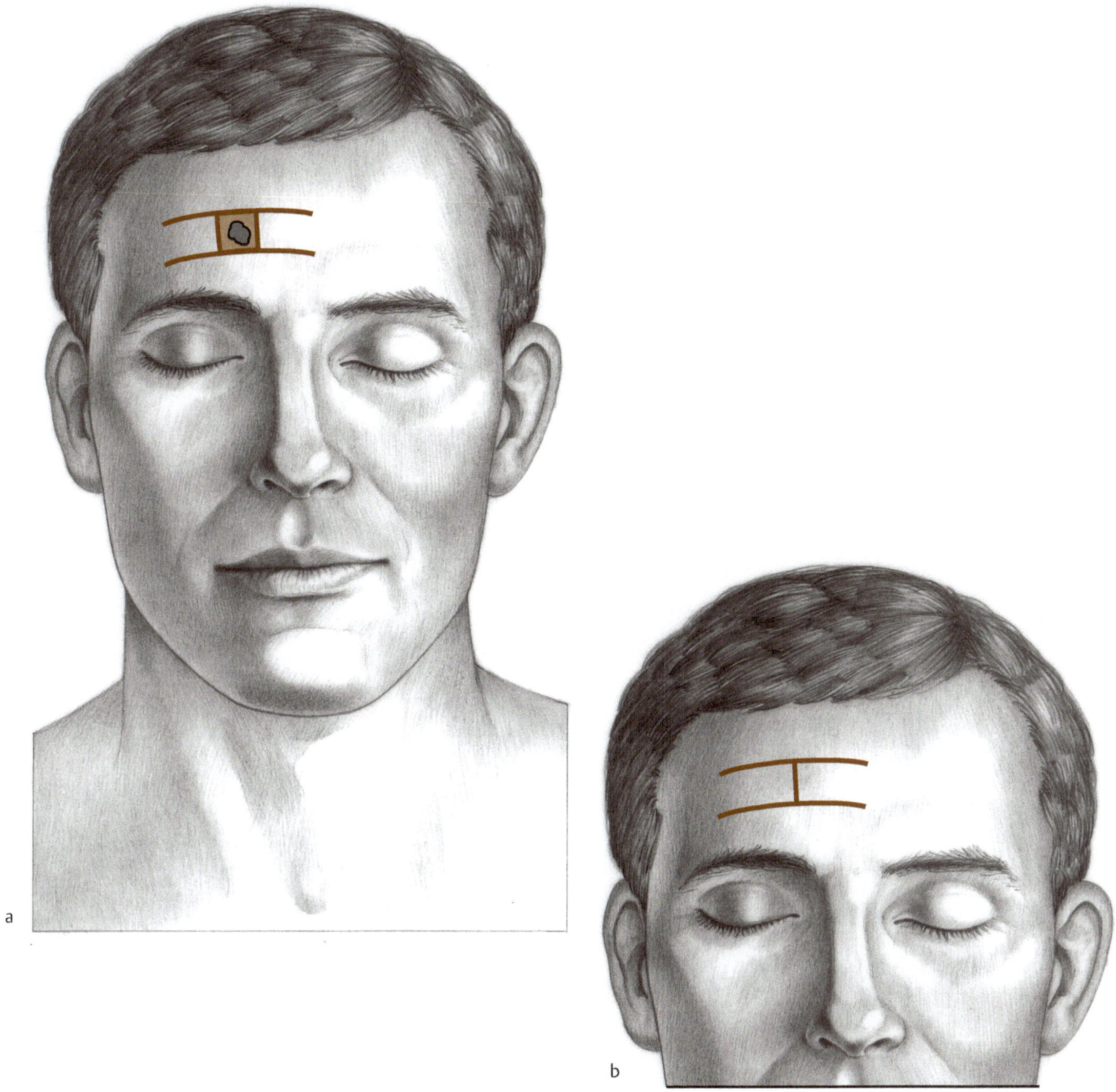

Fig. 4.4 (a, b) Bilateral advancement flaps of the forehead.

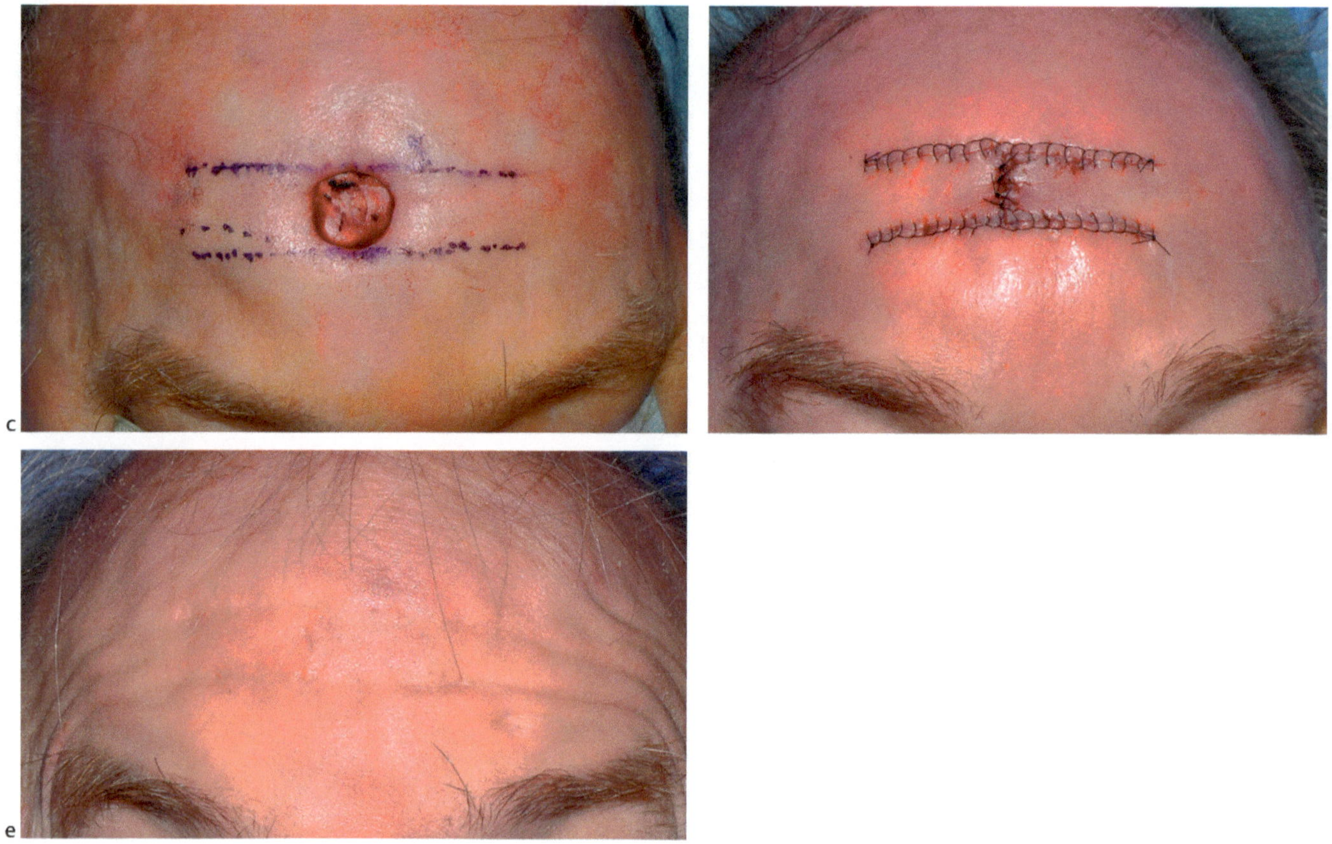

Fig. 4.4 (c) Defect of the forehead. (d) Forehead defect after closure. (e) Healed forehead advancement flaps.

Defects located near or adjacent to the hairline can be repaired with bilateral rotation flaps in an A-to-T fashion; this places one closure line in the hairline (**Fig. 4.5**). This flap design can also be used along the eyebrow (**Fig. 4.6**). The deep plane of dissection is just superficial to the frontalis muscle in the forehead and just superficial to the galea at and posterior to the hairline. If the defect extends deep to the galea, then the entire flap can be elevated deep to this layer. Care must be taken beyond the hairline to preserve the hair follicles. De-epithelializing a few millimeters of the scalp at the pretrichal region and beveling the flap incision will usually result in hair growing through the incision for better scar camouflage.

Single rotation flaps can also be used centrally (**Fig. 4.7**). A large cutback may be necessary to facilitate closure of small-to-medium defects secondary to the lack of tissue elasticity in the forehead skin.

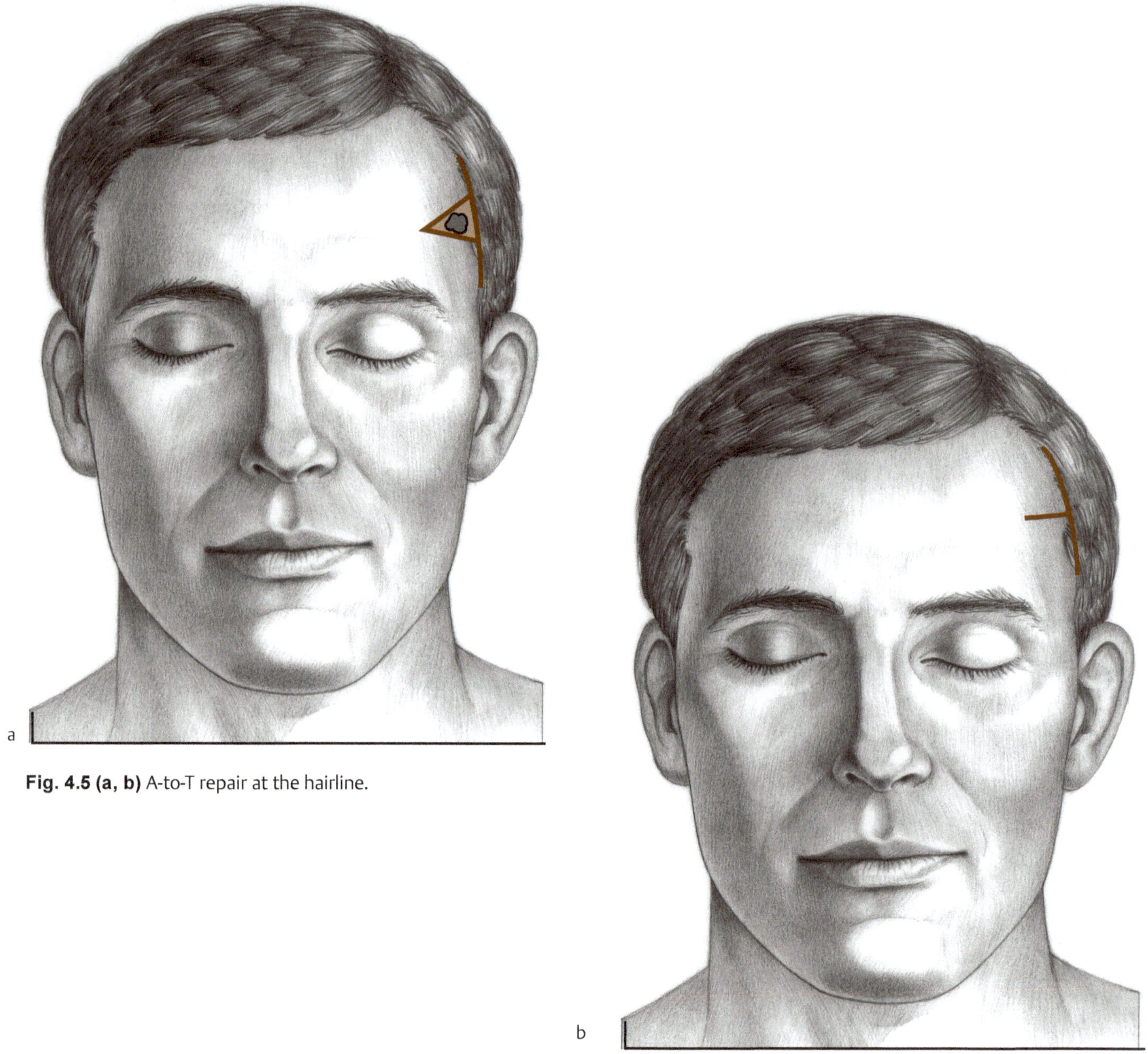

Fig. 4.5 (a, b) A-to-T repair at the hairline.

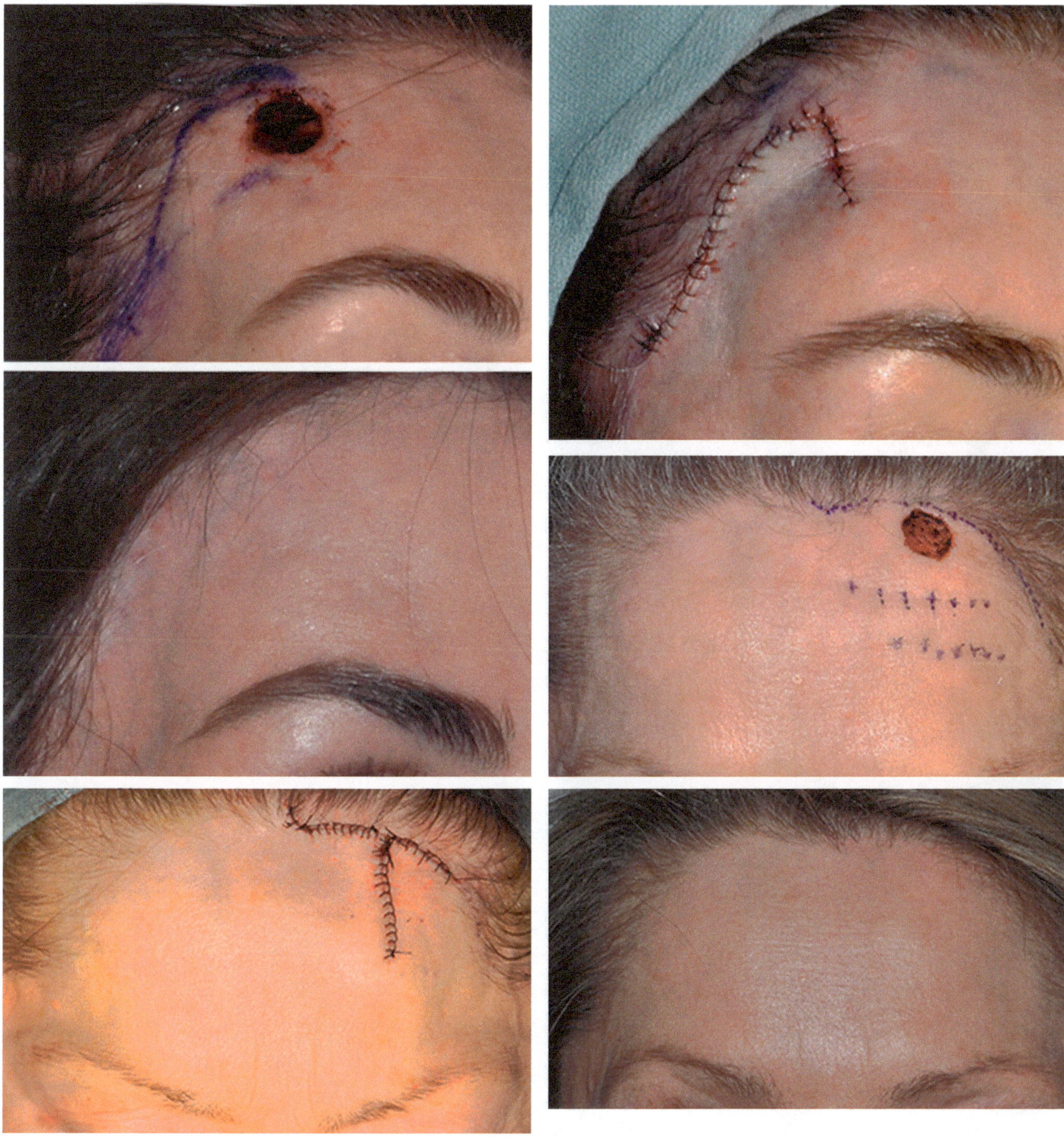

c d e f g h

Fig. 4.5 (c) Hairline defect. **(d)** Hairline rotation advancement flap. **(e)** Healed wound. **(f)** Hairline defect. **(g)** O-T advancement flap. **(h)** Healed wound.

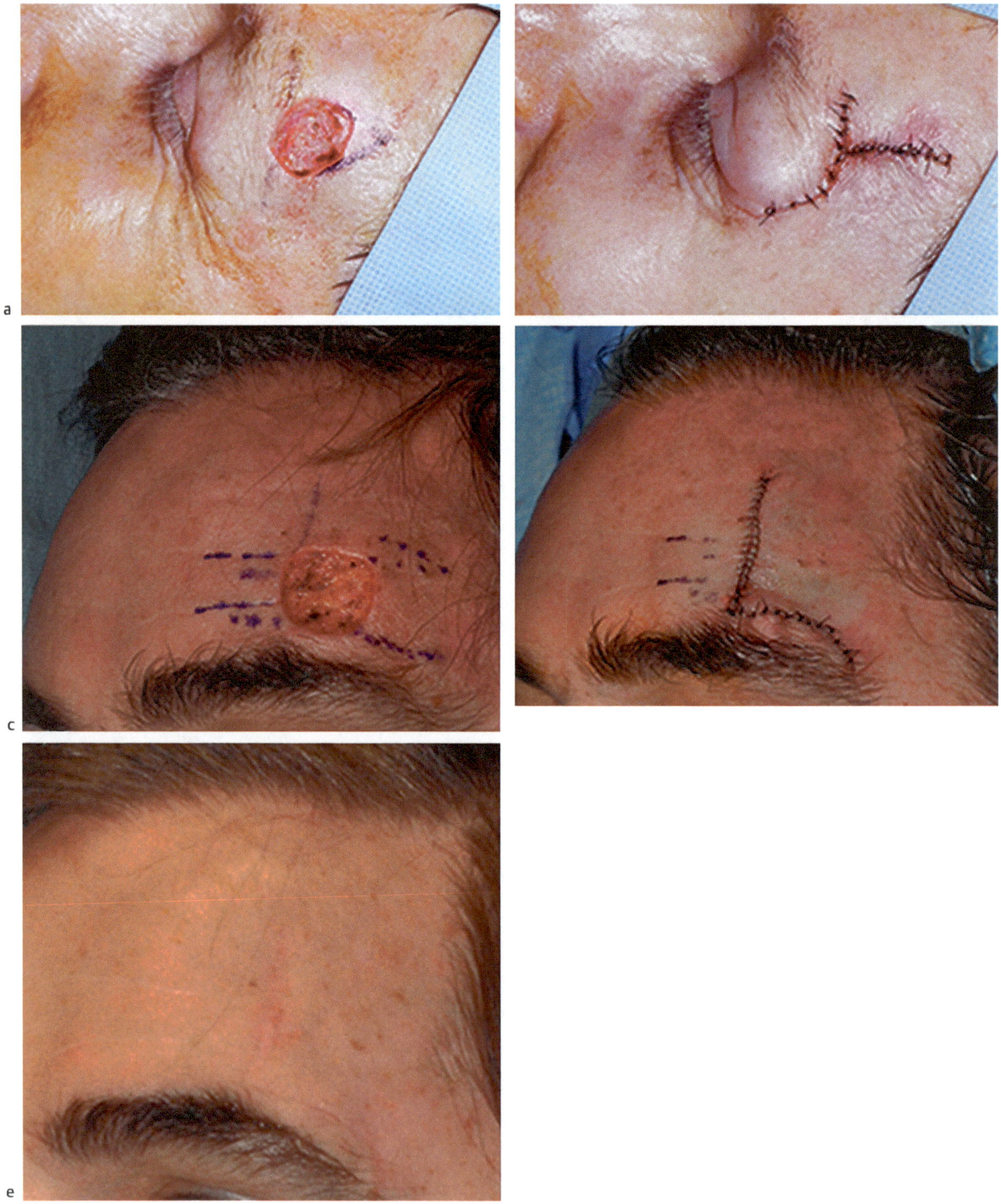

Fig. 4.6 (a) A-to-T flap at the eyebrow. **(b)** A-to-T flap closure at the eyebrow. **(c)** Eyebrow defect. **(d)** Eyebrow temporal advancement flap. **(e)** Healed wound.

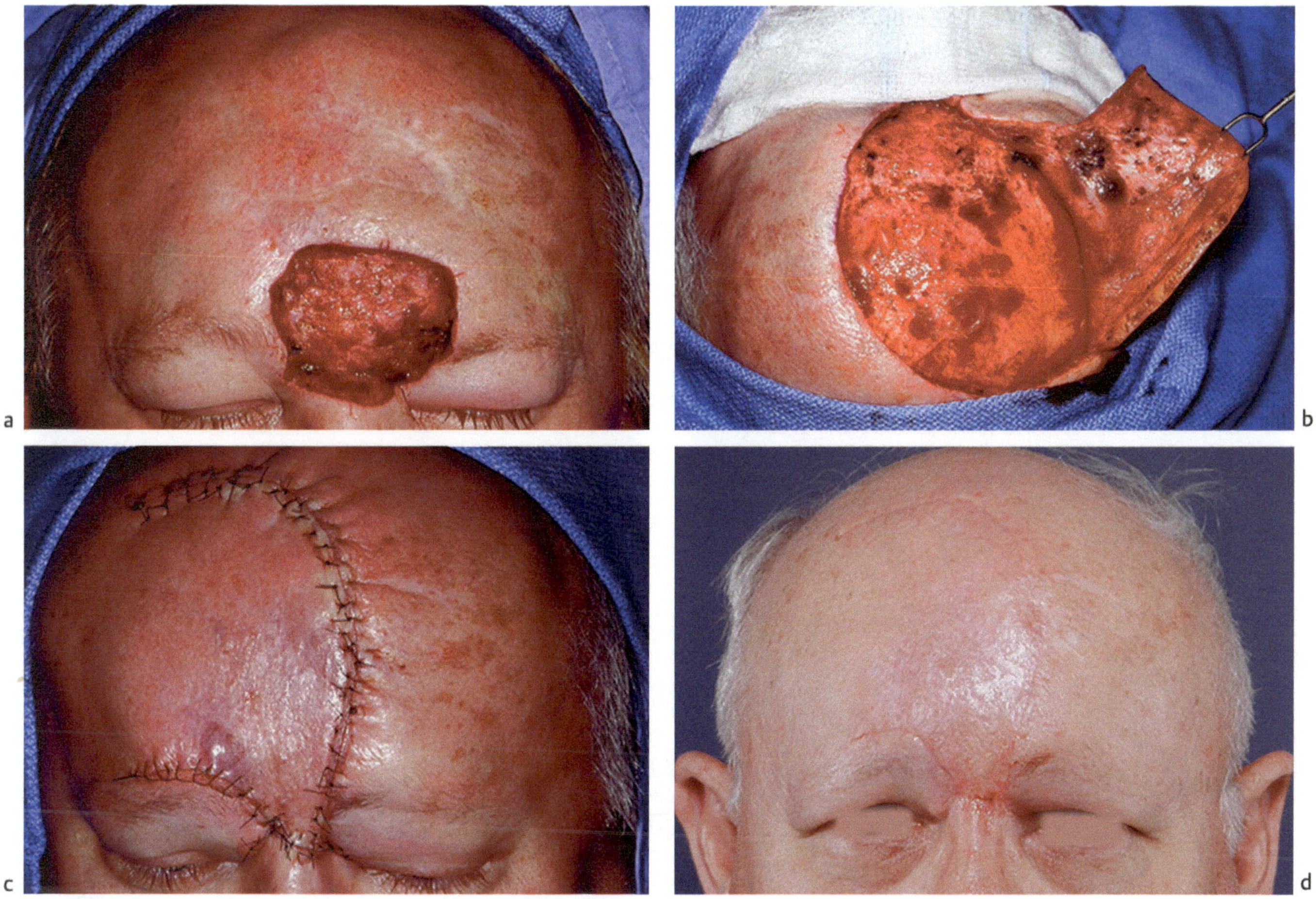

Fig. 4.7 (a) Central forehead defect. **(b)** Large rotation flap elevated in the subgaleal plane. **(c)** Large rotation flap closure using the eyebrow as camouflage for the inferior flap border. **(d)** Early flap result.

Single or double transposition flaps are useful in the temple, either to close smaller defects with the aesthetic subunit or to recruit tissue from the more lax cheek area for larger defects (**Fig. 4.8**). Bilobed flap designs are valuable when the donor site of a single transposition flap cannot be closed primarily. Bilobed flaps can be designed with the base oriented either anteriorly or posteriorly (**Fig. 4.9**). Flaps are raised in the subcutaneous level, and attention should be paid to the course of the temporal branch of the facial nerve to avoid injury.

A final consideration in the temporal forehead and in the central forehead near the hairline or in the glabellar concavity is the possibility of allowing wounds to heal by secondary intention. The wound is treated with a moist occlusive dressing during the healing phase. In many cases, lesions within the concave portion of the lateral forehead and close to the hairline will heal in a few weeks with acceptable scars.

Massive defects of the forehead can be addressed with a variety of techniques, including tissue expansion or skin grafting with later serial excision. If the patient is willing to allow the bed of the wound to granulate for 3 to 4 weeks, full-thickness skin grafts may be used with adequate results.

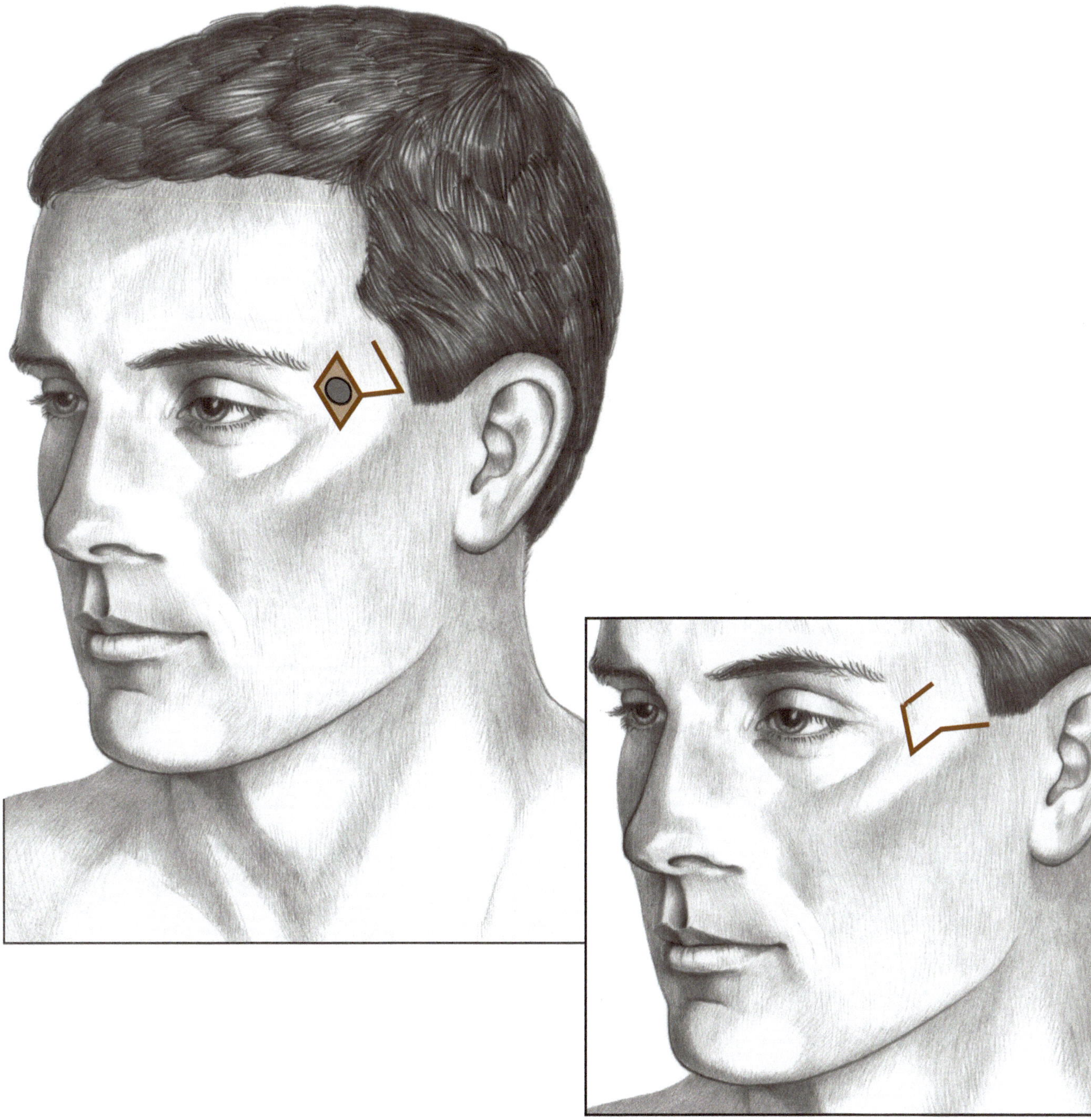

Fig. 4.8 Rhombic flap of the temple.

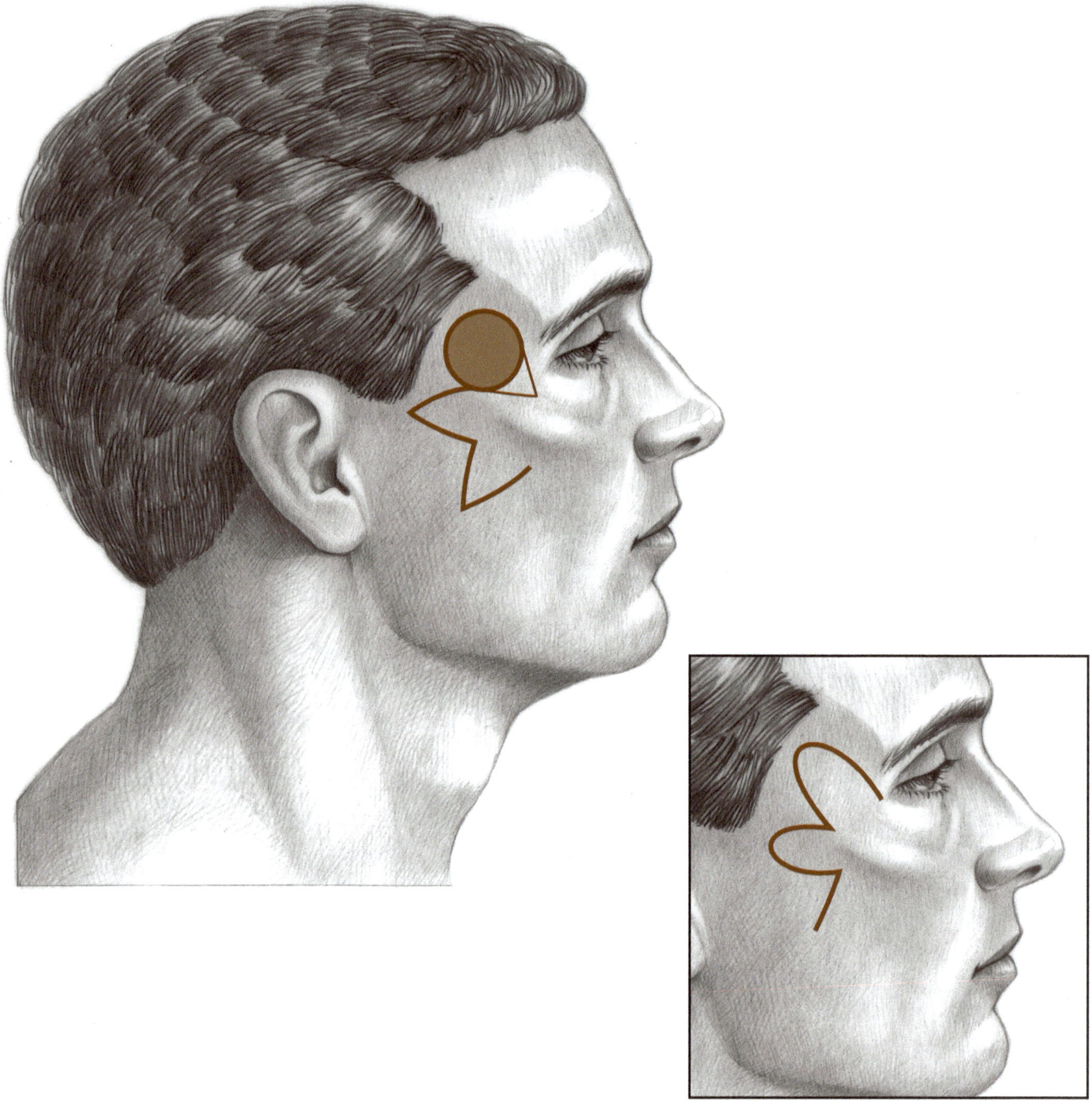

a

Fig. 4.9 (a) Anteriorly based bilobed flap of the temple.

b
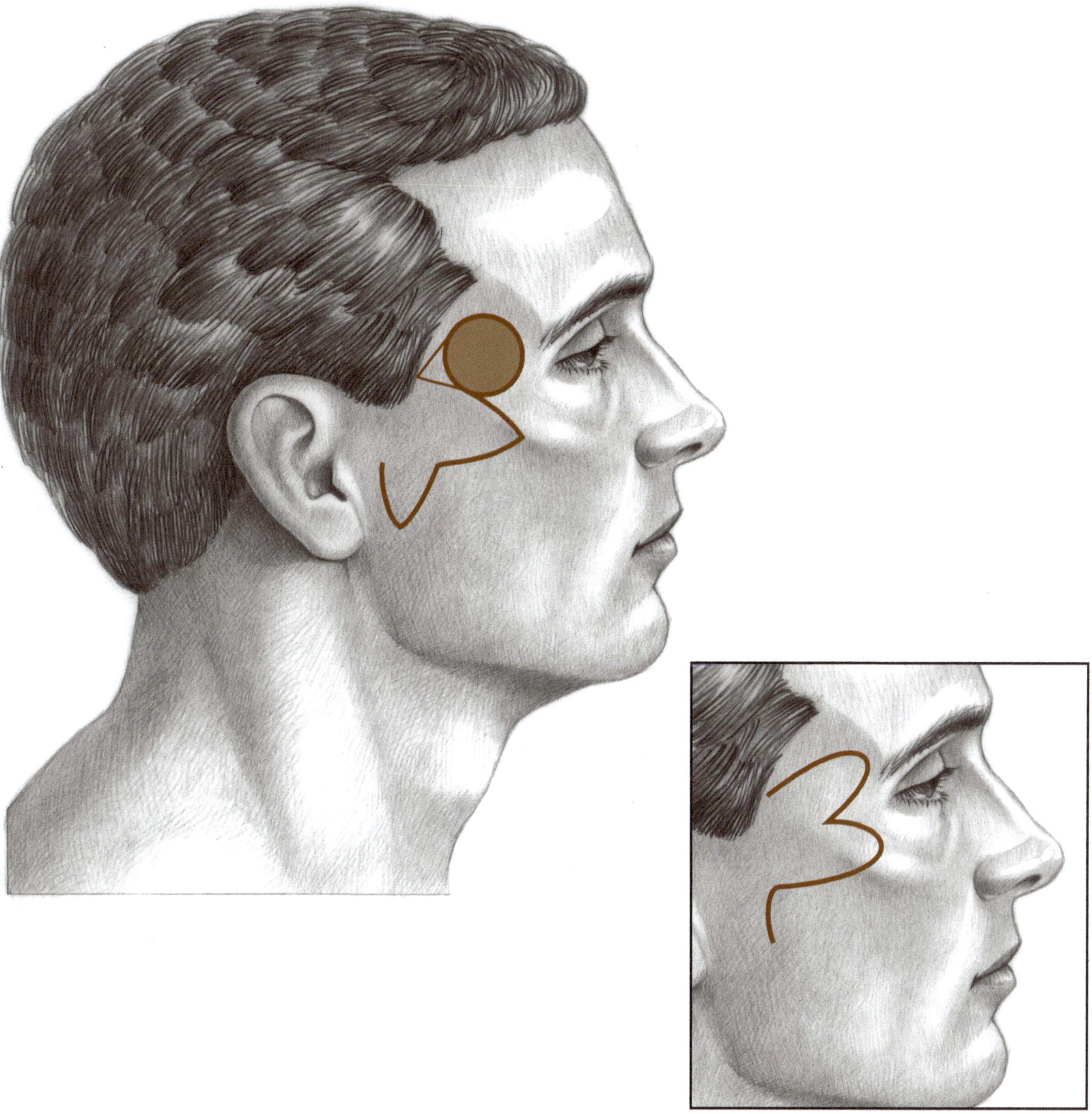

Fig. 4.9 (b) Posteriorly based bilobed flap of the temple.

Suggested Reading

Becker FF. Local flaps in facial plastic surgery. J Dermatol Surg Oncol 1988;14(6):635–647

Coleman DJ. Use of expanded temporal flaps to resurface the skin grafted forehead. Br J Plast Surg 1987;40(2):171–172

Fatah MF. Innervation and functional reconstruction of the forehead. Br J Plast Surg 1991;44(5):351–358

Field LM. The forehead V-to-T plasty (Dieffenbach's winged V-plasty). J Dermatol Surg Oncol 1986;12(6):560–562

Grekin RC, Schaler RE, Crumley RL. Cancer of the forehead and temple regions. Dermatol Clin 1989;7(4):699–710

Larrabee WF Jr. Design of local skin flaps. In: Thomas JR, ed. AAO-HNS Instructional Courses. Vol. 3. St. Louis: Mosby Year Book; 1990:252–273

Siegle RJ. Forehead reconstruction. J Dermatol Surg Oncol 1991;17(2):200–204

Sutton AE, Quatela VC. Bilobed flap reconstruction of the temporal forehead. Arch Otolaryngol Head Neck Surg 1992;118(9):978–982, discussion 983–984

Zitelli JA. Wound healing by secondary intention: a cosmetic appraisal. J Am Acad Dermatol 1983;9(3):407–415

5 Eyes

Summary

This chapter focuses on the principles and surgical techniques associated with reconstruction of defects involving the eye. Eyelid reconstruction seeks to provide adequate eyelid function and globe protection while maintaining acceptable cosmetic result. Eye reconstruction is broken up into subunits, with different treatment algorithms for upper compared to lower eyelid defects that are normally based on defect size. Of further importance, we discuss the evaluation of canthal tendon integrity and reconstruction with respect to lateral and medial canthal injuries.

Keywords: tarsus, canthal tendon, anterior lamella, posterior lamella, skin graft, cutler-beard flap, tarsal conjunctival flap, gray line, canthoplasty

♦ Introduction

In periocular reconstruction, the surgeon must provide adequate eyelid function, globe protection, and aesthetically acceptable results. The anatomical boundaries of the periocular aesthetic unit are the inferior border of the eyebrow, the lateral and inferior orbital rim, and the nasojugal groove (**Fig. 5.1**). The periocular region can be divided into four subunits: the lower eyelid, the upper eyelid, the medial canthal region, and the lateral canthal region. The upper and lower eyelids are divided superficially deep into the anterior lamella, containing skin and the orbicularis oculi muscle, as well as the posterior lamella of the conjunctiva, tarsi, and lid retractors. The medial canthal subunit is concave and contains the lacrimal drainage system and the medial canthal tendon. The lateral canthal subunit is slightly concave and contains the lateral canthal tendon. The eyebrow is treated as a subunit of the forehead, as its skin thickness, elasticity, and contour better match this region.

♦ Upper and Lower Eyelids

The upper and lower eyelids are separated into four categories for repair: anterior lamellar defects, and full-thickness defects involving <25% of the lid, 25–50% of the lid, and >50% of the lid. Full-thickness defects of the upper and lower eyelids must be reconstructed in multiple layers for optimal function and appearance. Each category will be discussed in detail for the upper and lower lids, along with the medial and lateral canthus.

♦ Upper Eyelid

Anterior Lamellar Defects

A partial-thickness defect of the upper or lower eyelid <0.5 cm in diameter heals well by secondary intention (**Fig. 5.2**). A defect <50% of the anterior lamella of the upper eyelid can be closed with a variety of local flaps. Upper eyelid defects are best closed with flaps incised parallel to the natural creases of the eyelid (**Fig. 5.3**). The orbicularis muscle is removed from the deep surface of the defect. The flaps are harvested as skin–muscle flaps. Care must be taken to avoid excessive tension on the closure. The muscle is closed with 6–0 or 7–0 buried absorbable sutures, and the skin is closed with a 6–0 or 7–0 monofilament suture. If excess tension causes lagophthalmos or ectropion, other tissues must be brought into the area for proper reconstruction.

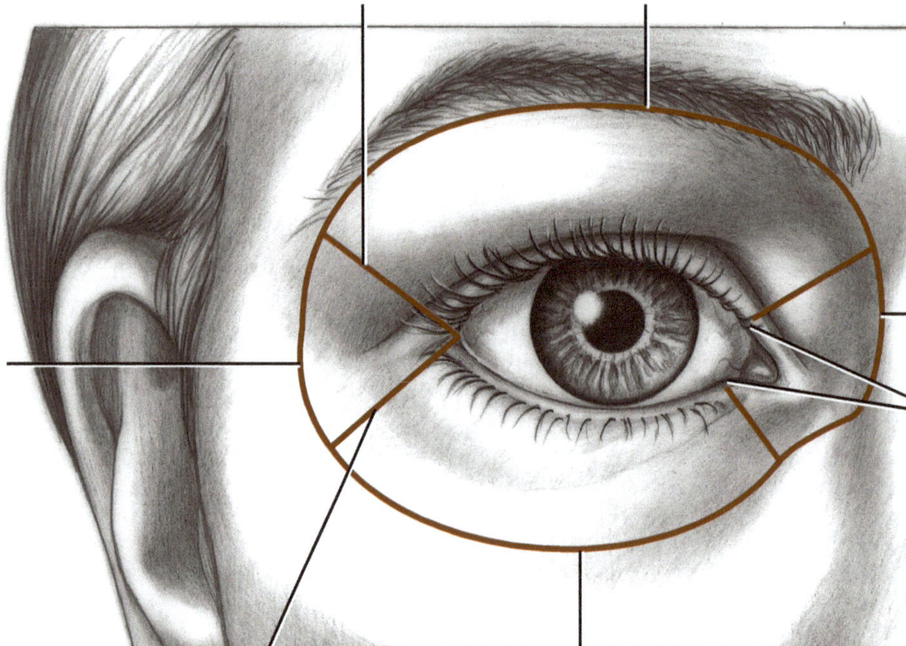

Fig. 5.1 Aesthetic subunits of the periocular region.

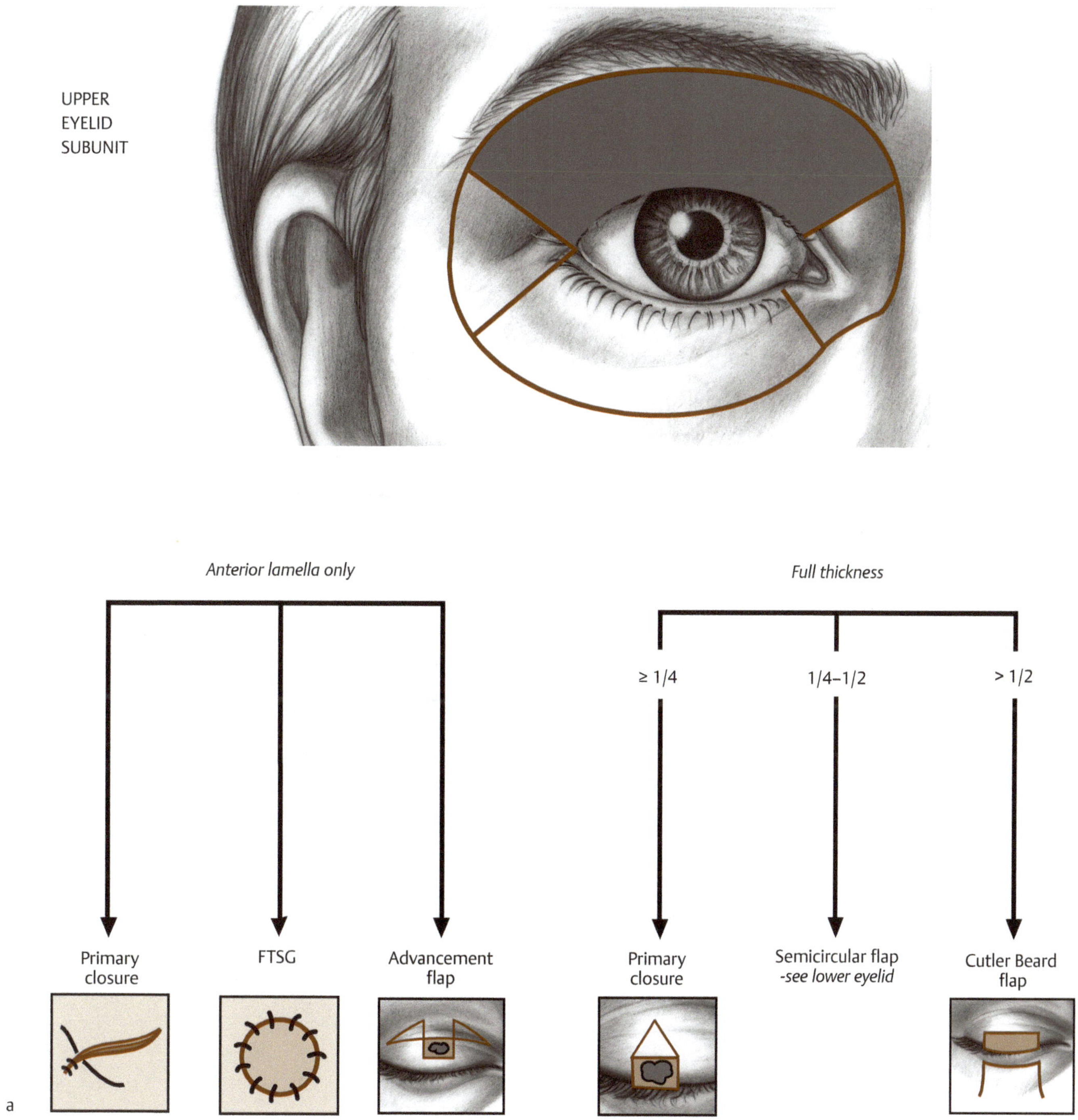

Fig. 5.2 (a) Upper eyelid subunit.

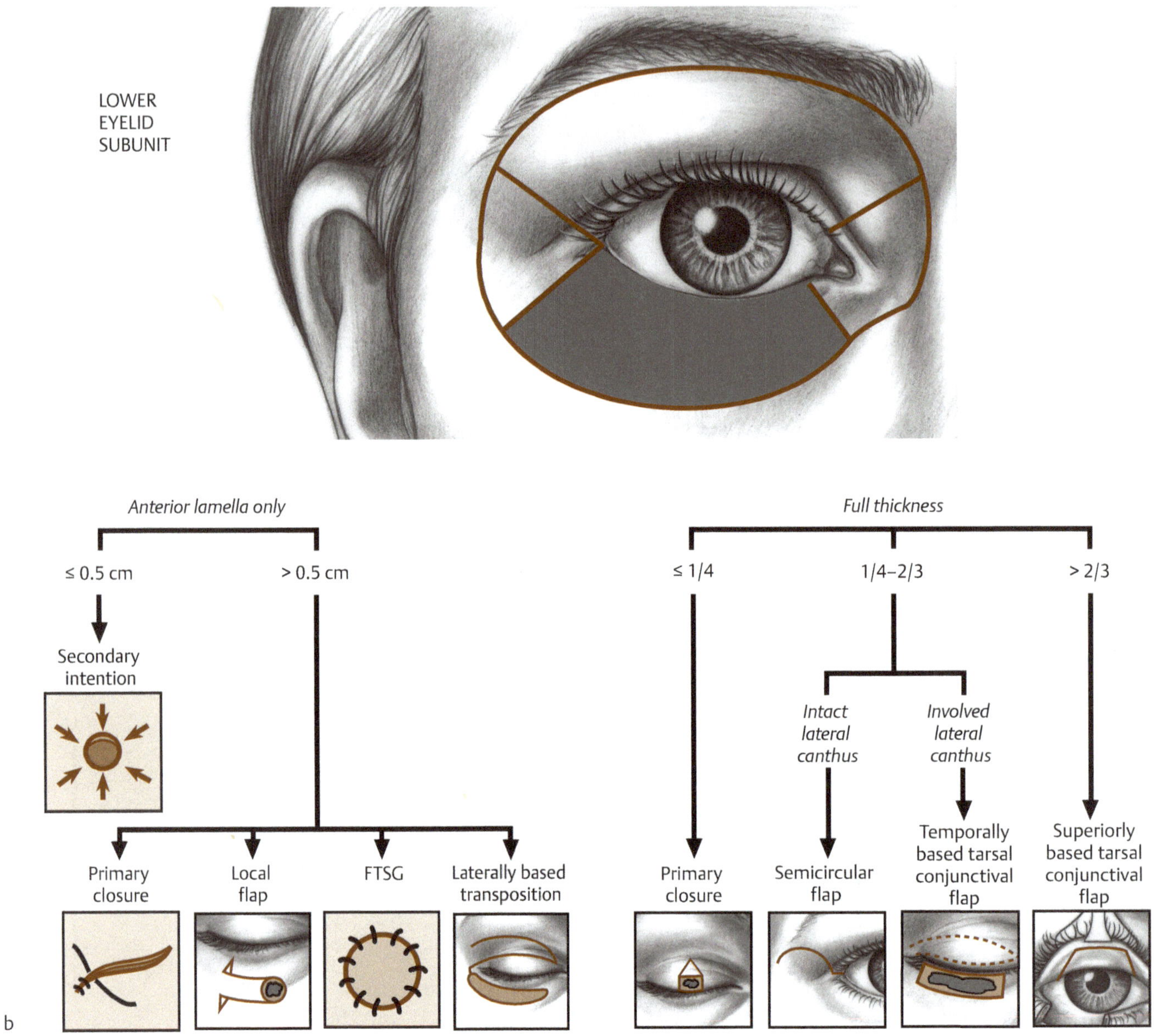

Fig. 5.2 (b) Lower eyelid subunit. FTSG, full-thickness skin graft.

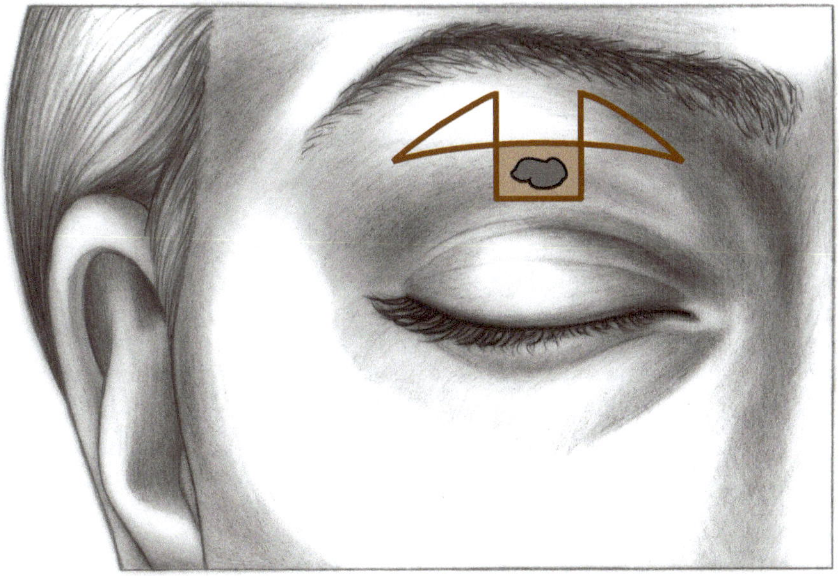

a

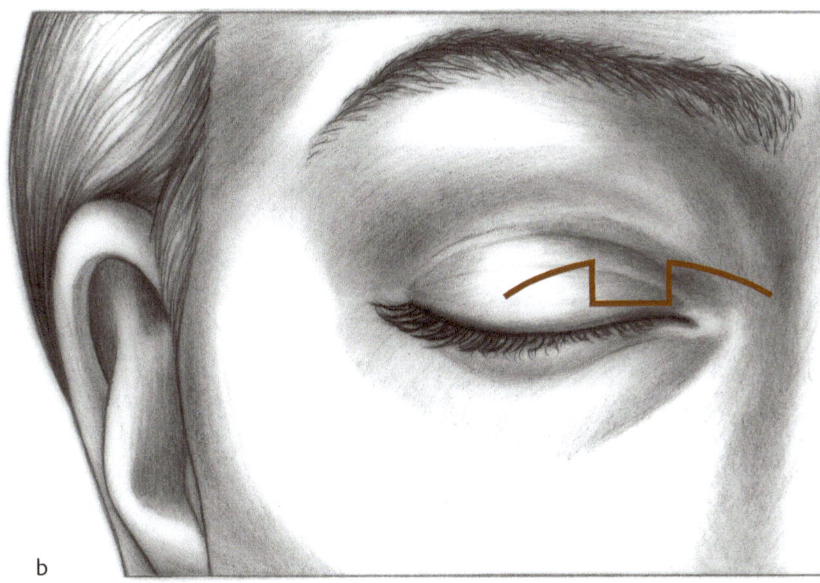

b

Fig. 5.3 (a, b) Advancement flap of the upper eyelid.

The excess skin usually present in the upper eyelid aids in reconstruction of both the upper and lower eyelid subunits. If excess tension causes lagophthalmos (as in defects >50% of the upper lid), a full-thickness skin graft (FTSG) from the opposite upper eyelid or the postauricular region is a good alternative to primary closure.

Full Thickness < 25%

Defects up to 25% of the upper or lower eyelid can be closed primarily (**Fig. 5.4, Fig. 5.5,** and **Fig. 5.6**). The incision through the tarsal plate is perpendicular to the lid margin. A full-thickness Burow triangle is incised away from the edge of the tarsal plate, farthest from the lid margin. The first suture of 6–0 silk is placed precisely at the lid margin ("gray line"), entering the skin 3 mm from the cut edge, to a depth of 3 mm, and exiting 3 mm from the opposite cut skin edge. Two or three 6–0 absorbable sutures with the knots superficial are then used to approximate the tarsus. The anterior lid margin is closed with 6–0 silk sutures left long, so they can be tied away from the lid margin under the most distal suture. An alternative is to use a buried mattress absorbable suture at the margin. The skin sutures are removed in 4 or 5 days and the lid margin sutures in 7 to 10 days.

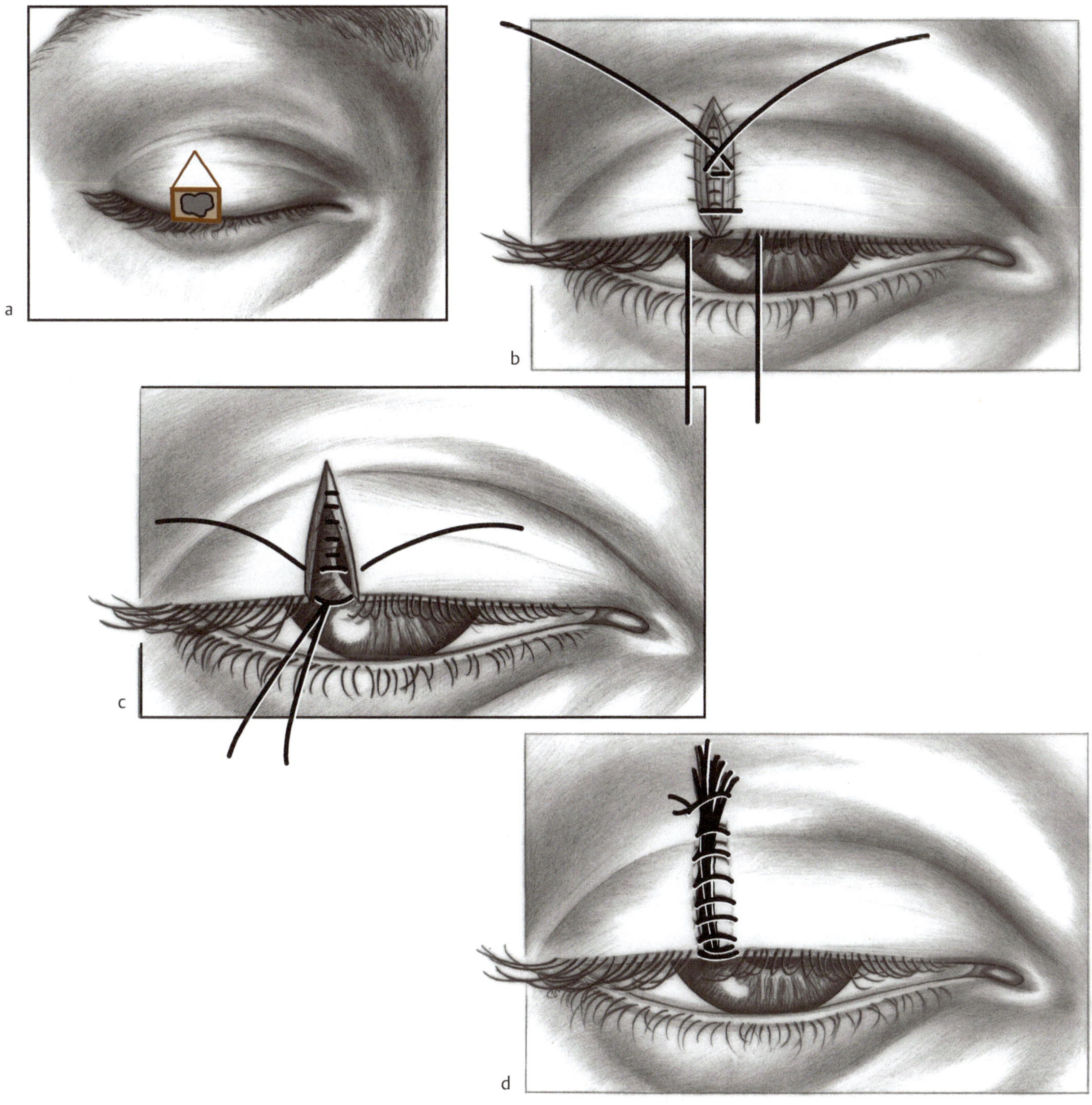

Fig. 5.4 (a–d) Primary repair of a full-thickness upper eyelid defect.

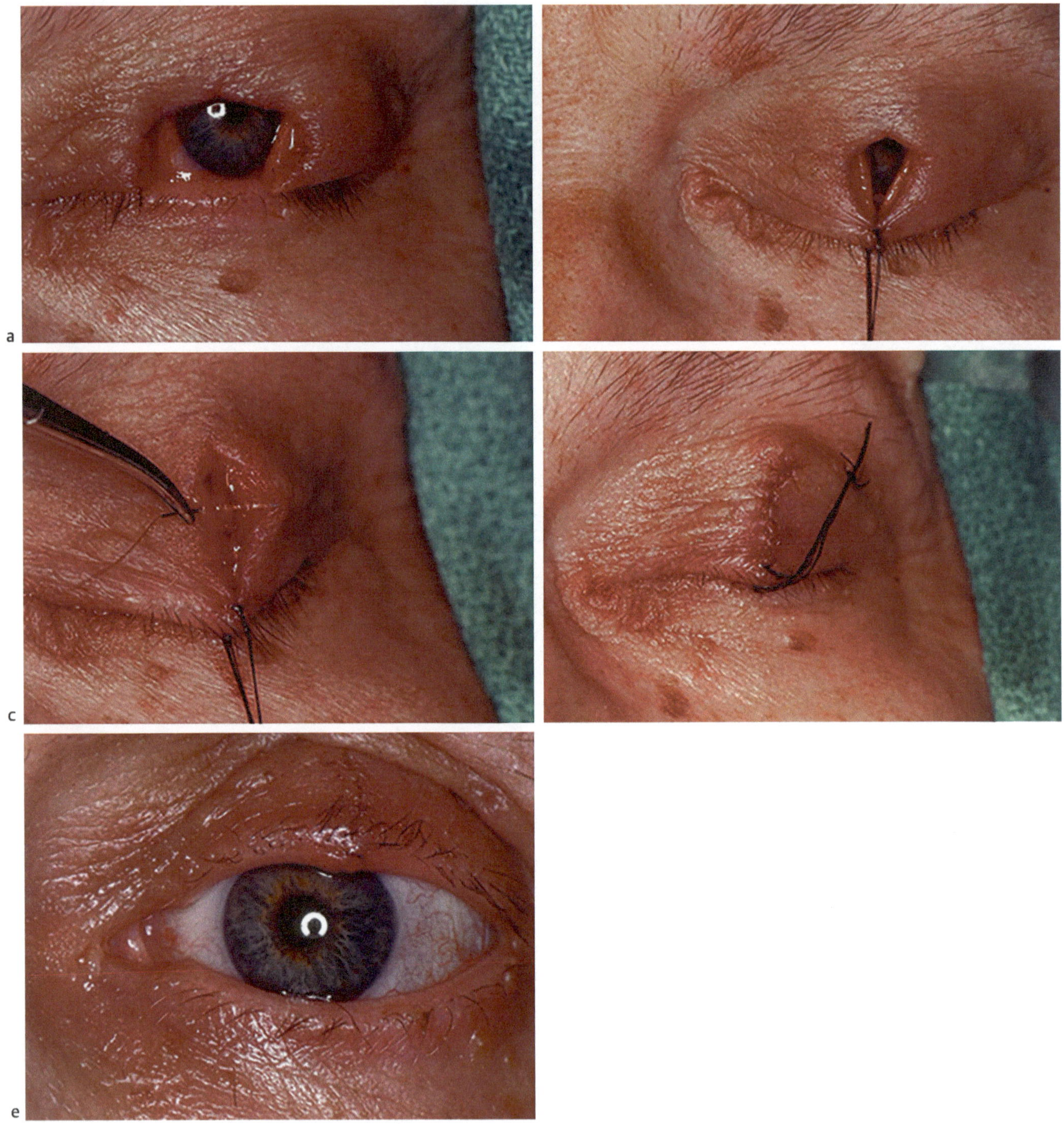

Fig. 5.5 **(a)** Full-thickness upper eyelid defect (<25%). **(b)** Primary closure of the eyelid with the first suture placed at the lid margin. **(c)** Approximation of the tarsus. **(d)** Closure of the anterior lid margin. **(e)** Early postoperative appearance.

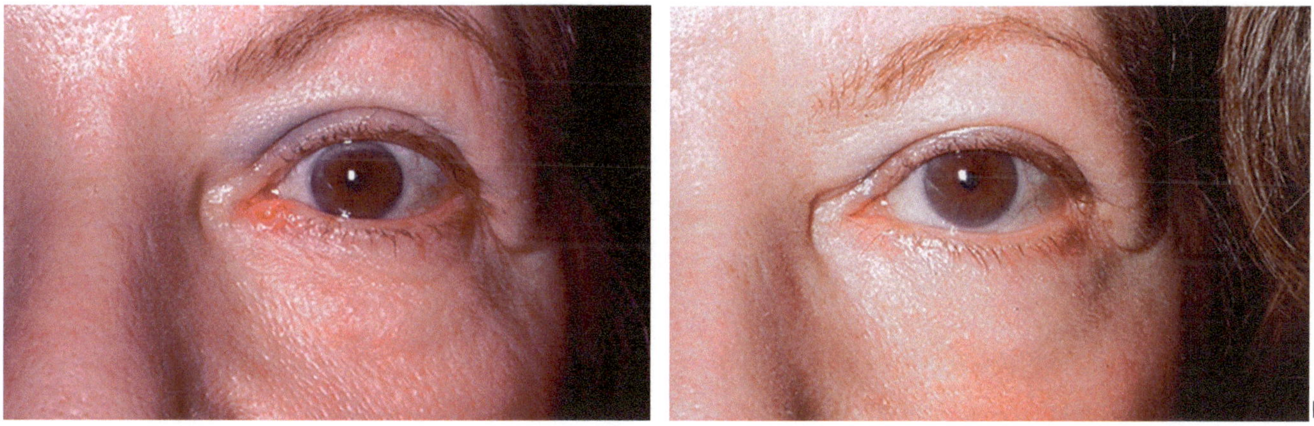

a b

Fig. 5.6 (a) Basal cell carcinoma of the left medial lower eyelid. **(b)** One year after full-thickness primary lower lid closure.

Full Thickness 25–50%

Up to one-half of the upper lid can be closed with the semicircular flap (**Fig. 5.7** and **Fig. 5.8**). The lateral canthus must be intact for utilization of this flap. The defect site is prepared, as in the primary closure case, with a Burow triangle excision at the base of the defect ("inverted house"), away from the tarsus. A semicircle, starting at the lateral canthus, and in the opposite direction from the lid involved, is drawn. For the lower lid, the semicircle is kept within the outlines of a line that would be an inferior continuation of the eyebrow. A skin flap is incised to the depth of the lateral orbital rim periosteum. The lateral canthal tendon is identified, and the limb to the involved eyelid is cut at the orbital rim. The defect edges are then approximated by pulling on the cut edges with skin hooks. Upper eyelid defects should be repaired with less tension, or ptosis will result.

If there is excessive tension at the first approximation of wound edges, then the orbital septum, lid retractors, and conjunctiva can be sequentially cut to relieve tension. Once appropriate tension is obtained, the primary defect site is closed, as previously described, for primary closure of full-thickness defects. The lateral canthus is reformed with a vertical mattress 5–0 or 6–0 monofilament suture tied over a bolster. This suture is placed beginning at the skin surface of the normal lid and passing full thickness through first the normal and then the involved lid. The short limb of the vertical mattress suture is passed from the involved lid to the normal lid and includes the intact limb of the lateral canthal tendon. This suture is left in place 7 to 10 days. The rest of the semicircular flap is closed, using the principle of halving, with vertical mattress sutures.

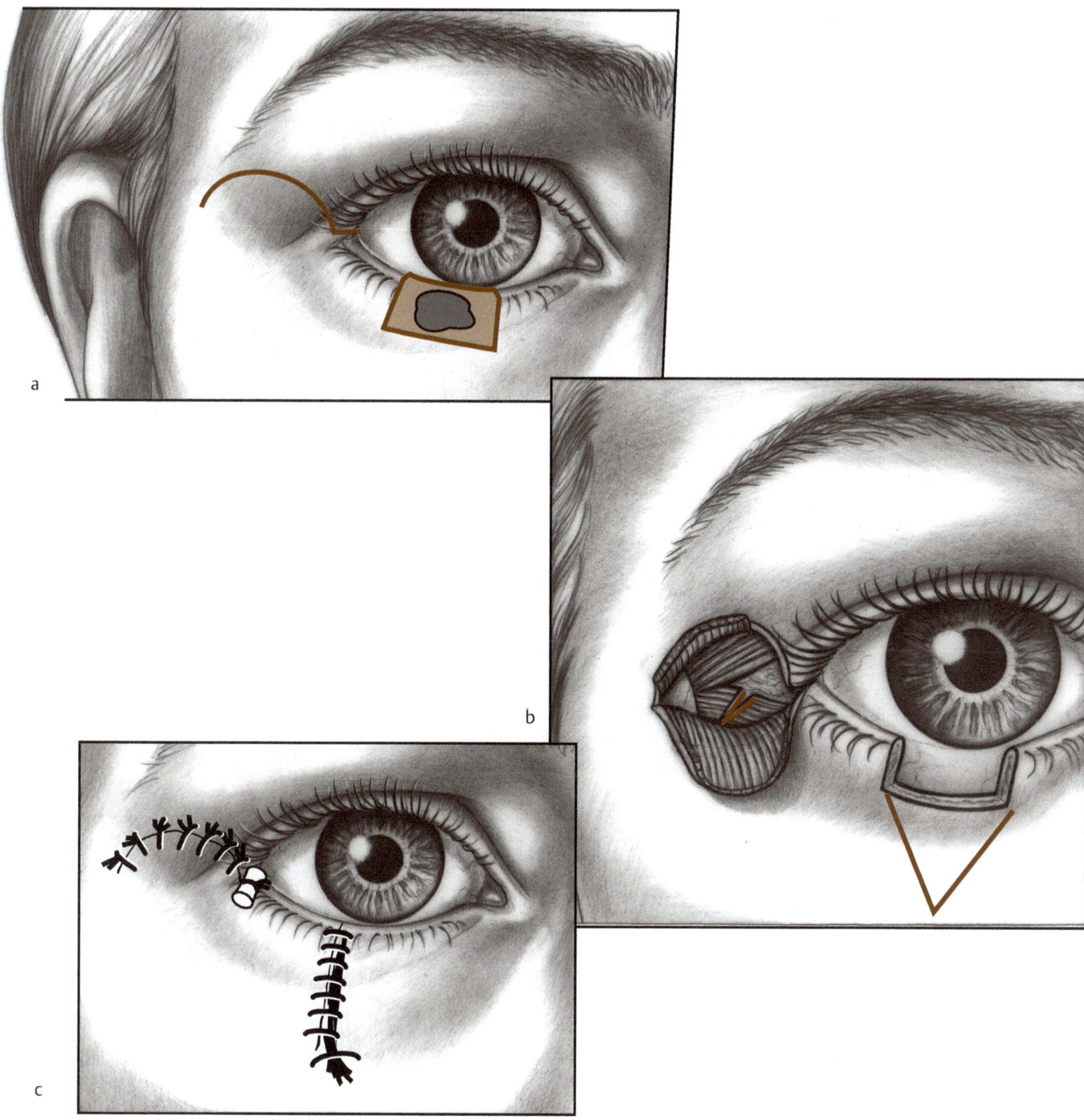

Fig. 5.7 (a–c) Lower lid semicircular flap.

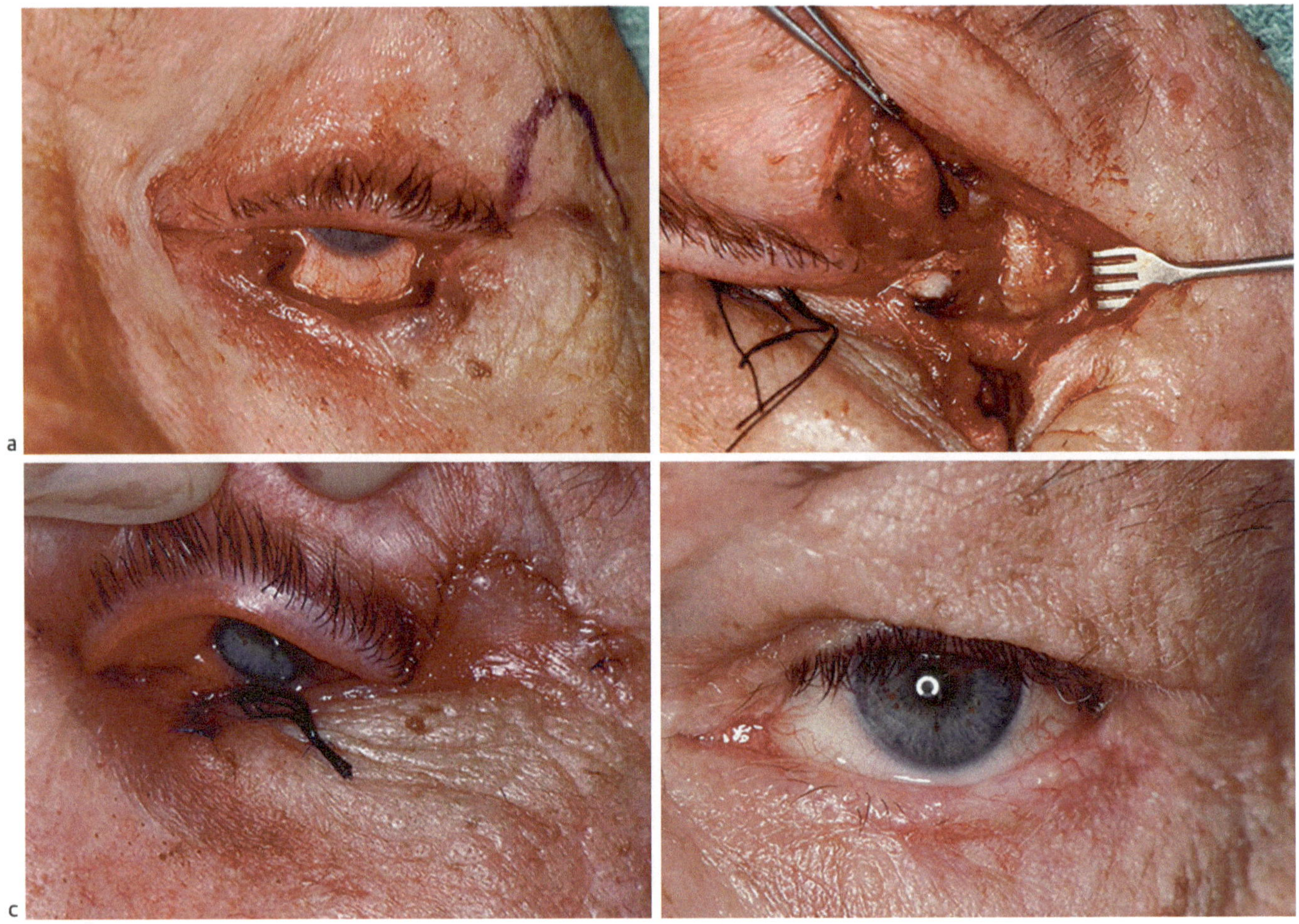

Fig. 5.8 (a) Lower eyelid defect (<two-thirds) with planned semicircular flap. **(b)** Skin flap created, and lateral canthal tendon identified and cut. **(c)** Closure of flap and defect. **(d)** Appearance postoperatively.

Full Thickness > 50%

More than 50% of the upper eyelid is reconstructed with the Cutler–Beard flap (**Fig. 5.9** and **Fig. 5.10**). A full-thickness horizontal incision, just inferior to the lower tarsus and of appropriate length corresponding to the defect, is made. Full-thickness vertical incisions are made in an inferior direction from the ends of the horizontal incision. The flap is pulled into place under the intact lower tarsal bridge. The upper lid tarsal remnants are fixed to the lower lid conjunctiva and retractors with partial-thickness 6–0 or 7–0 absorbable sutures with the knots tied away from the conjunctiva. The muscle layer and skin layer are then closed. The eye is protected until flap division with an external eye shield.

The eye is reopened in 6 to 8 weeks. The upper eyelid is contoured to match the opposite upper eyelid. The conjunctiva is left 1 to 2 mm long on the upper eyelid side at division. This tissue is wrapped around the edge of the newly formed upper lid margin. The inferior edge of the lower tarsal bridge is sharply opened, and the flap remnant is contoured for proper, no-tension closure at the fresh border. The wound is closed in layers.

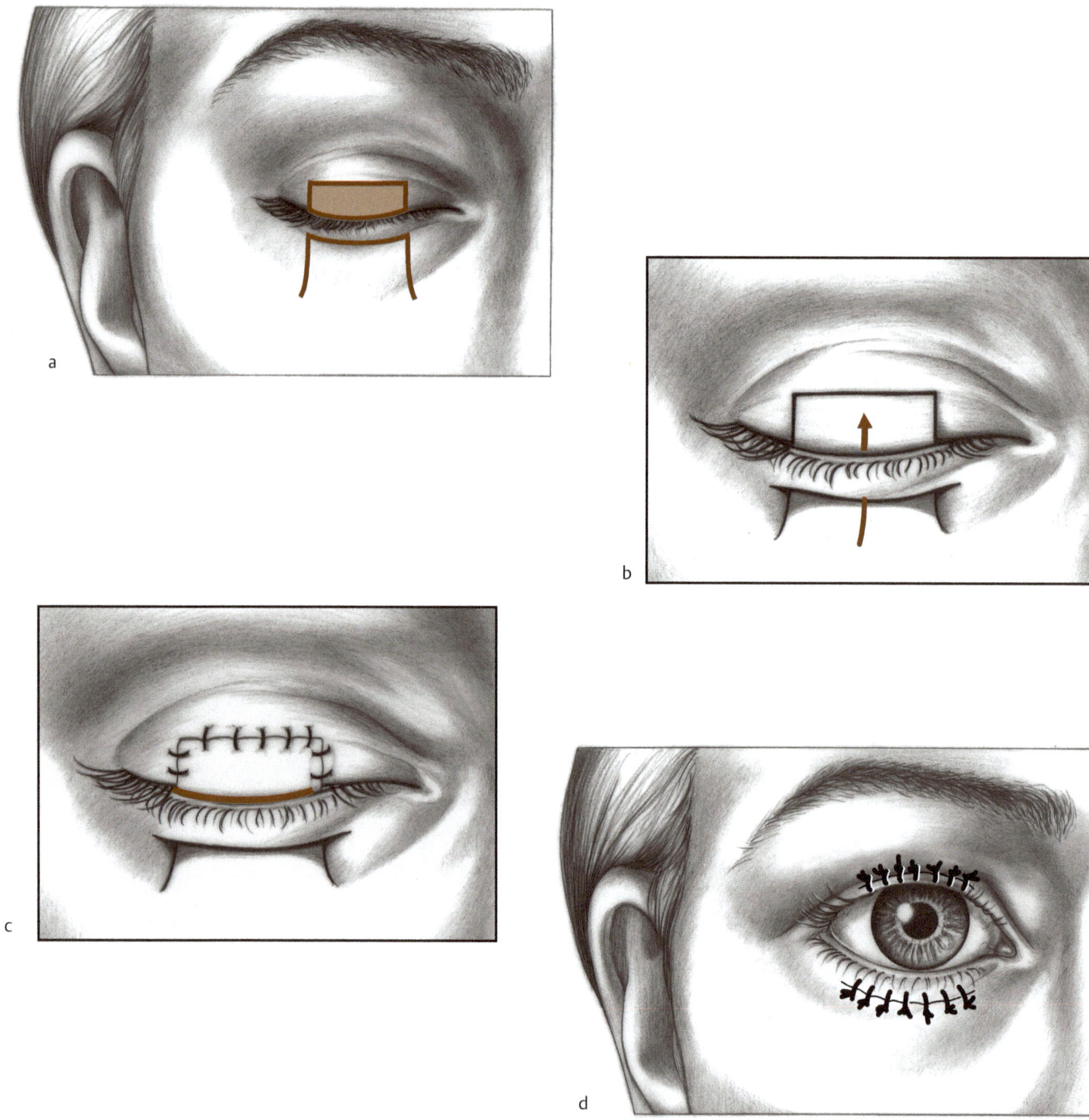

Fig. 5.9 (a–d) Cutler–Beard flap.

a 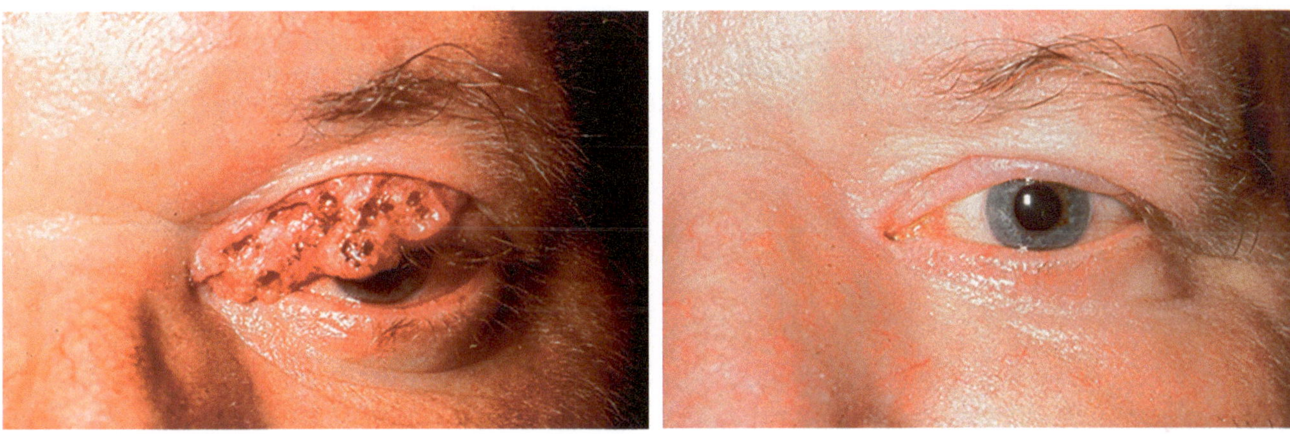 b

Fig. 5.10 (a) Large squamous cell carcinoma of the upper eyelid. **(b)** One year after Cutler–Beard flap reconstruction of the upper eyelid.

♦ Lower Eyelid

Anterior Lamellar Defects

A partial-thickness defect of the lower eyelid <0.5 cm in diameter heals well by secondary intention (**Fig. 5.2**). A defect <50% of the anterior lamella of the lower eyelid can be closed with a variety of local flaps, such as rectangular advancement flaps (**Fig. 5.11**). In lower eyelid reconstruction, maximal tension should be oriented in a plane parallel to the lower eyelid to prevent ectropion. Rotation flaps of lower eyelid skin are an excellent choice for many anterior lamellar defects (**Fig. 5.12**). In either case, the orbicularis muscle is removed from the deep surface of the defect. The flaps are harvested as skin–muscle flaps. Care must be taken to avoid excessive tension on the closure. The muscle is closed with 6–0 or 7–0 buried absorbable sutures, and the skin is closed with a 6–0 or 7–0 monofilament suture. If excess tension causes lagophthalmos or ectropion, other tissues must be brought into the area for proper reconstruction.

The excess skin usually present in the upper eyelid aids in reconstruction of both the upper and lower eyelid subunits. A partial-thickness defect >50% of the lower eyelid skin can be reconstructed with an FTSG of upper eyelid or postauricular skin. Alternatively, the upper eyelid skin–muscle layer can be transferred into a lower eyelid anterior lamella defect as a laterally based transposition flap (**Fig. 5.13**). The inferior incision of the flap is placed in the supertarsal crease. The donor site is closed primarily, and the flap is inset with 6–0 or 7–0 absorbable muscle sutures and 6–0 or 7–0 monofilament skin sutures. Blepharoplasty is usually performed on the opposite upper eyelid to maintain symmetry. If there is concern for future need of skin for grafting, then the contralateral blepharoplasty is deferred.

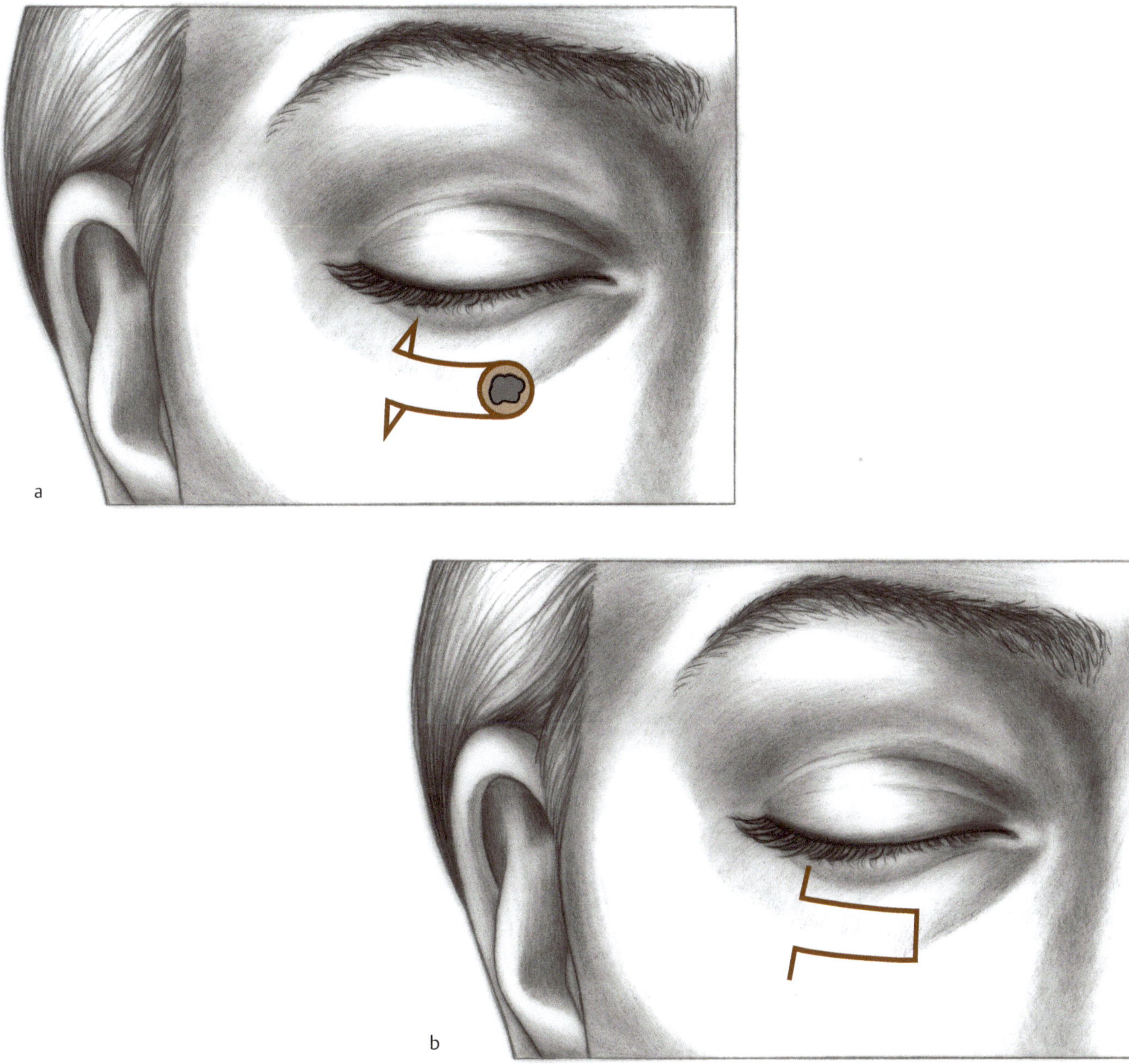

Fig. 5.11 (a, b) Advancement flap of the lower eyelid.

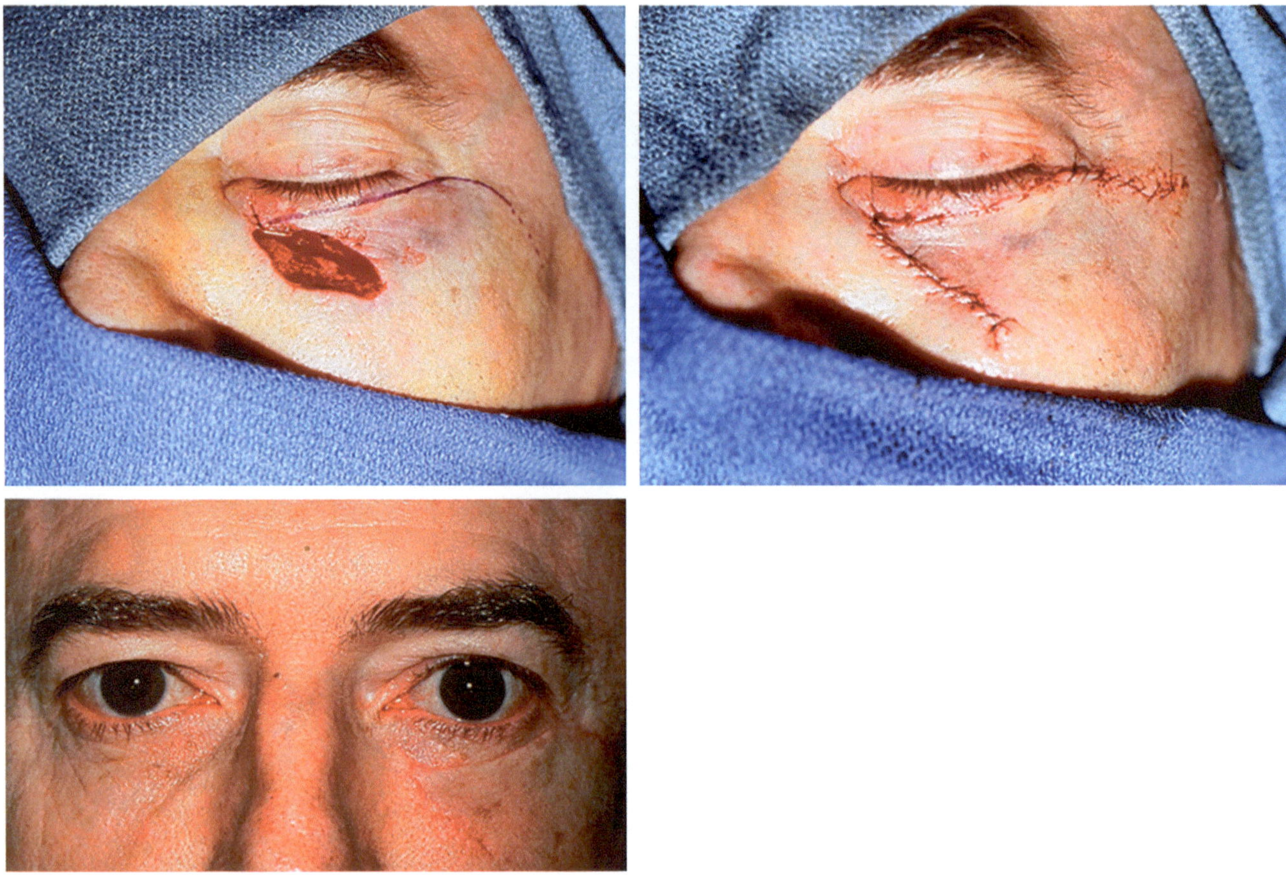

a b c

Fig. 5.12 (a) Planned rotation flap for lower eyelid closure. **(b)** Flap closure of the lower eyelid. **(c)** Early result for lower eyelid reconstruction.

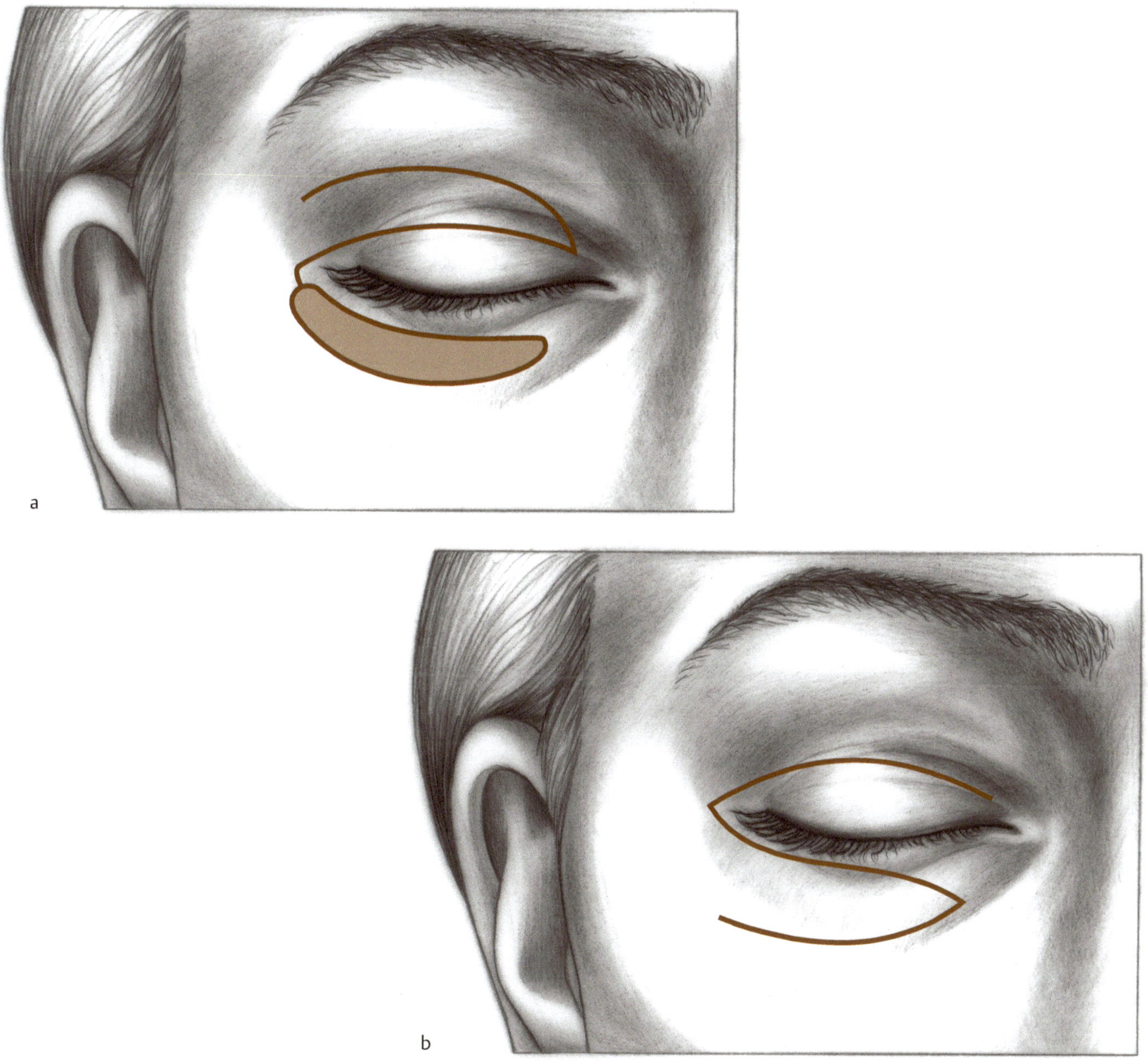

Fig. 5.13 (a, b) Laterally based upper lid myocutaneous flap.

Full Thickness <25%

See "Full Thickness <25%" for upper eyelids in previous pages of this chapter.

Full Thickness 25–50%

Up to two-thirds of the lower lid can be closed with the semicircular flap (**Fig. 5.7** and **Fig. 5.8**). The lateral canthus must be intact for utilization of this flap. The closure is comparable to that of the upper eyelid for "Full Thickness 25–50%" as illustrated above. Lower lid defects should be reconstructed so that the lower lid margin is tight against the globe to prevent ectropion.

Full Thickness > 50%

A defect involving up to two-thirds of the lower lid and the lateral canthus is reconstructed with the temporally based tarsal-conjunctival flap (**Fig. 5.14** and **Fig. 5.15**). The flap is incised on the conjunctiva of the everted upper eyelid, staying 3 to 4 mm from the lid margin. Müller muscle is left in place. The flap is left temporally hinged on a 4-mm pedicle and is rotated into place. The flap is fixed to the lower lid conjunctiva and lid retractor remnants with 8–0 chromic suture. The lower lid remnant is split at the gray line for 2 to 3 mm. The distal end of the flap is sandwiched into this area and the suture fixated with a full-thickness mattress suture of 6–0 silk. The anterior lamella is reconstructed with either an advancement flap or lower eyelid skin, or a laterally based myocutaneous flap from the upper eyelid.

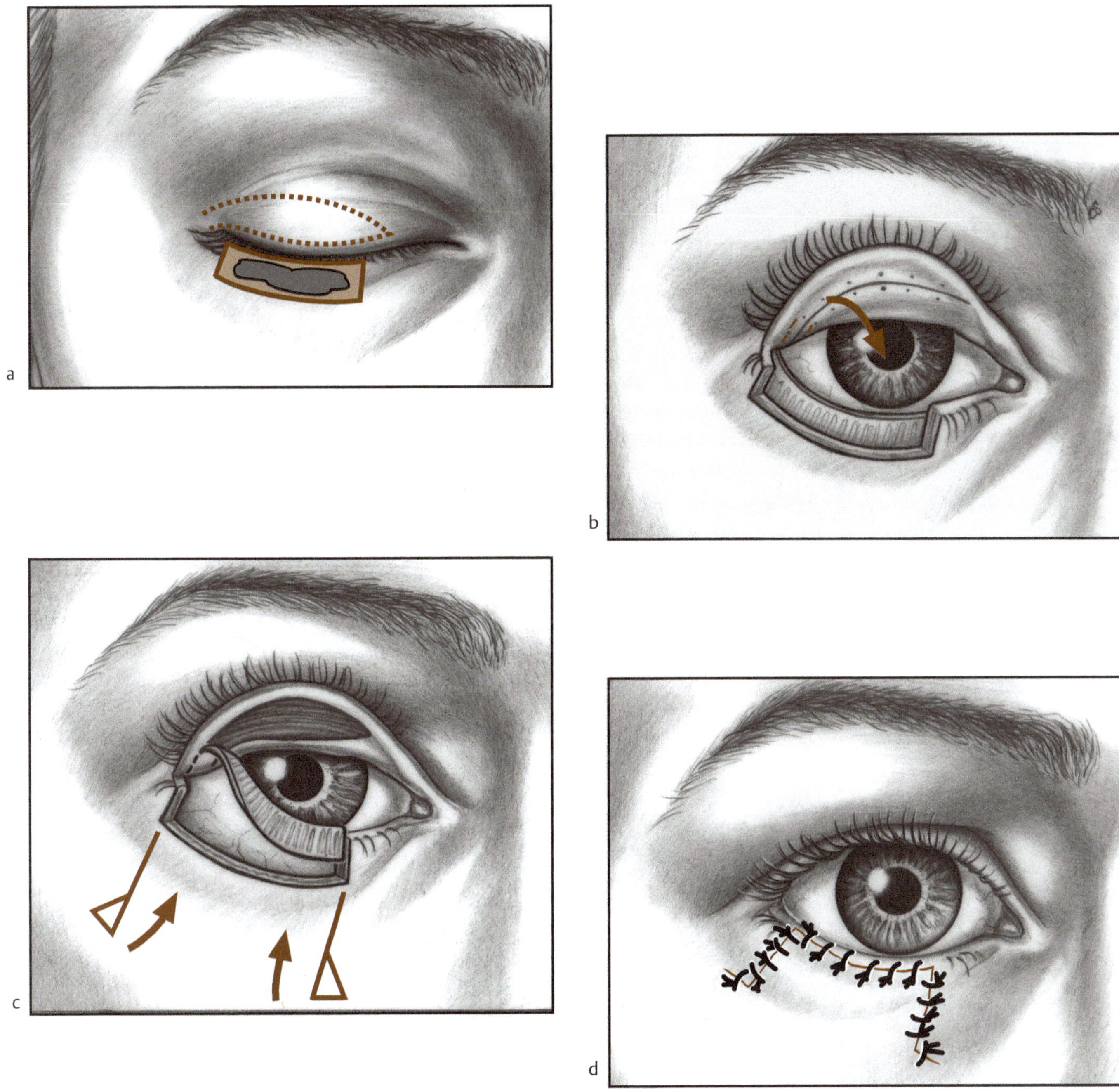

Fig. 5.14 (a–d) Temporally based tarsal conjunctival flap.

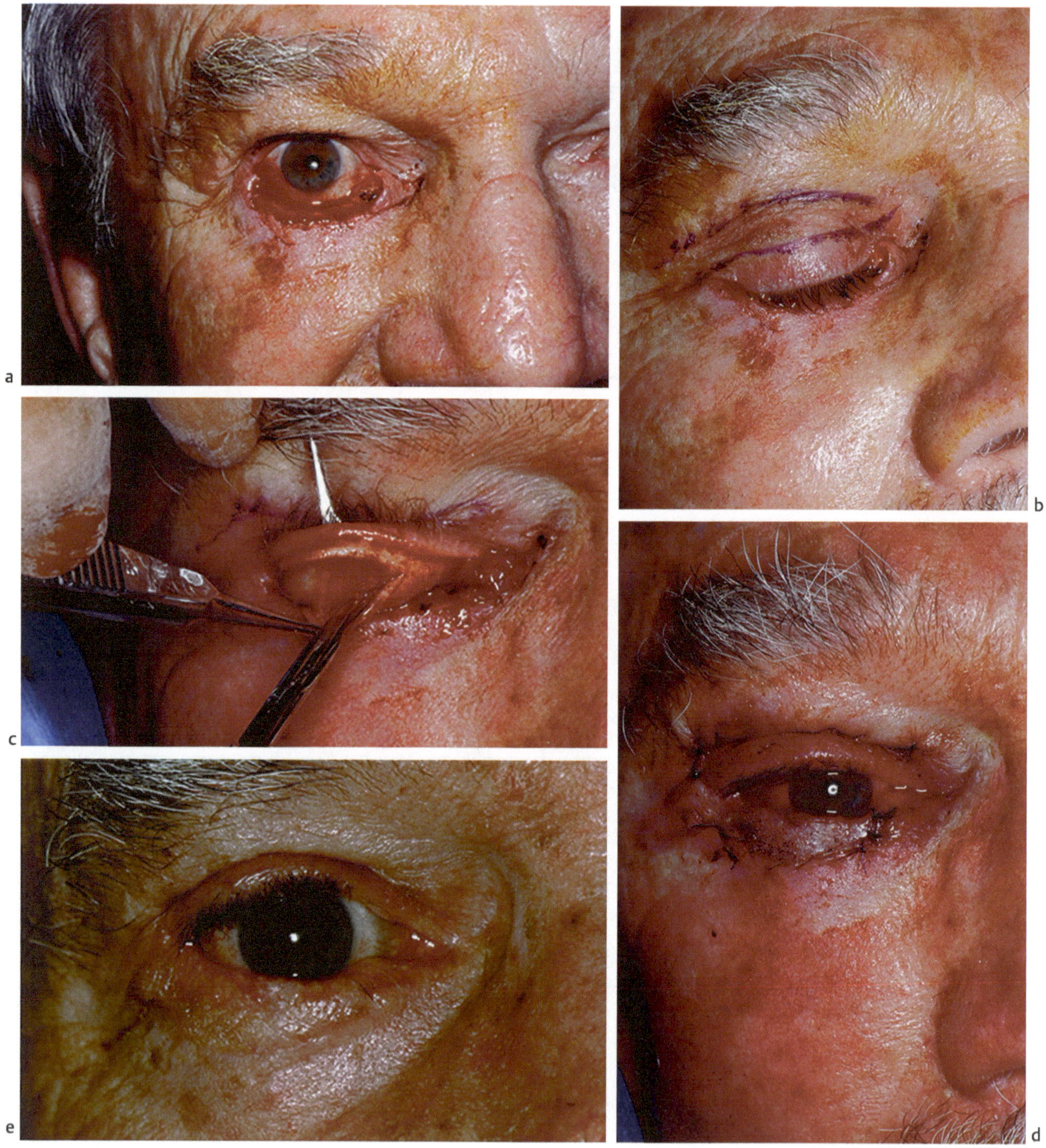

Fig. 5.15 (a) Large full-thickness defect of the lower eyelid. **(b)** Planned laterally based myocutaneous flap of the upper eyelid. **(c)** Temporally based tarsal conjunctival flap being elevated from the upper eyelid. **(d)** Closure in place. **(e)** Postoperative result.

A larger lower eyelid defect is reconstructed with the superiorly based tarsal-conjunctival flap, combined with a local advancement flap, an FTSG, or a laterally based myocutaneous flap from the upper eyelid (**Fig. 5.16, Fig. 5.17, Fig. 5.18** and **Fig. 5.19**). The rectangular-shaped tarsal-conjunctival flap is outlined on the everted eyelid. The flap is incised, with the anterior edge at least 3 mm from the lid margin. Müller muscle is not included in the flap. The portion of the flap that will overlie the pupil is incised and each side tubed upon itself with 7–0 Vicryl suture. The intact leading edge of the flap is inset into the defect and fixed in place with 8–0 chromic suture. The edges of the defect are split at the gray line, and the flap is sandwiched in with 6–0 silk mattress sutures. The inferiormost corners are reinforced with 7–0 silk mattress sutures, tied over bolsters. The anterior lamella is reconstructed as previously described with local tissue or a skin graft.

The flap is divided in 6 weeks, with 1 to 2 mm of excess conjunctiva left on the lower pedicles. The excess conjunctiva is wrapped over the fresh skin edge and is inset with 8–0 chromic suture. The donor upper eyelid is compared with the opposite upper eyelid for contour. If there is elevation or notching, the eyelid is everted, and scar bands are incised until the eyelids match. Although the reconstructed lower eyelid has no eyelashes, the eyelids both retain their normal length. This is a major advantage of this technique over the Mustarde technique that borrows tissue from the upper lid to reconstruct the lower lid.

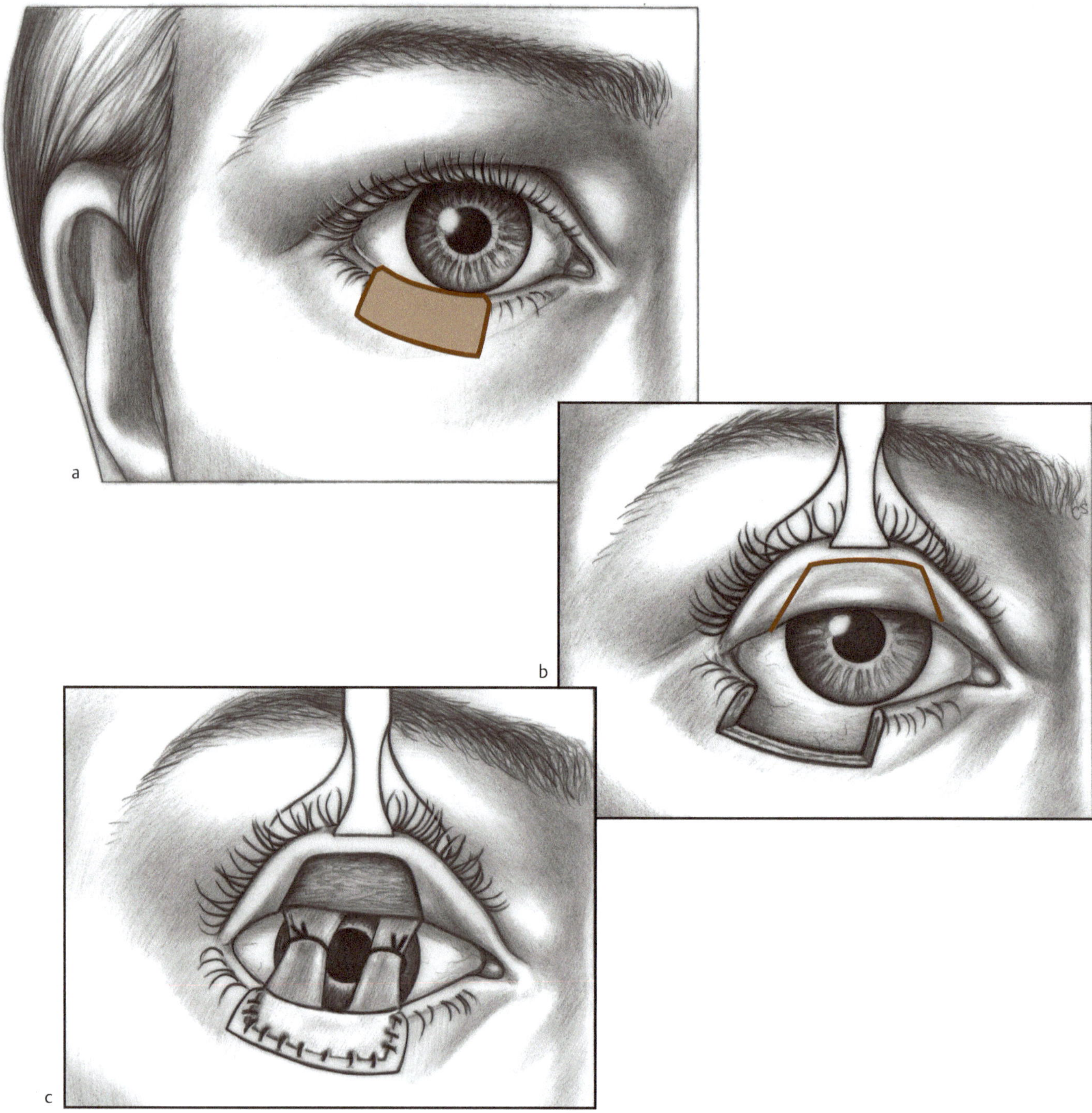

Fig. 5.16 (a–c) Superiorly based bipedicled tarsal conjunctival flap with full-thickness skin graft for the anterior lamella.

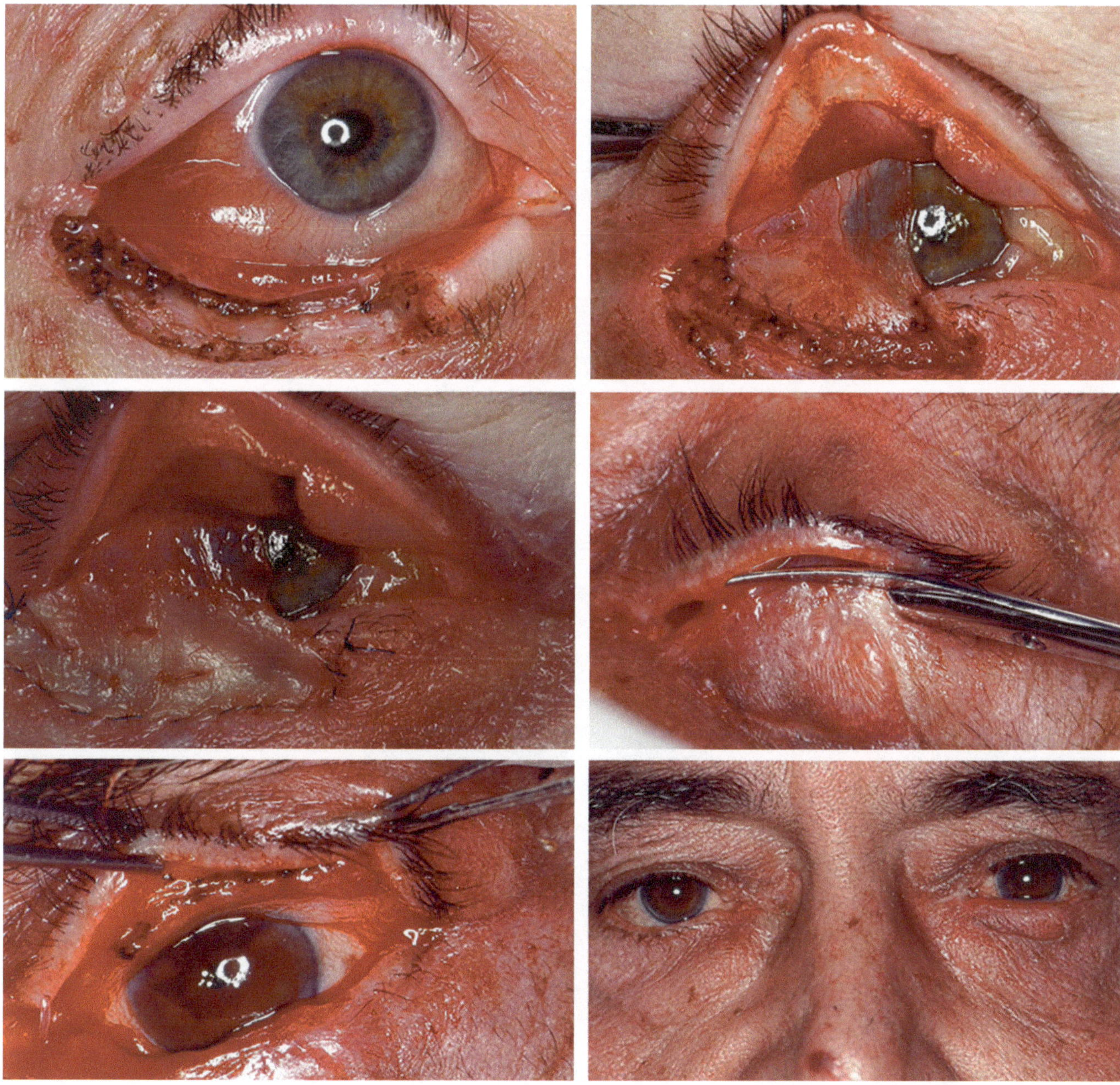

a b c d e f

Fig. 5.17 (a) Defect involving two-thirds of the lower lid and lateral canthus. **(b)** Incision of the conjunctiva of the everted upper eyelid and creation of a temporally based tarsal conjunctival flap. **(c)** Fixation of the flap to the lower lid conjunctiva and lid retractor remnants. **(d)** Advancement of the lower eyelid tissue and releasing of the tarsal conjunctival flap. **(e)** Closure of the upper eyelid conjunctiva. **(f)** Appearance postoperatively.

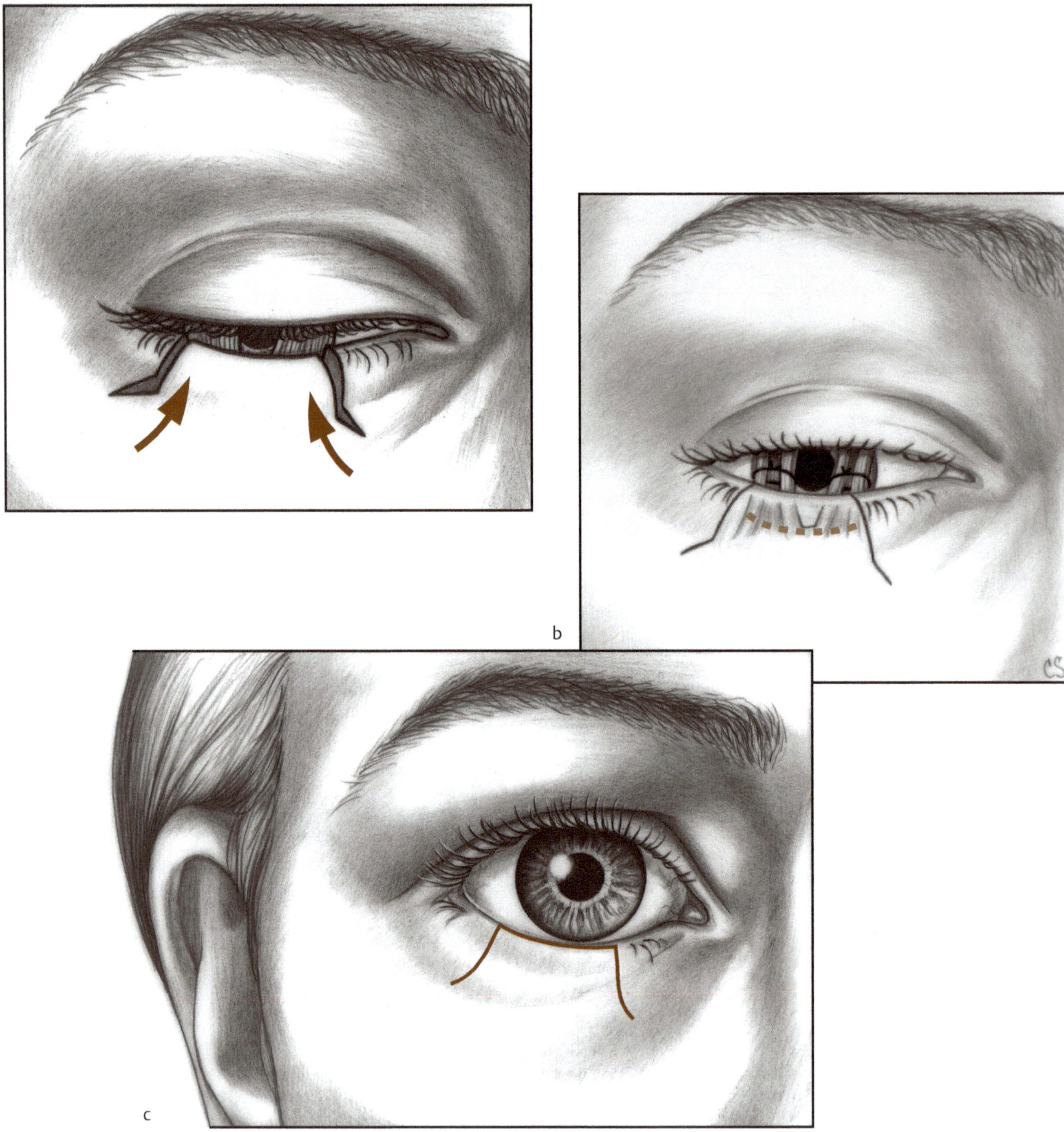

Fig. 5.18 (a–c) Bipedicled tarsal conjunctival flap with lower lid advancement flap closure.

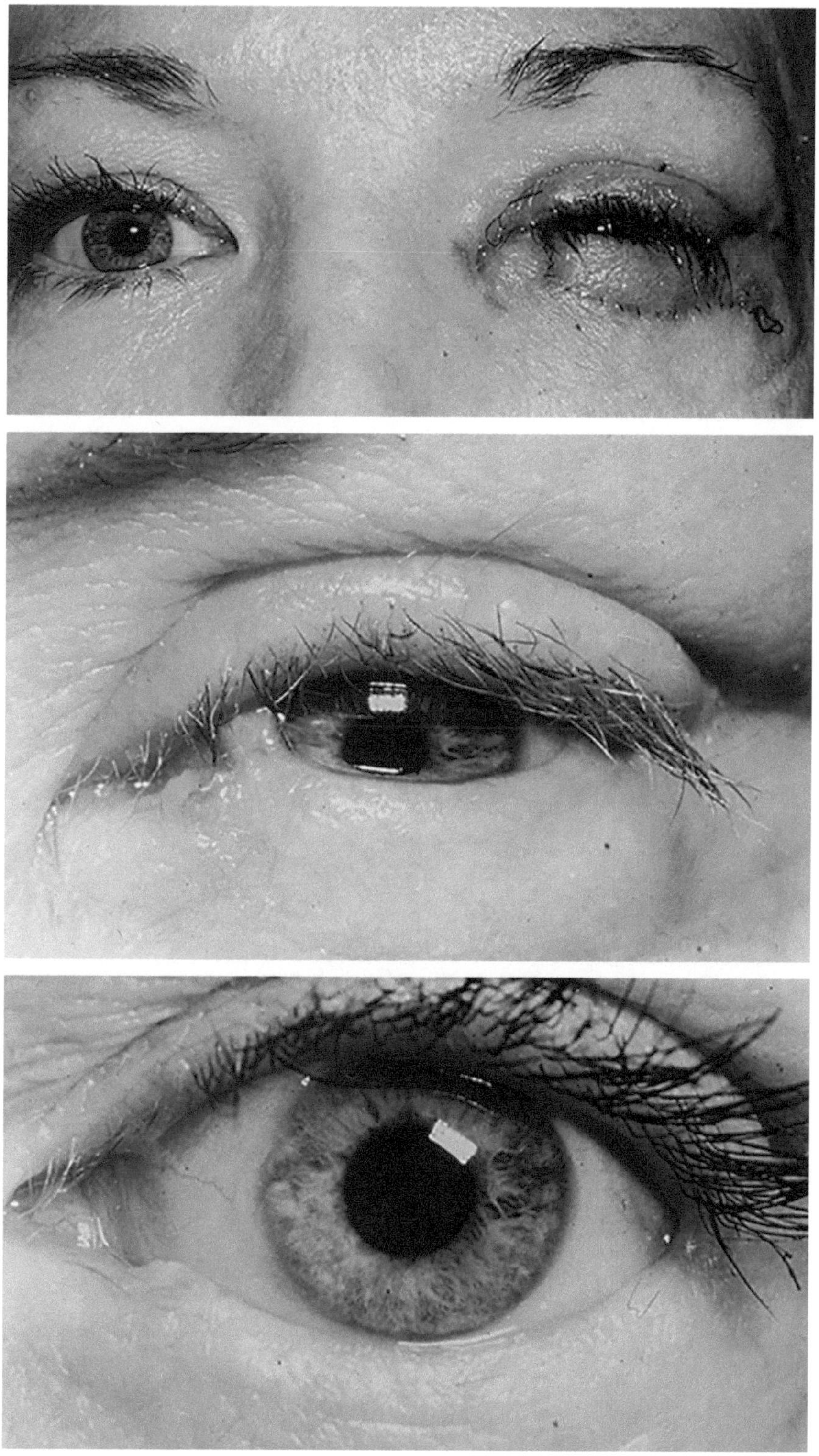

a b c

Fig. 5.19 (a) Wound of the left lower lid closed with a laterally based myocutaneous upper lid flap and bipedicled tarsal conjunctival flap. **(b)** Prior to pedicle division of the bipedicled tarsal conjunctival flap. **(c)** Late postoperative appearance.

♦ Medial Canthus

The lacrimal drainage system is routinely probed and intubated to ensure competence in medial canthal defects. If there is a defect of this system, lacrimal intubation with Silastic stents is placed for 1 to 3 months postoperatively.

Next, the medial canthal tendon is examined. The posterior limb of this tendon is imperative for holding the eyelid tightly against the globe. If the tendon has been damaged, it is reconstituted with 5–0 monofilament horizontal mattress sutures from the anterior and posterior limb remnant, to the anterior and posterior lacrimal crest periosteum, respectively.

Skin-only defects of up to 1 cm in diameter, and centered in the concave medial canthal region, heal well by secondary intention (**Fig. 5.20**). Larger defects are reconstructed with a FTSG from the opposite upper eyelid or retroauricular region, a glabellar flap, or a small paramedian forehead flap (**Fig. 5.21** and **Fig. 5.22**). If a forehead flap is used, then it must be aggressively thinned prior to inset (**Fig. 5.23**). Refer to Chapter 6 for more detail on the forehead flap procedure. Combined defects of the medial canthus, orbit, maxilla, nose, and cheek can be reconstructed with combinations of paramedian forehead flaps and cheek flaps, with or without calvarial bone grafts. Refer to the combined defect section in Chapter 7.

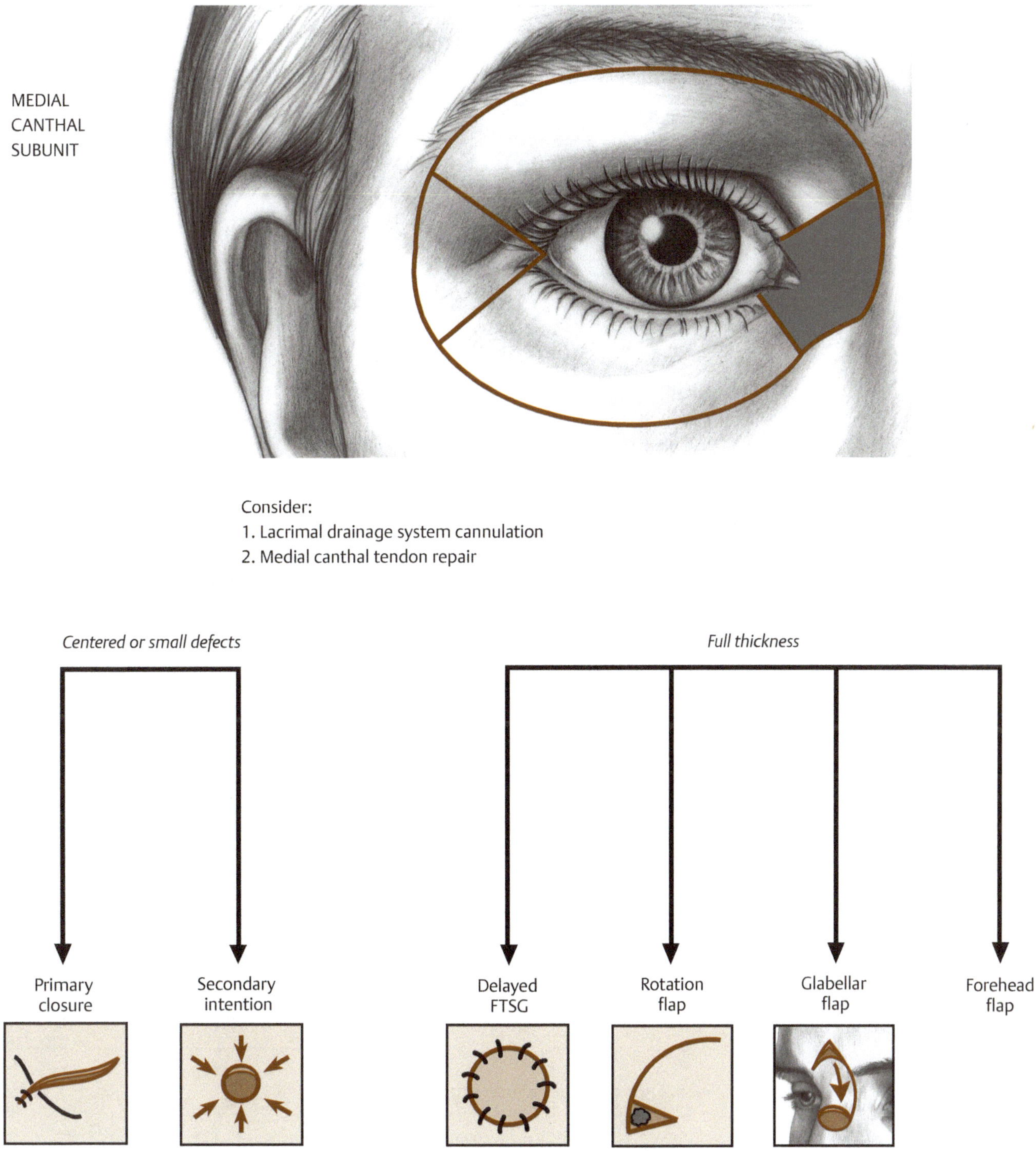

Fig. 5.20 Medial canthal subunit. FTSG, full-thickness skin graft.

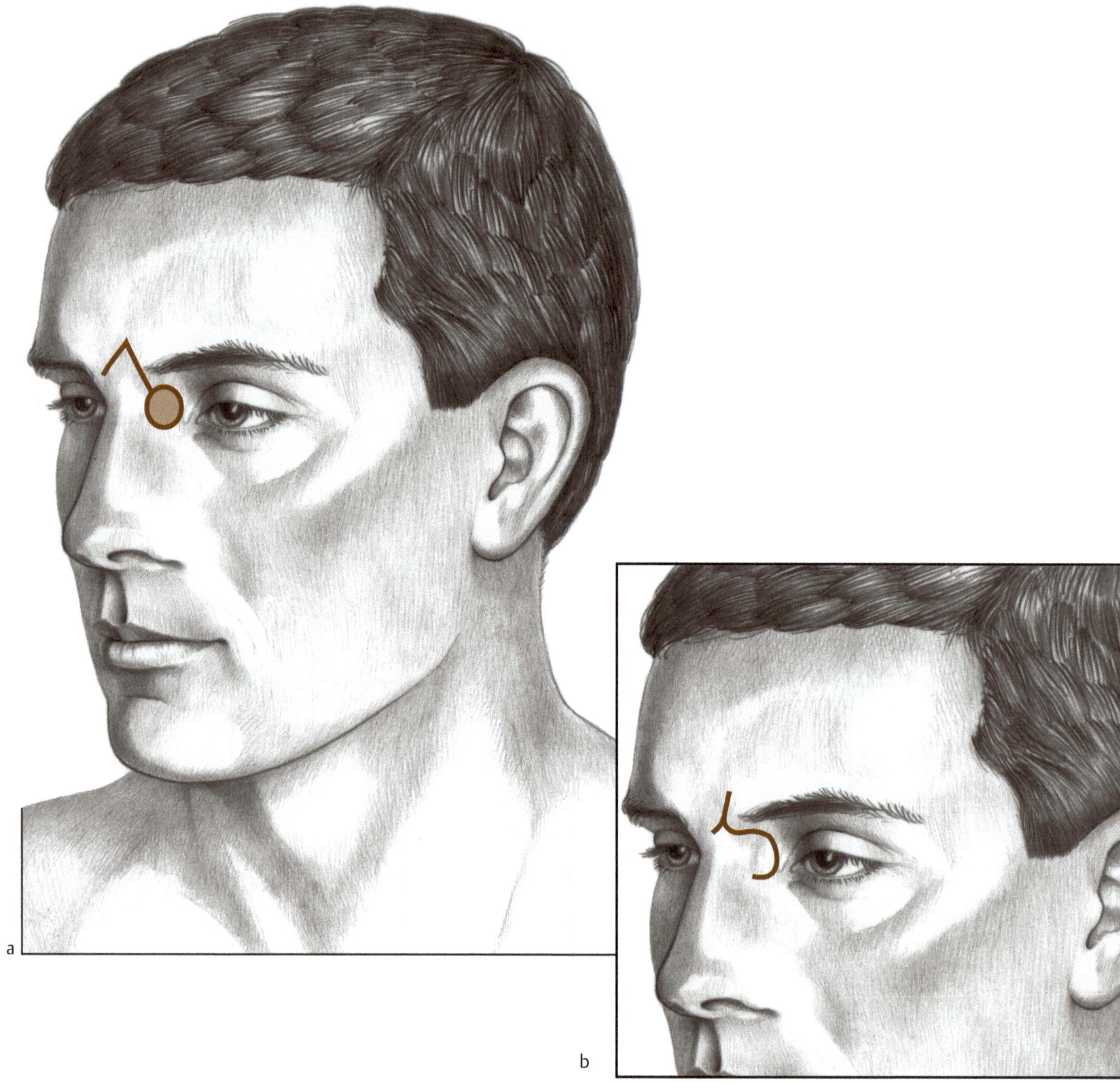

Fig. 5.21 (a, b) Glabellar flap to the medial canthus.

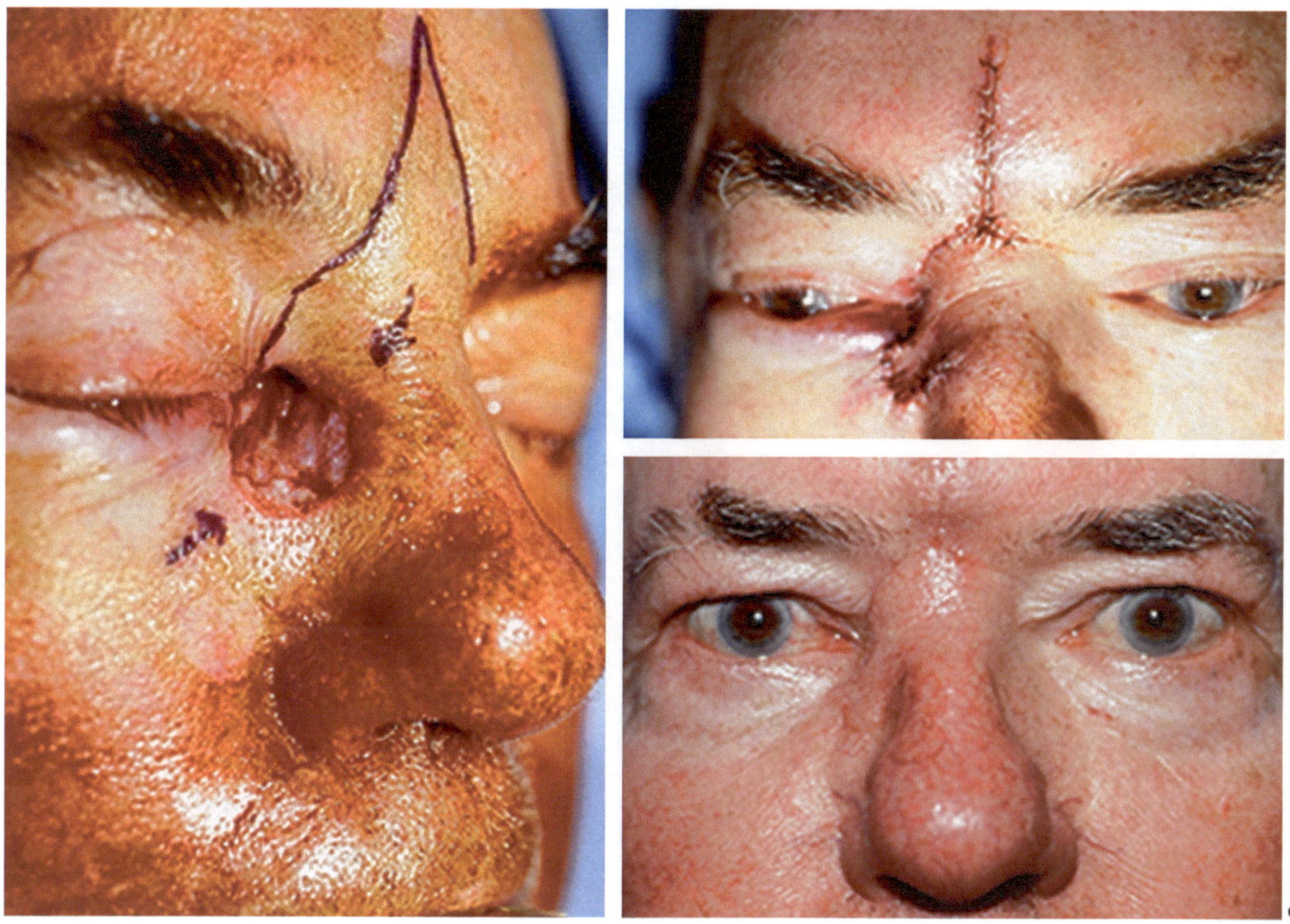

a b c

Fig. 5.22 (a) Glabellar flap planned for a medial canthal defect. **(b)** Flap closed. **(c)** Early postoperative result.

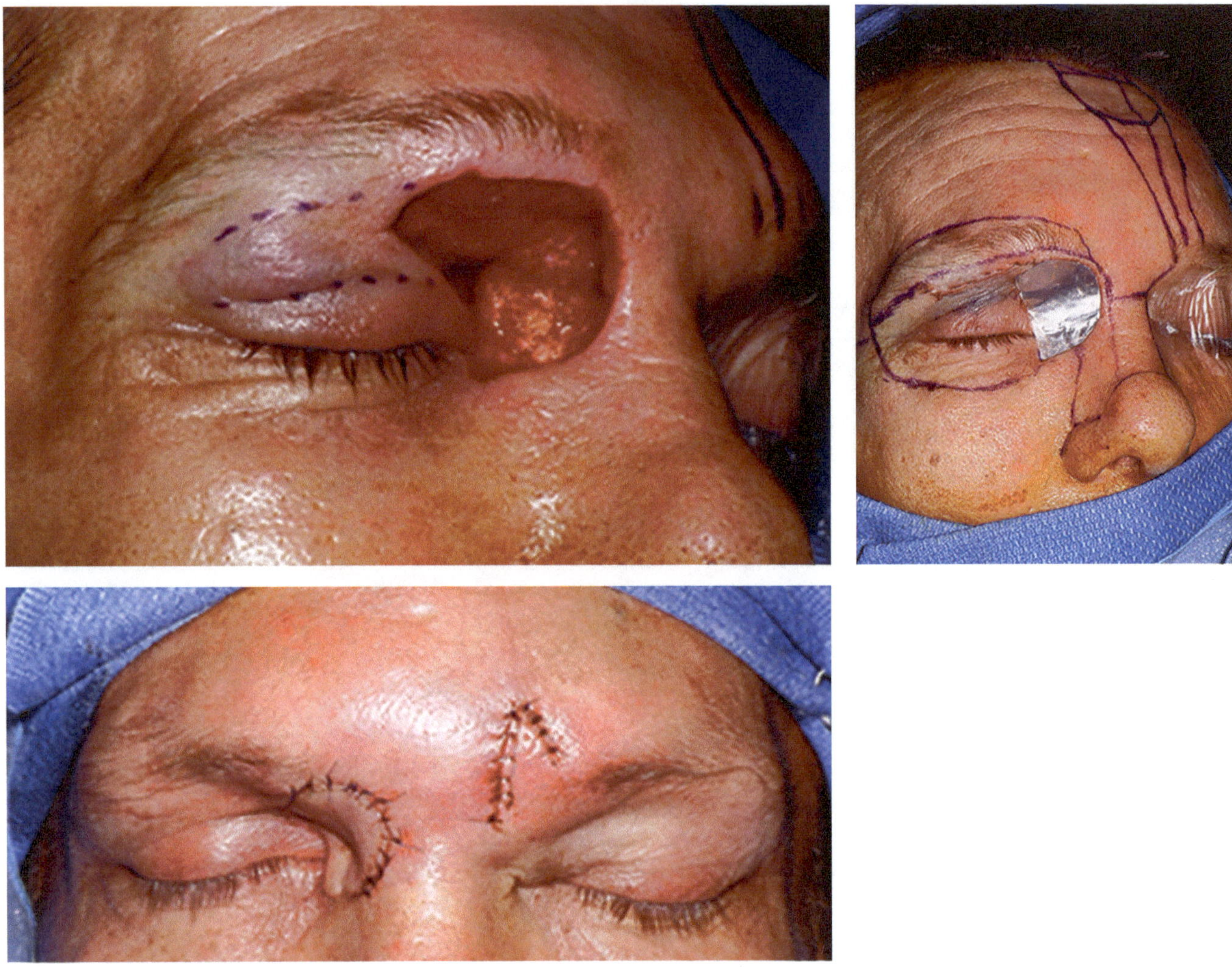

Fig. 5.23 (a) Large medial canthal and nasal defect. **(b)** Forehead flap planned for a medial canthal defect. **(c)** After pedicle inset procedure.

♦ Lateral Canthus

The lateral canthal tendon must be examined for competence in defects of this region (**Fig. 5.24**). If the tendon is damaged, it should be reconstructed with buried 5–0 monofilament horizontal mattress sutures to the inner periosteum of the lateral orbital rim. If there is lower lid laxity noted at the time of reconstruction, then the lower limb of the lateral canthal tendon should be plicated in mild cases, or shortened in moderate-to-severe cases near its attachment to the orbital rim, and reconstituted with 5–0 monofilament mattress sutures. The skin is reconstructed with a cheek or temple rotation advancement flap, elevated just deep to the subdermal plexus (**Fig. 5.25** and **Fig. 5.26**). Buried 5–0 long-lasting absorbable sutures from the inferior flap to the orbital rim periosteum help maintain the flap position and prevent ectropion.

Combined defects involving both the upper and lower eyelids and the lateral canthus require more complex reconstruction, typically involving a bipedicle superiorly based tarsal-conjunctival flap, cheek rotation advancement, and lateral canthal tendon reconstruction.

LATERAL
CANTHAL
SUBUNIT

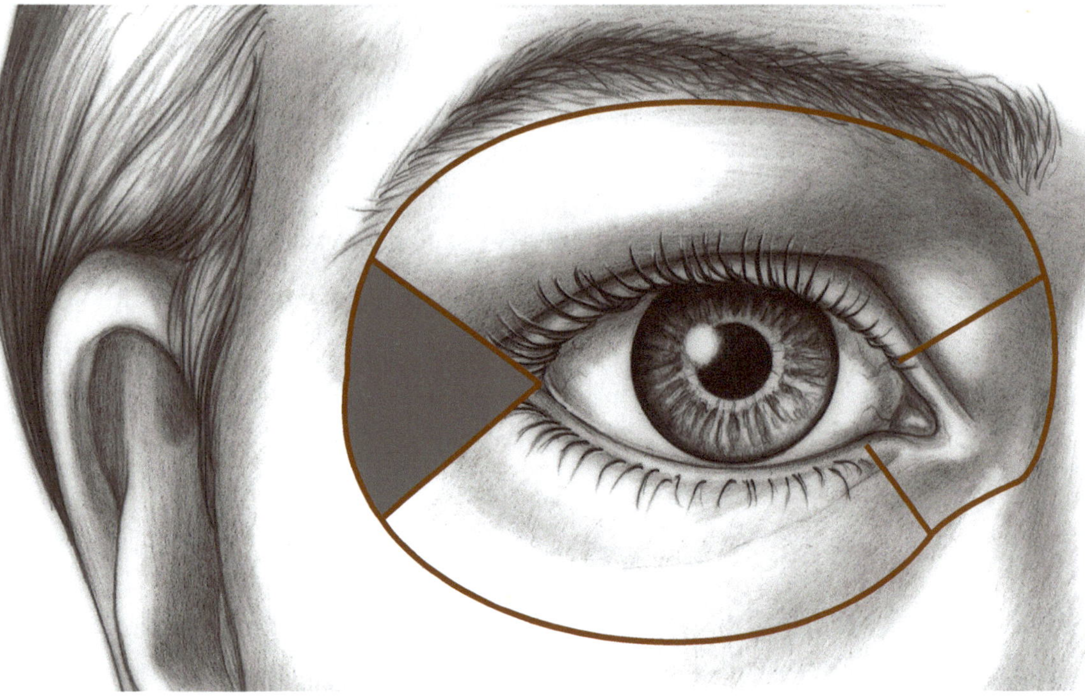

Consider:

1. Lateral canthal tendon repair

Secondary intention
(fair)

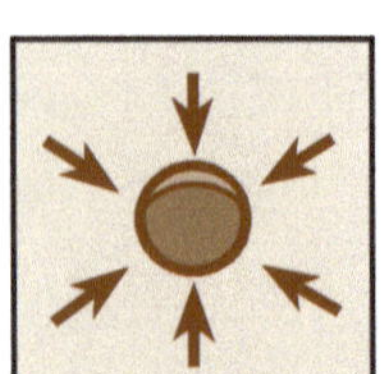

Primary
closure

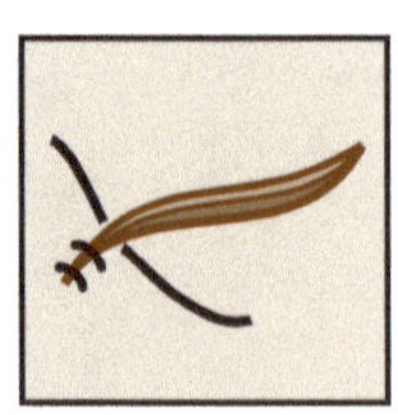

Local flap from temple or
cheek

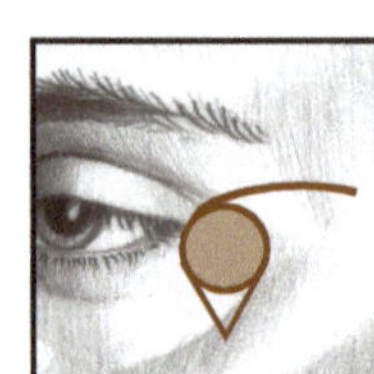

Fig. 5.24 Lateral canthal subunit.

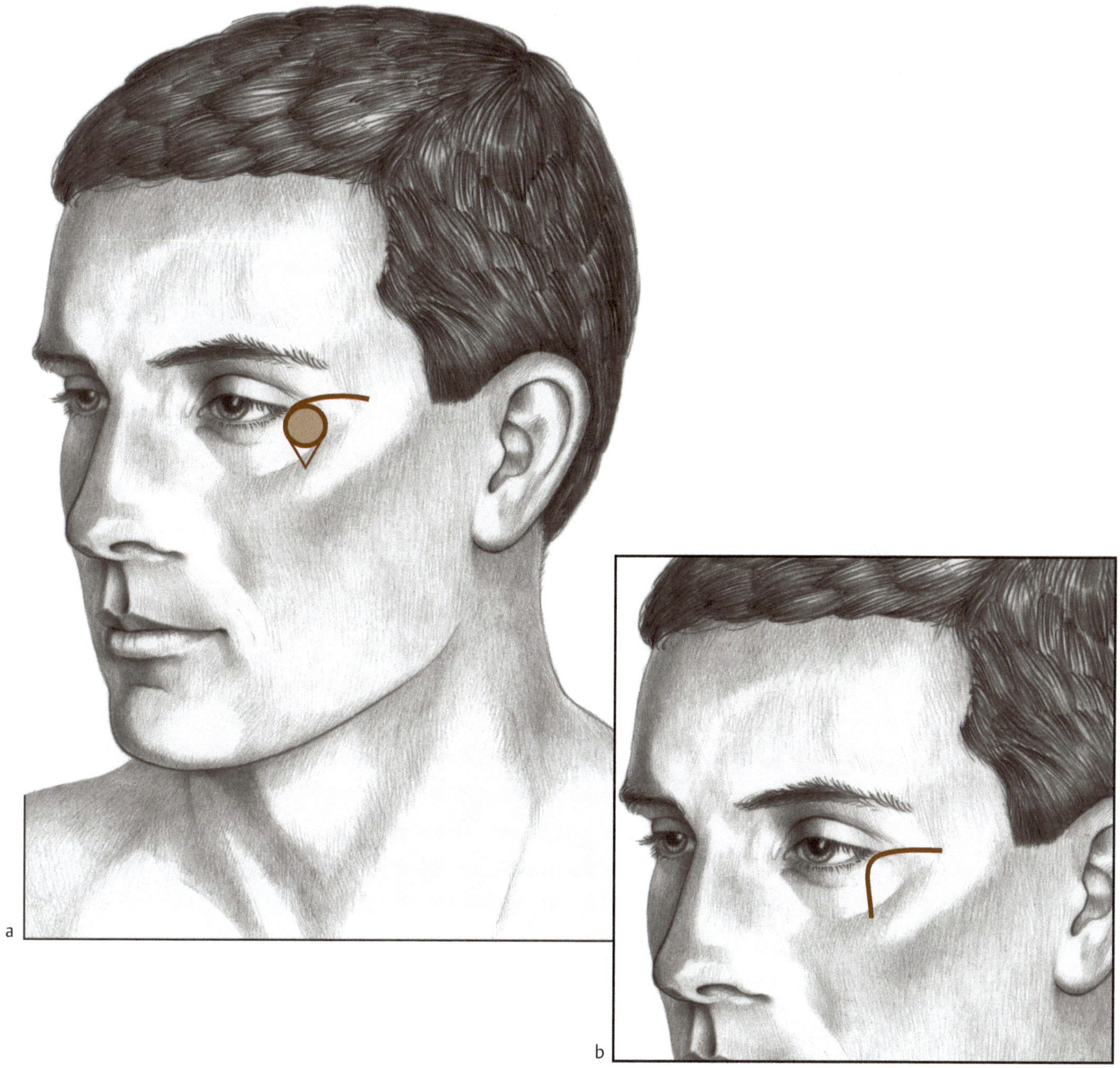

Fig. 5.25 (a, b) Cheek rotation flap to lateral canthus.

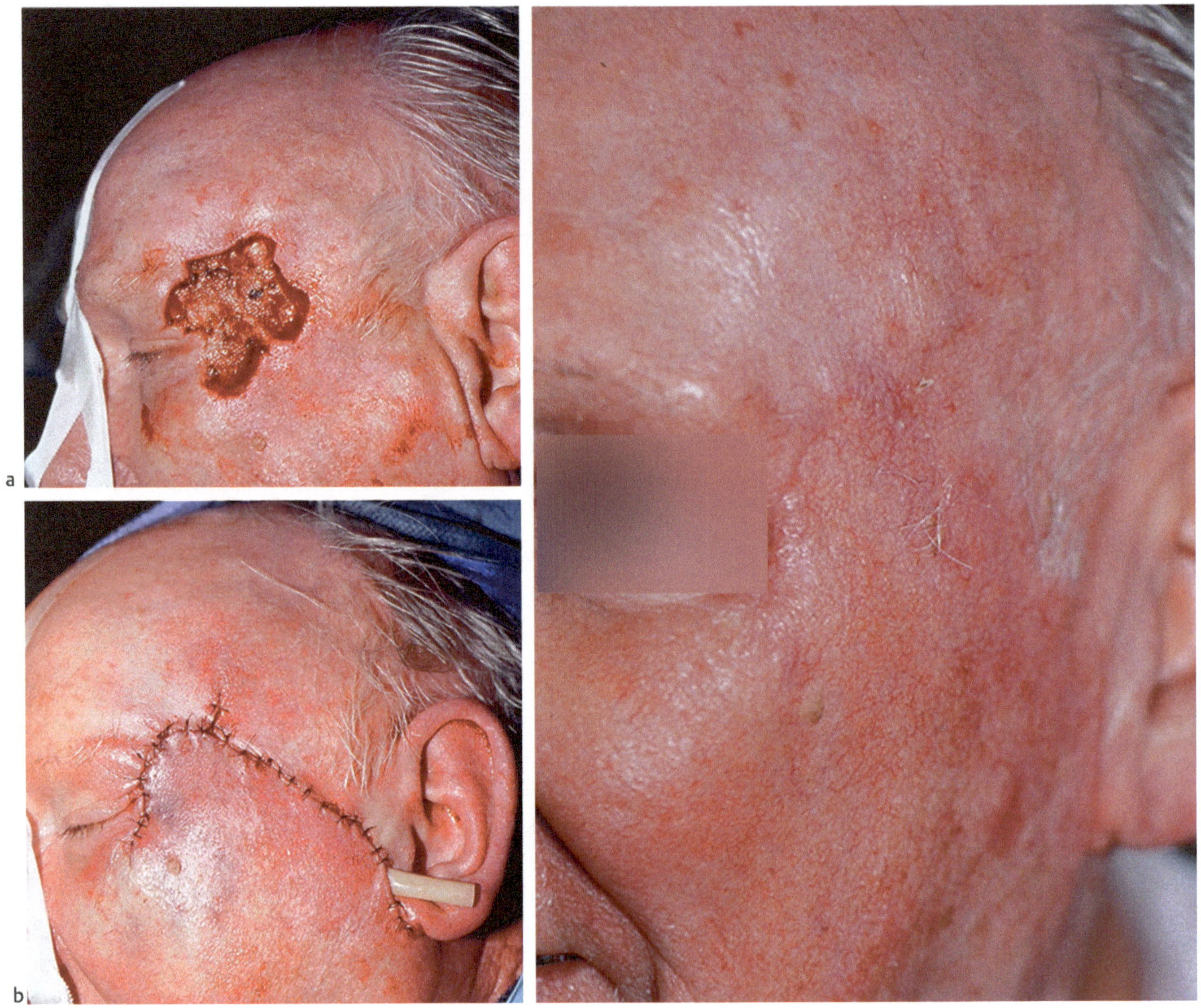

Fig. 5.26 **(a)** Large lateral canthal defect. **(b)** Cheek rotation flap in place. **(c)** Postoperative result.

Suggested Reading

Becker FF. Reconstructive surgery of the mental canthal region. Ann Plast Surg 1981;7(4):259–268

Cutler NL, Beard C. A method for partial and total upper lid reconstruction. Am J Ophthalmol 1955;39(1):1–7

Hargiss JL. Bipedicle tarsoconjunctival flap. Ophthal Plast Reconstr Surg 1989;5(2):99–103

Price DL, Sherris DA, Bartley GB, Garrity JA. Forehead flap periorbital reconstruction. Arch Facial Plast Surg 2004;6(4):222–227

Sherris DA, Heffernan JT. Techniques in periocular reconstruction. Facial Plast Surg 1994;10(2):202–213

Sherris DA, Murakami CS. Five things oculoplastic surgeons should know about facial plastic surgery. Ophthal Plast Reconstr Surg 1999;15(4):229–231

Smith BC, Della Rocca RL, Nesi FA, Lisman RD. Ophthalmic plastic and reconstructive surgery. St. Louis: CV Mosby; 1987

Spinelli HM, Jelks GW. Periocular reconstruction: a systematic approach. Plast Reconstr Surg 1993;91(6):1017–1024, discussion 1025–1026

Tenzel RR. Orbit and oculoplastics. In: Podos SM, Yanoff M, eds. Textbook of Ophthalmology. Vol. 4. New York: Gower Medical Publishing; 1993

Tenzel RR. Ophthalmic plastic surgery. In: Clayman HM, ed. Atlas of Contemporary Ophthalmic Surgery. St. Louis: CV Mosby; 1990

Tenzel RR. Reconstruction of the central one half of an eyelid. Arch Ophthalmol 1975;93(2):125–126

6 Nose

Summary

This chapter focuses on subunit reconstruction of nasal defects. Nasal subunits are important in preoperative planning for reconstruction and can guide treatment decisions. We discuss the importance of cartilage grafting as well as reconstruction of internal nasal lining in defects that involve such components. Specific attention is also given to larger defects that require transposition flaps such as melolabial and paramedian forehead flap reconstruction.

Keywords: nasal subunits, ala, paramedian forehead flap, septal lining, melolabial flap, composite graft, columella, skin graft harvest

♦ Introduction

The complex contours of the nose reflect the underlying structure and variations in the thickness of the skin/soft tissue envelope. In general, the three layers of the nose—skin, bony or cartilaginous framework, and mucosal lining—should each be reconstructed separately. The skin itself is thick and sebaceous over the nasal tip and ala, and thin over the nasal dorsum and sidewalls. Th e skin is more mobile over the superior two-thirds of the nose. The shapes of the nasal bones, dorsal septum, and upper lateral cartilages define the shape of the upper two-thirds of the nose. The shape and strength of the lower lateral cartilages primarily define the shape of the tip. The summation of all these factors creates the nasal aesthetic subunits (**Fig. 6.1**).

These aesthetic subunits have shadowed valleys and lighted ridges at their natural boundaries. The nose can be divided into nine subunits: two sidewalls, dorsum, two alae, tip, two soft tissue triangles, and columella. The medial canthal area is considered in this chapter as the superior aspect of the sidewall subunit. Incisions in the subunit boundaries along relaxed skin tension lines or in the midline of the nose heal with less perceptible scars.

Because the subunits tend to be either somewhat convex or somewhat concave, reconstructions are least noticeable when they assume these same configurations. For example, the pincushioning frequently seen with melolabial flaps can be an advantage when reconstructing the convex ala. When defects assume most of an aesthetic subunit, it is better to resect the remainder and to reconstruct the entire subunit as a totality.

Defects frequently do not follow clear schemata and may involve parts of several subunits. It is occasionally desirable to combine different techniques for these complex defects, using a different flap or graft for each of two aesthetic subunits. In difficult cases, where the defect involves only skin and subcutaneous tissue, a full-thickness skin graft (FTSG) alone can be used to resurface a large area with an acceptable, though not optimal, result. The forehead flap, however, is used for reconstruction of most significant nasal defects.

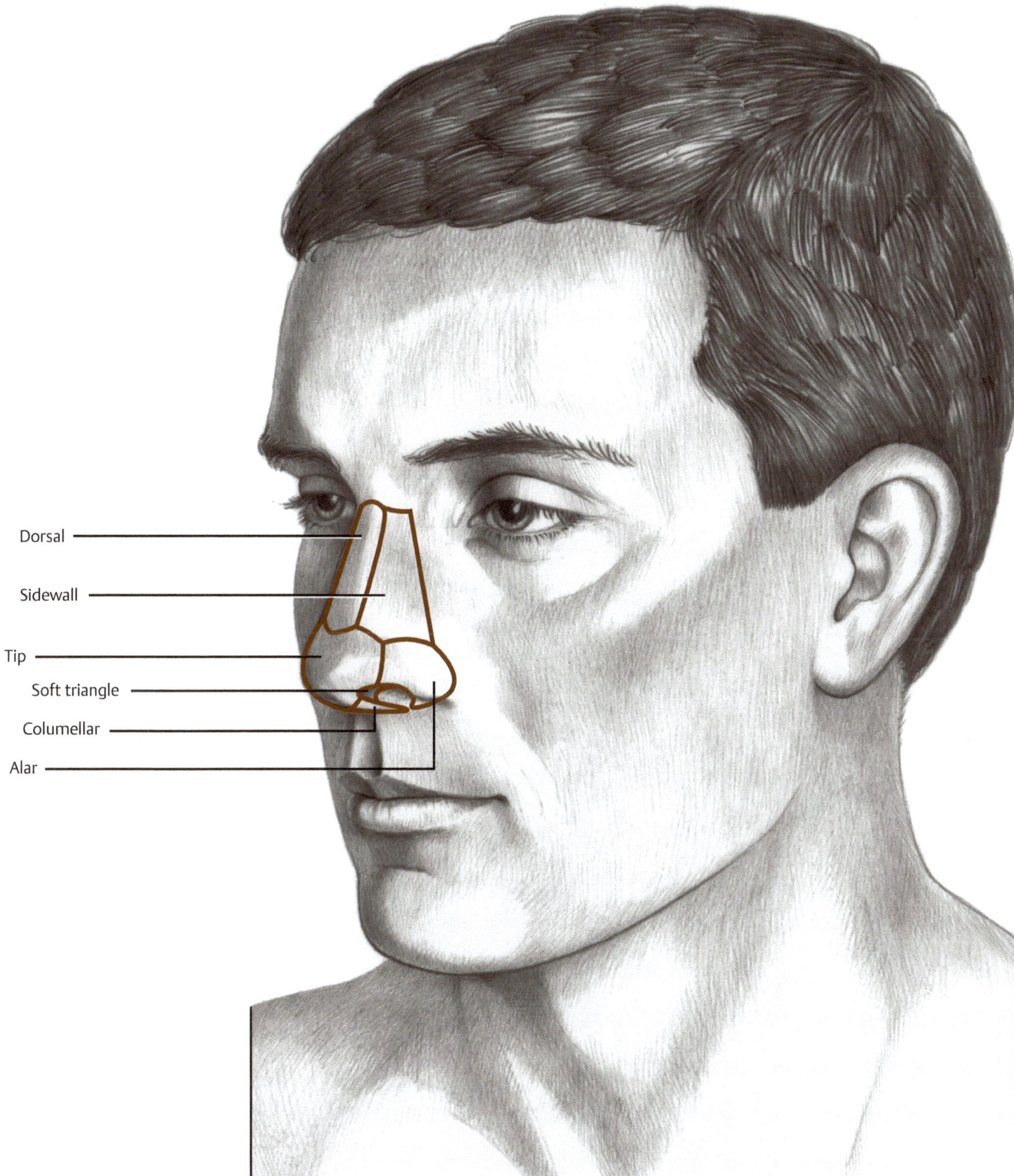

Fig. 6.1 Nasal subunits.

Alar retraction can be an unfortunate sequela of reconstructing defects near the alar margin. Transposition flaps should be designed to avoid tension on the ala. Any flap-closing tension should ideally be in the midline so the tip is elevated symmetrically rather than raising one or the other ala. Cartilaginous defects of the upper or lower lateral cartilages must be repaired with septal or auricular cartilage, to provide support and prevent retraction of the skin–soft tissue envelope.

Pincushioning or a "trapdoor deformity" can result from even well-designed flap repairs on the nose. Wide undermining of the nasal skin–soft tissue envelope in the plane just superficial to the periosteum and perichondrium, as well as flap incisions in the same deep plane, will help to avoid the problem at the time of primary surgery. If pincushioning does occur, it is treated early in the postoperative course with a subcutaneous steroid injection. A typical injection is 0.2 to 0.3 mL of triamcinolone acetate (10 mg/mL). These injections are begun as early as 3 weeks postoperatively and repeated at monthly intervals, as needed. In some cases, secondary revision with defatting and wide undermining may be necessary, but it is usually delayed for 6 months to allow maturation of the wound.

♦ Dorsal and Sidewall Subunits

Skin-only defects of the dorsum and sidewall can be repaired using an FTSG with adequate, though sometimes suboptimal, results (**Fig. 6.2** and **Fig. 6.3**). Healing by secondary intention works well only in the medial canthal area. Secondary intention healing is most appropriate for defects whose geometric center is approximately at the level of the medial canthus on the nasal sidewall. Defects that are centered below the medial canthus may heal with contraction of the lower lid. Similarly, defects centered above the medial canthus may heal with contracture of the upper eyelid.

For defects that are more superior or horizontally oriented, the glabellar rotation flap can be used (**Fig. 6.4** and **Fig. 6.5**). This flap requires significant length of incisions and a large mobilization of tissue for a relatively small defect, but the incisions are well camouflaged.

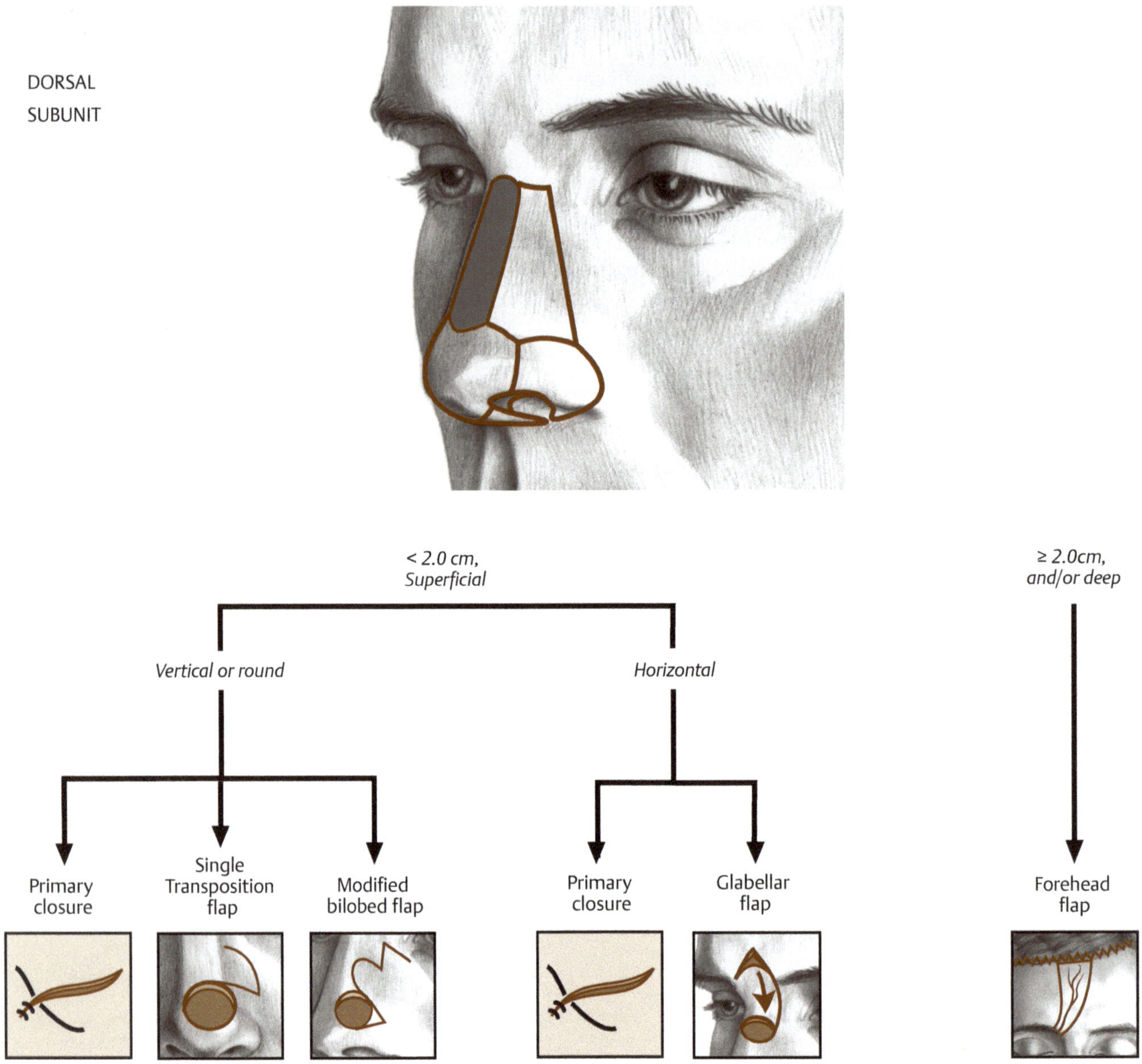

Fig. 6.2 Dorsal subunit.

SIDEWALL
SUBUNIT

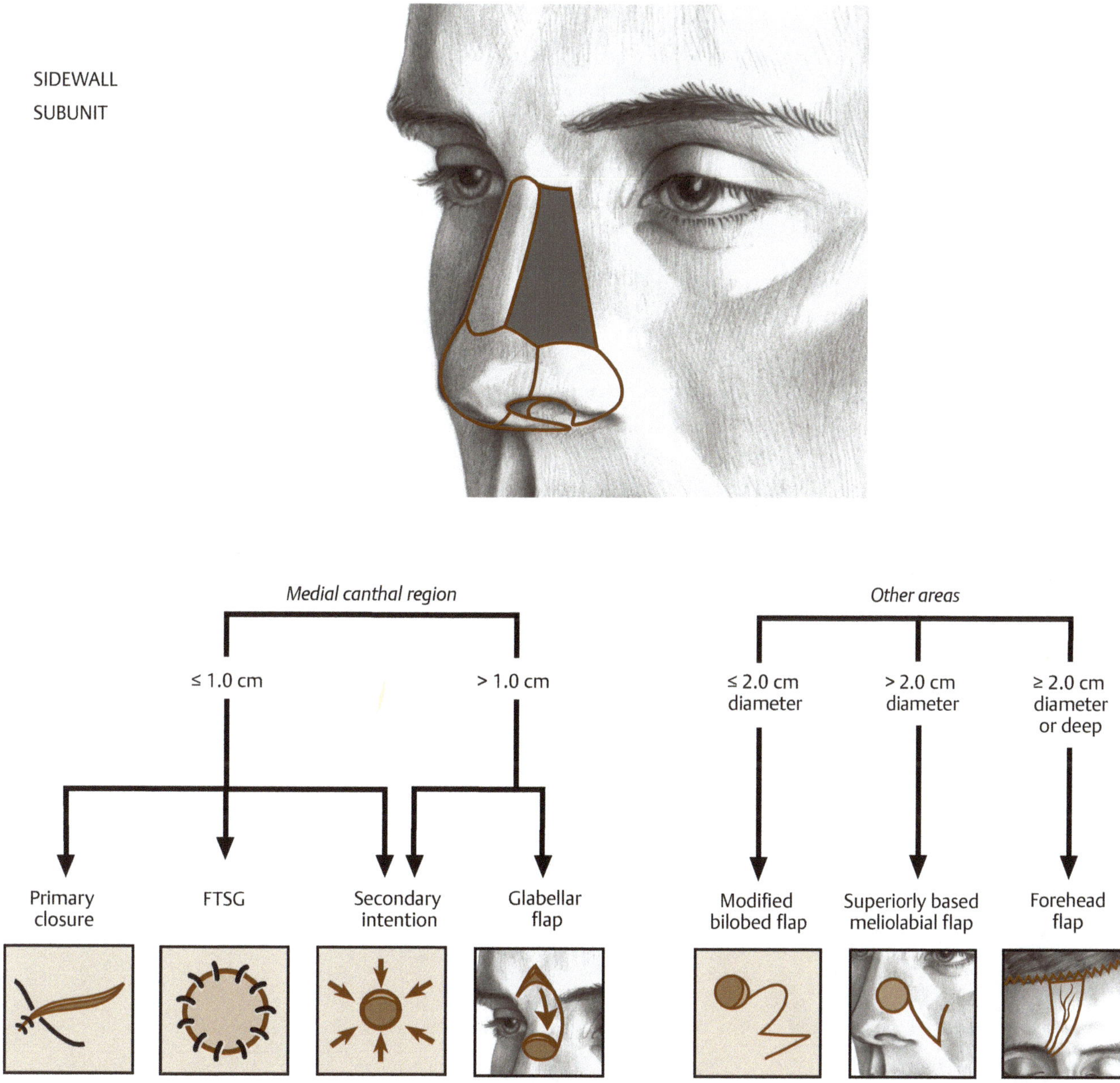

Fig. 6.3 Sidewall subunit. FTSG, full-thickness skin graft.

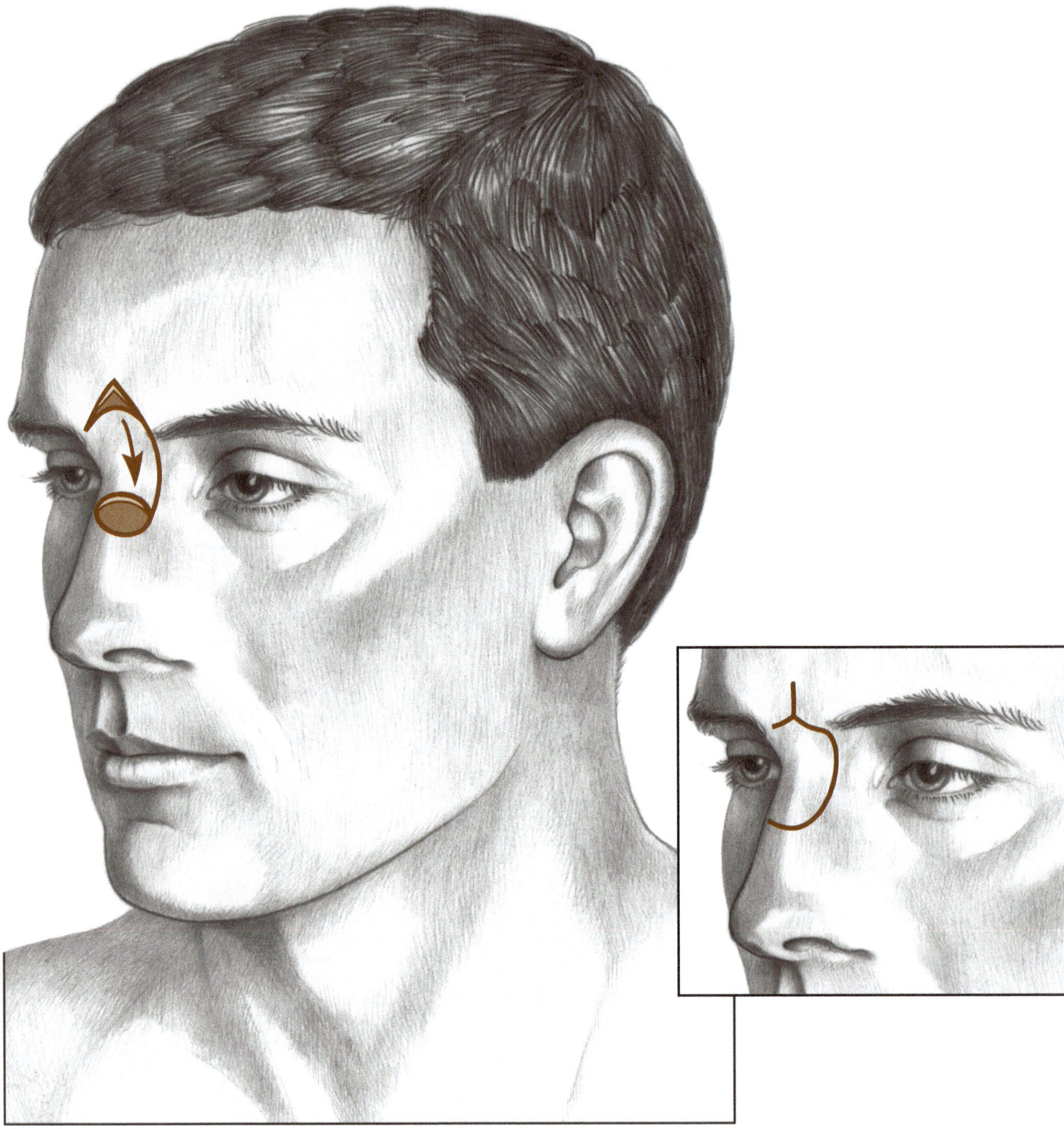

Fig. 6.4 Glabellar flap.

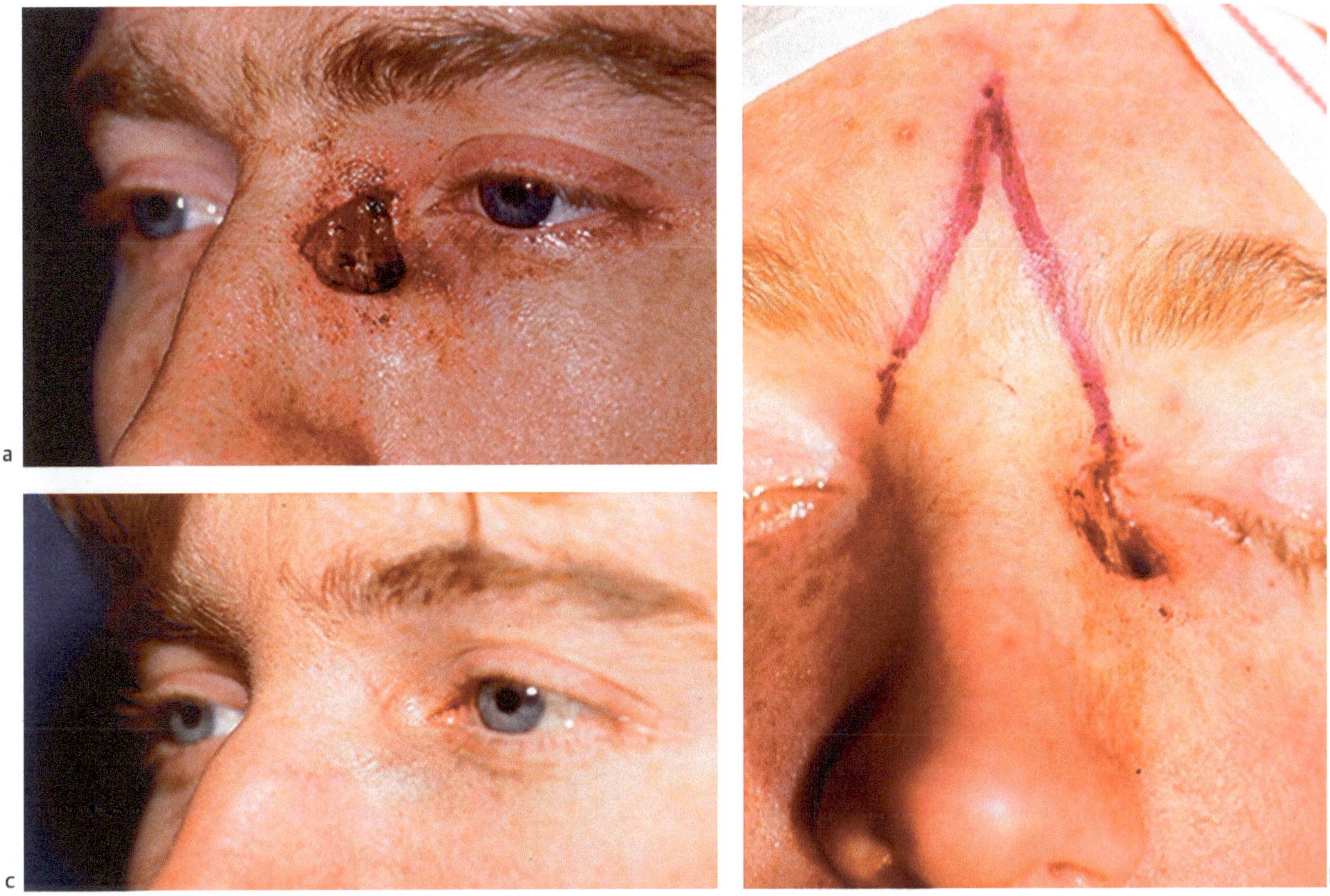

Fig. 6.5 (a) High nasal sidewall defect. **(b)** Glabellar flap planned. **(c)** Postoperative result.

Small defects of the dorsal midline can be closed primarily or with single or double transposition flaps. Primary closure can be accomplished in either the vertical or the horizontal plane, as long as it does not result in distortion of the nasal tip or ala (**Fig. 6.6**). Single transposition flaps are planned so that the closure site is placed in the alar crease when possible (**Fig. 6.7**).

Flap closure can occasionally be facilitated by removing a preexisting dorsal hump after elevation of the skin–soft tissue envelope. If the closing tension of a single transposition flap causes alar elevation, then a double transposition flap (bilobed) is selected.

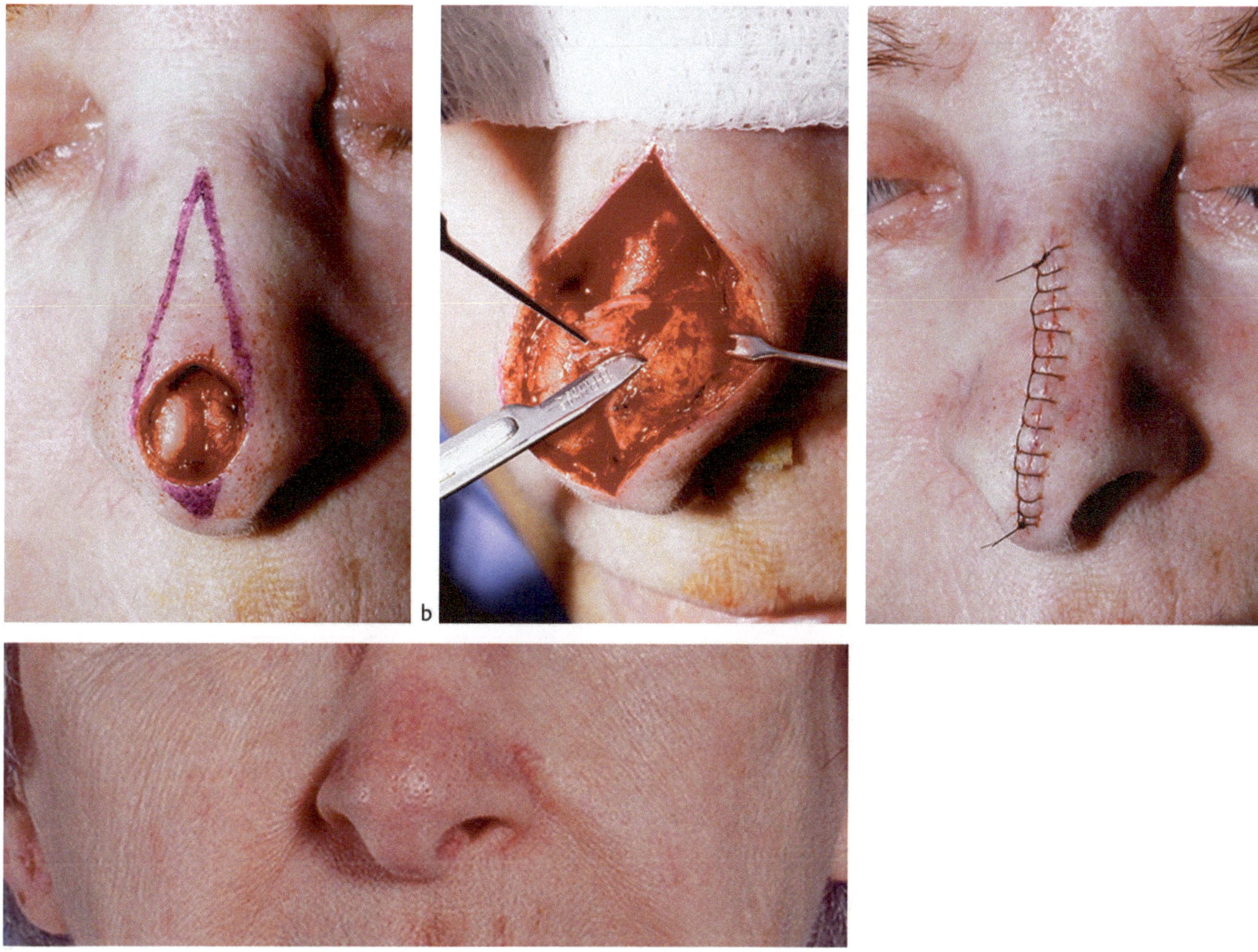

a b c d

Fig. 6.6 (a) Planned primary closure of a midline nasal defect with dog-ear excisions. **(b)** Tip cartilages are shaved to facilitate primary closure. **(c)** After closure. **(d)** Late postoperative result.

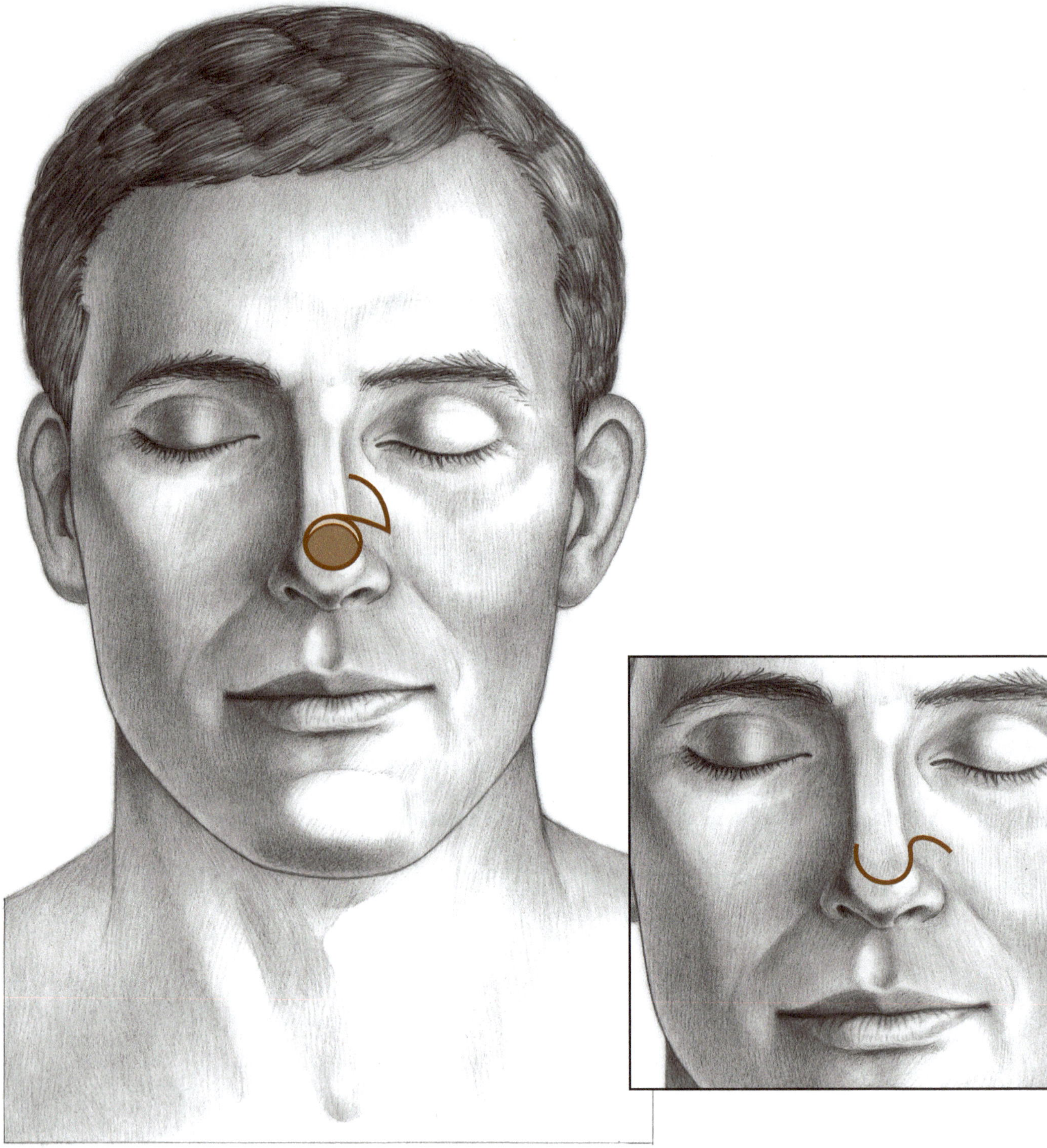

a

Fig. 6.7 (a) Single transposition flap to the nasal tip.

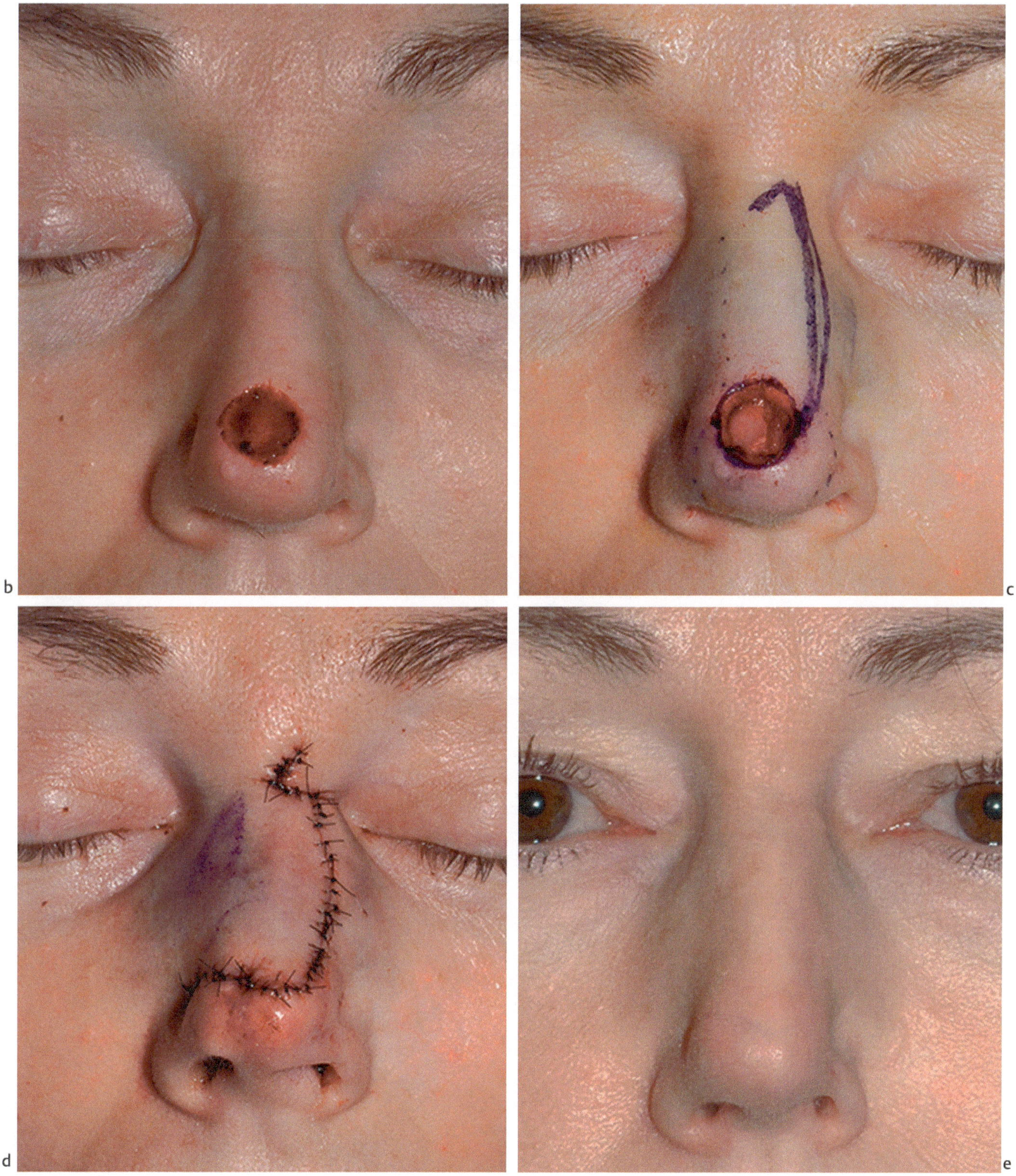

Fig. 6.7 **(b)** Nasal defect. **(c)** Defect with dorsal nasal sliding advancement flap template. **(d)** Flap closed. **(e)** Wound healed.

The modified bilobed flap is chosen for cases of nasal reconstruction because this design creates less of a standing cone formation than the standard bilobed design (**Fig. 6.8, Fig. 6.9,** and **Fig. 6.10**). The Zitelli-modified bilobed flap is designed with the total arc of rotation of 100 degrees or less, and each limb of the flap rotates 45 to 50 degrees. The flap can be either medially or laterally based. The first limb is designed the same size or just slightly smaller than the defect size, and the second limb is typically one-half to three quarters of the size of the primary limb. This flap design takes advantage of the less adherent skin and subcutaneous tissue of the dorsal and sidewall subunits for reconstruction of defects.

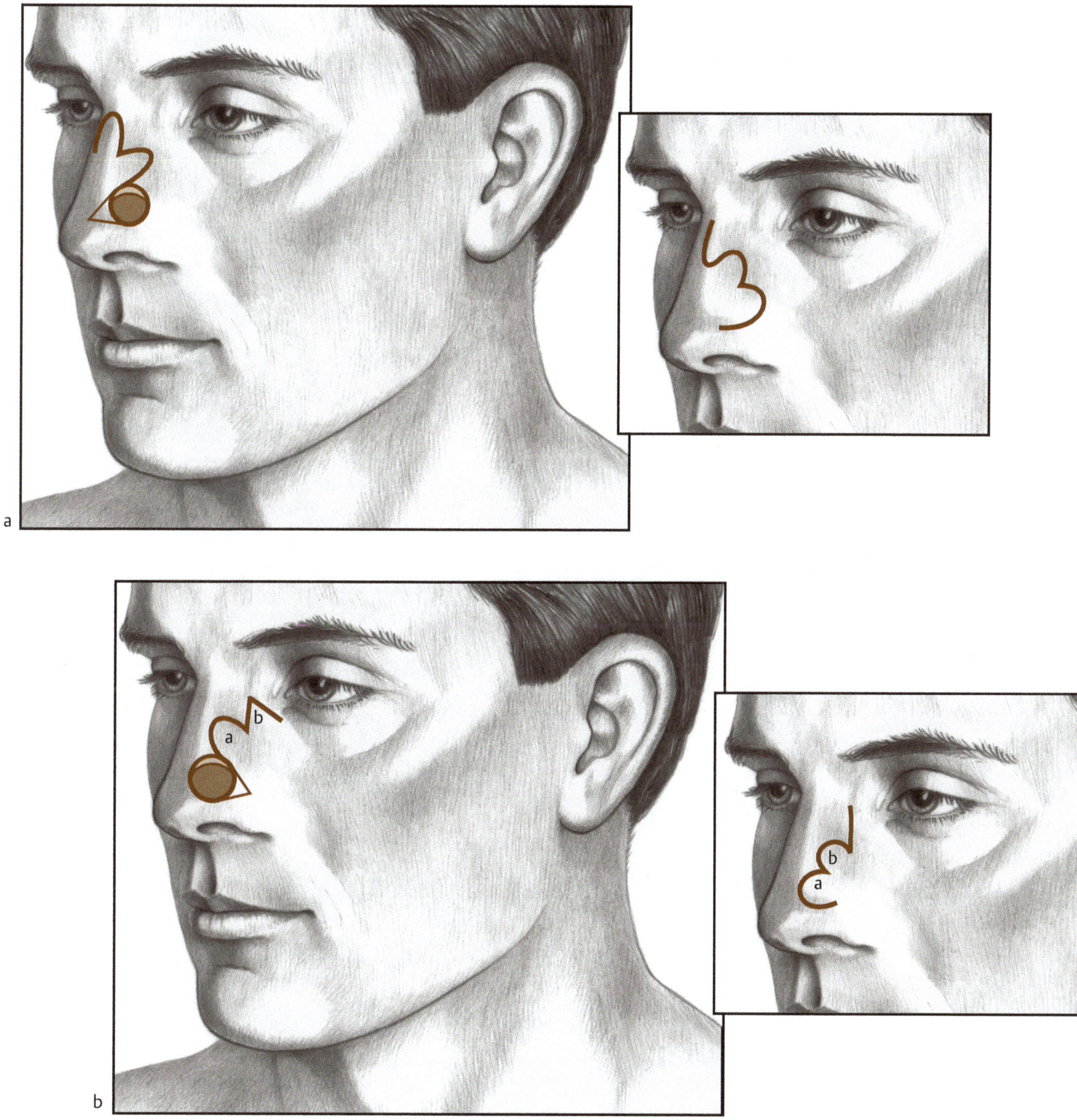

Fig. 6.8 (a) Medial based and **(b)** laterally based bilobed flap (Zitelli modification).

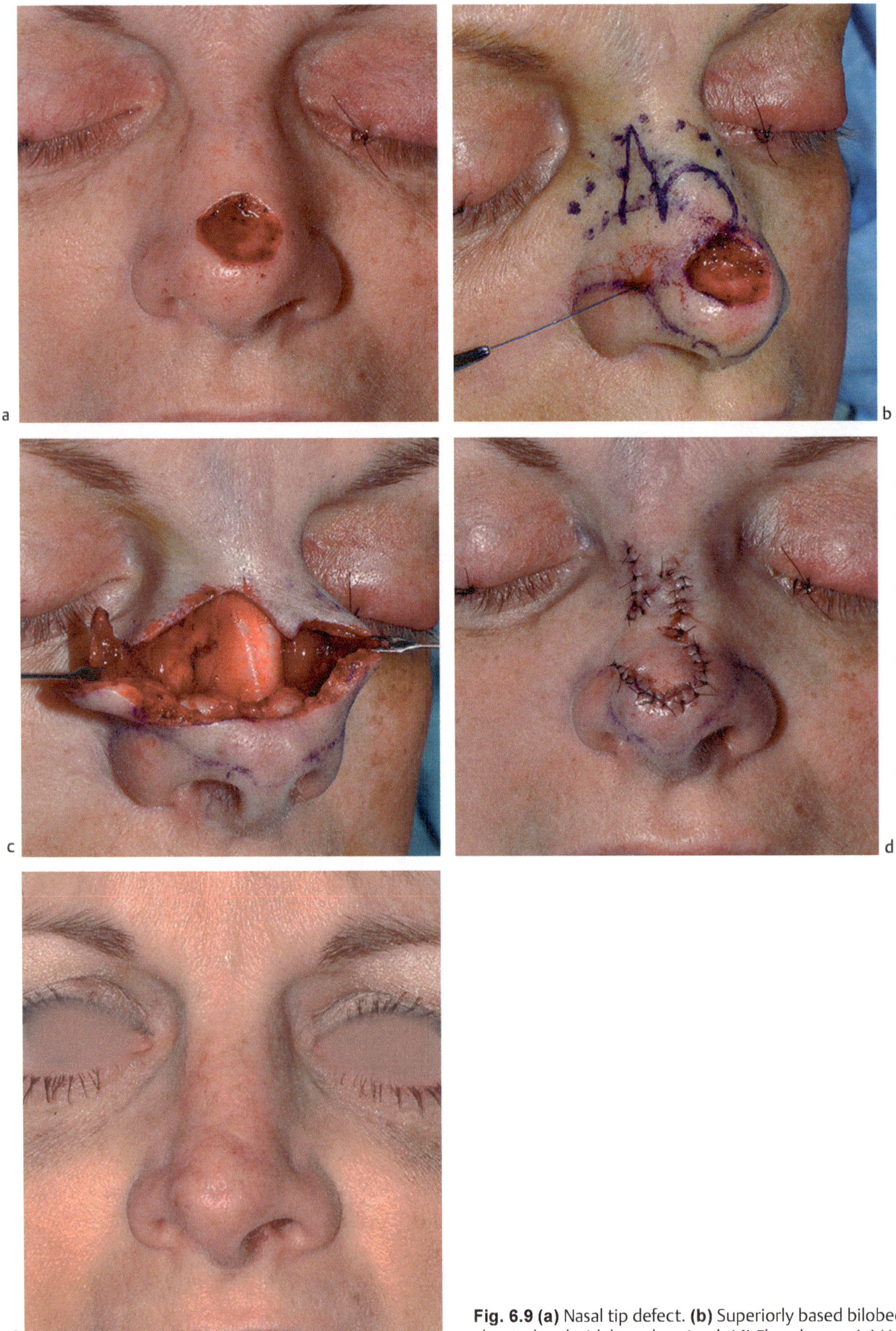

Fig. 6.9 (a) Nasal tip defect. **(b)** Superiorly based bilobed flap. **(c)** Flap elevated and widely undermined. **(d)** Flap closure. **(e)** Healed wound.

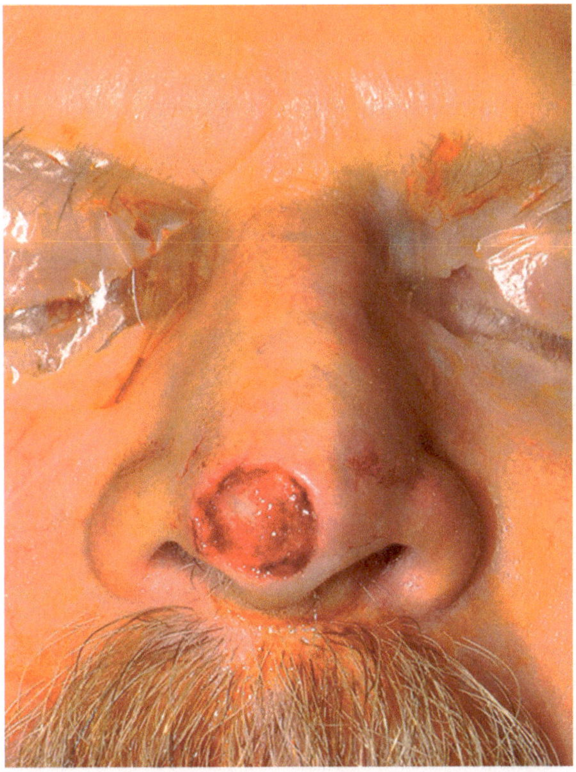

a

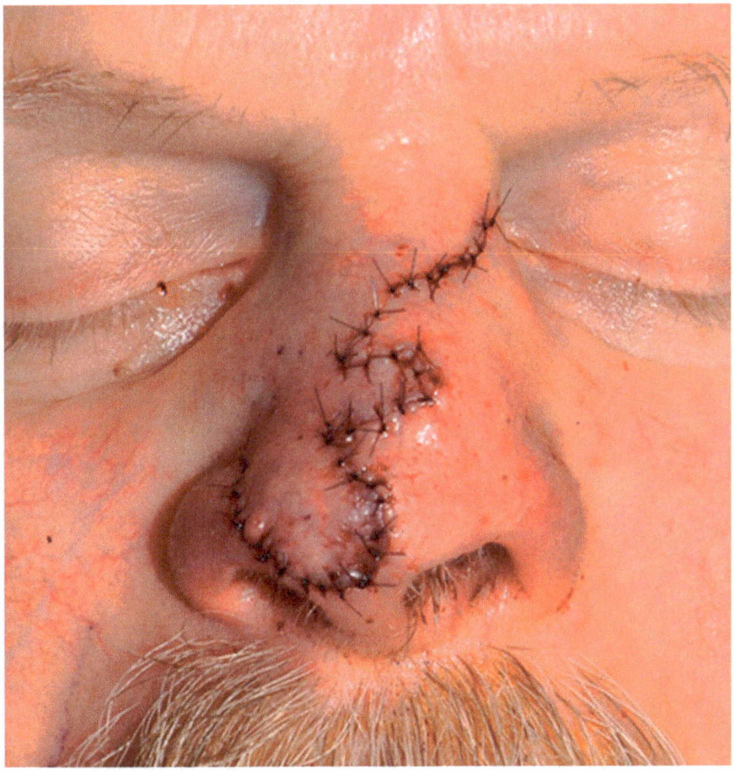

b

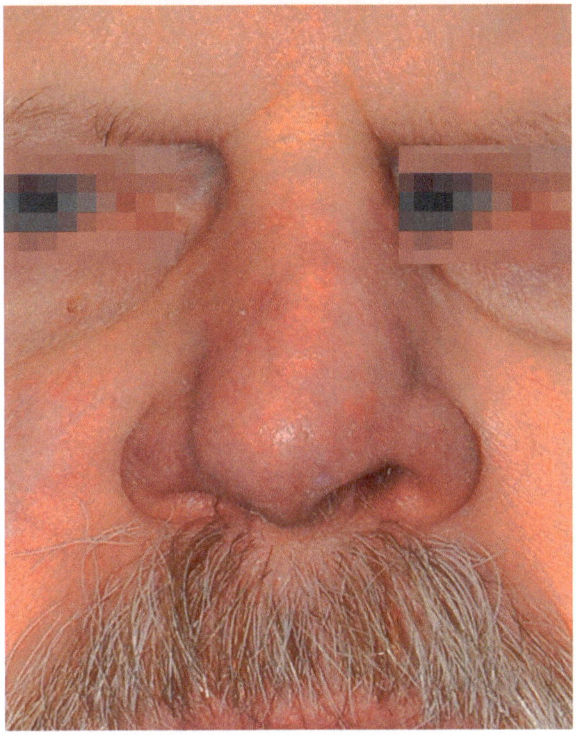

c

Fig. 6.10 (a) Nasal tip defect. **(b)** Flap in place. **(c)** Wound healed.

Large defects of the dorsum and combined defects of the dorsum and sidewall usually require a melolabial flap or a forehead flap for adequate closure. The nasal lining and structural framework of the nose also commonly demand reconstruction in these cases. Skin-only defects of the sidewall can be replaced with a melolabial flap with pexing sutures from the dermis of the flap to the underlying periosteum to re-create the nasofacial groove (**Fig. 6.11** and **Fig. 6.12**).

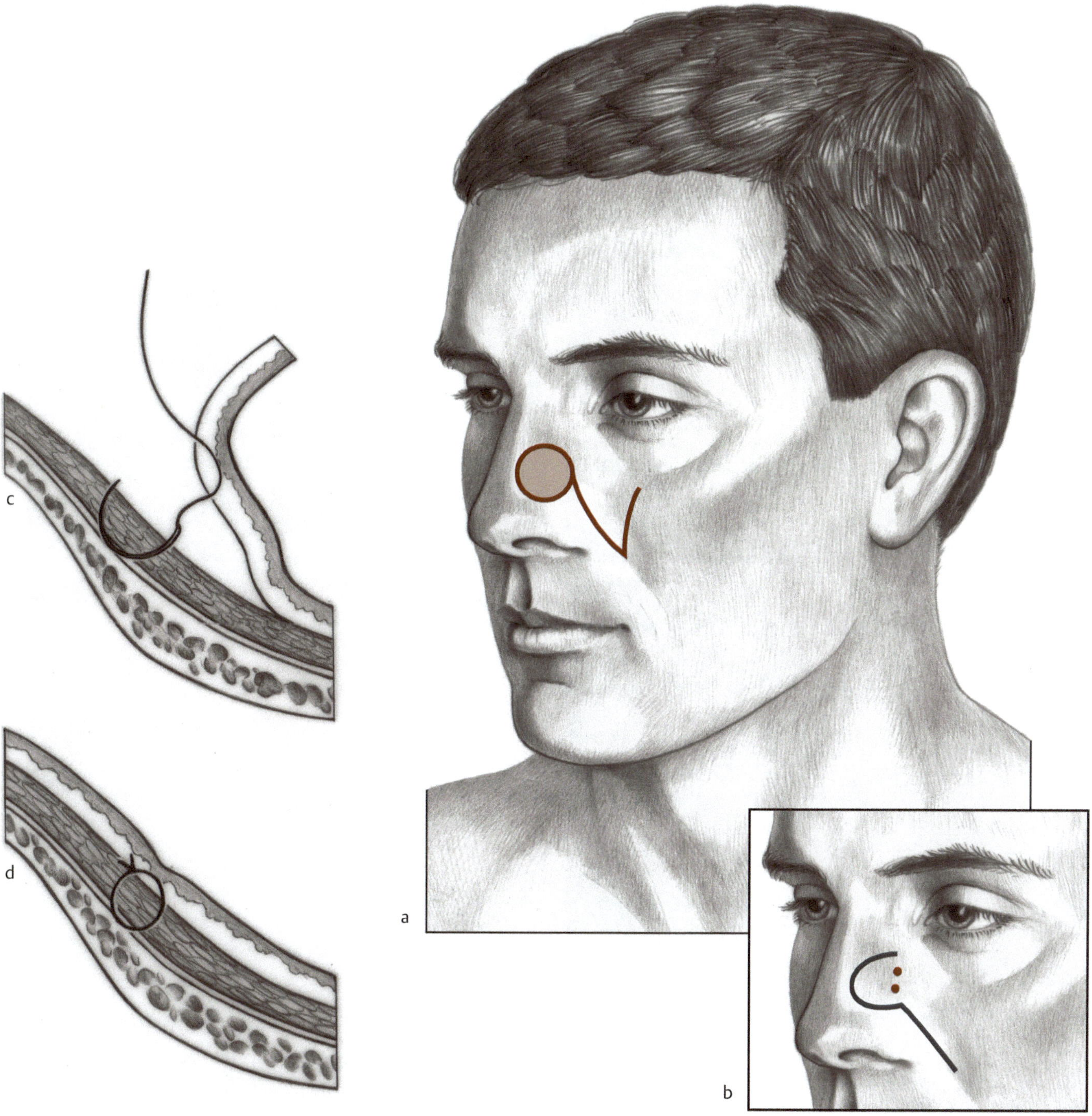

Fig. 6.11 (a–d) Melolabial and cheek flap with pexing sutures to re-create the nasofacial groove.

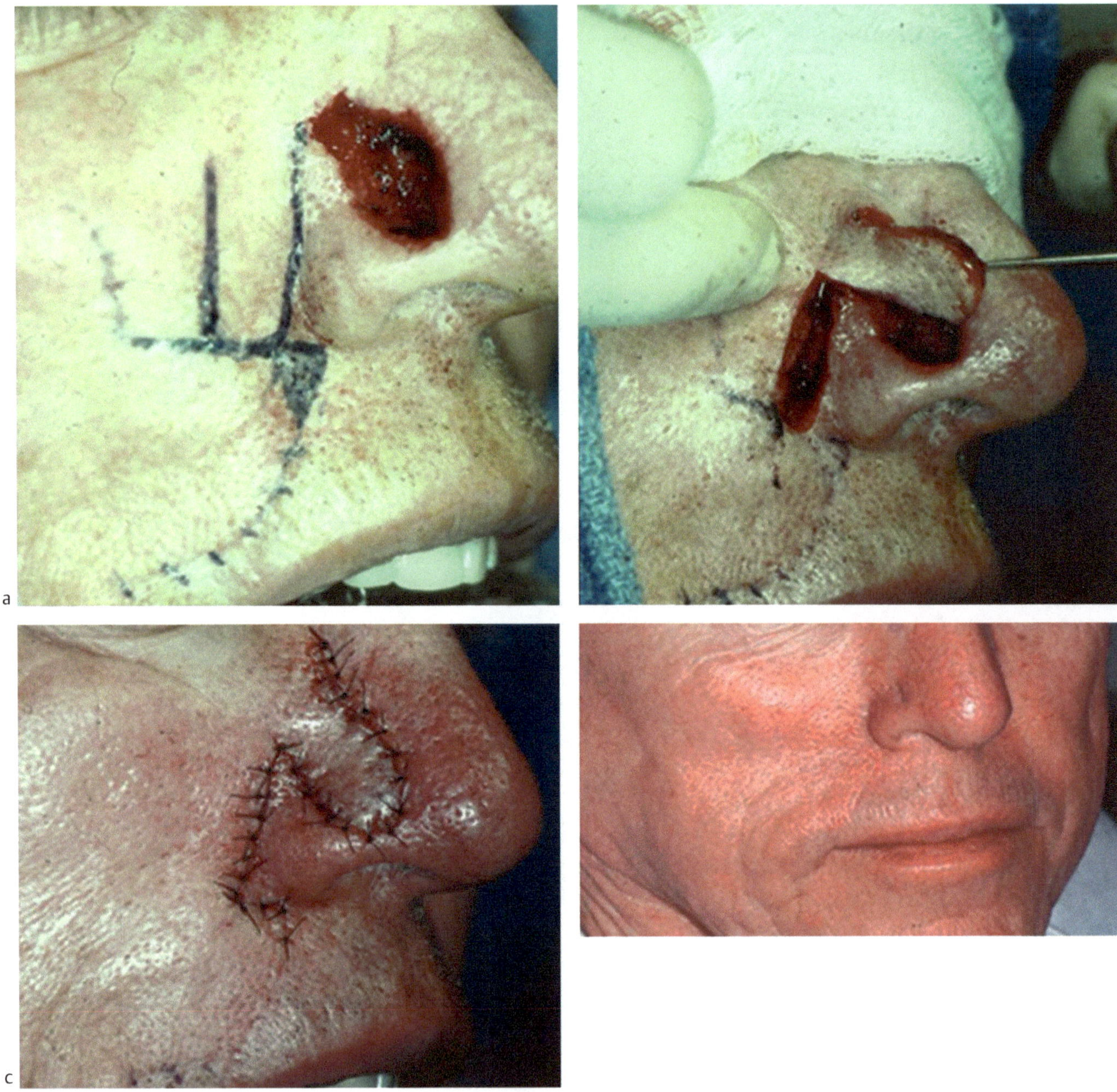

a b c d

Fig. 6.12 (a) Right nasal defect and planned superiorly based transposition flap of cheek to nose. **(b)** Flap elevated. **(c)** Flap in place. **(d)** Late postoperative result.

♦ Tip Subunit

The skin in the tip is thicker, more sebaceous, and more tightly adherent to the underlying framework than the skin of the upper nose. Tissue can be transposed from the more mobile superior areas, but transposition flaps within the tip or alar subunits are not practical (**Fig. 6.13**). For small defects of the tip alone, an FTSG can be used with adequate results (**Fig. 6.14** and **Fig. 6.15**). These results can be improved in deeper defects by allowing the bed of the wound to granulate for 2 to 3 weeks and thereby fill from below. Donor sites should be selected to match nasal skin thickness, color, and skin texture as closely as possible. Preauricular skin is a good choice, particularly in older individuals where the donor site can be closed in the preauricular crease. If the color match is good, the skin on the posterior aspect of the earlobe is elastic and has a texture similar to that of the tip.

Tip defects and those defects involving both the tip and adjacent supratip areas are best closed with a bilobed flap. The Zitelli modification is chosen because it transfers each lobe 45 to 50 degrees, rather than 90 degrees, thus minimizing standing cone formation. The flap can be either medially or laterally based, depending on the position of the defect.

Large defects involving the tip and ala, or the tip and part of the sidewall, can sometimes be repaired with a large melolabial flap, but they usually require a forehead flap (see Forehead Flap section). Superficial (skin-only) extensions of a defect from the tip onto the columella can be repaired with a large FTSG, but more extensive columellar defects require a staged, superiorly based melolabial flap or a composite graft (see the following section).

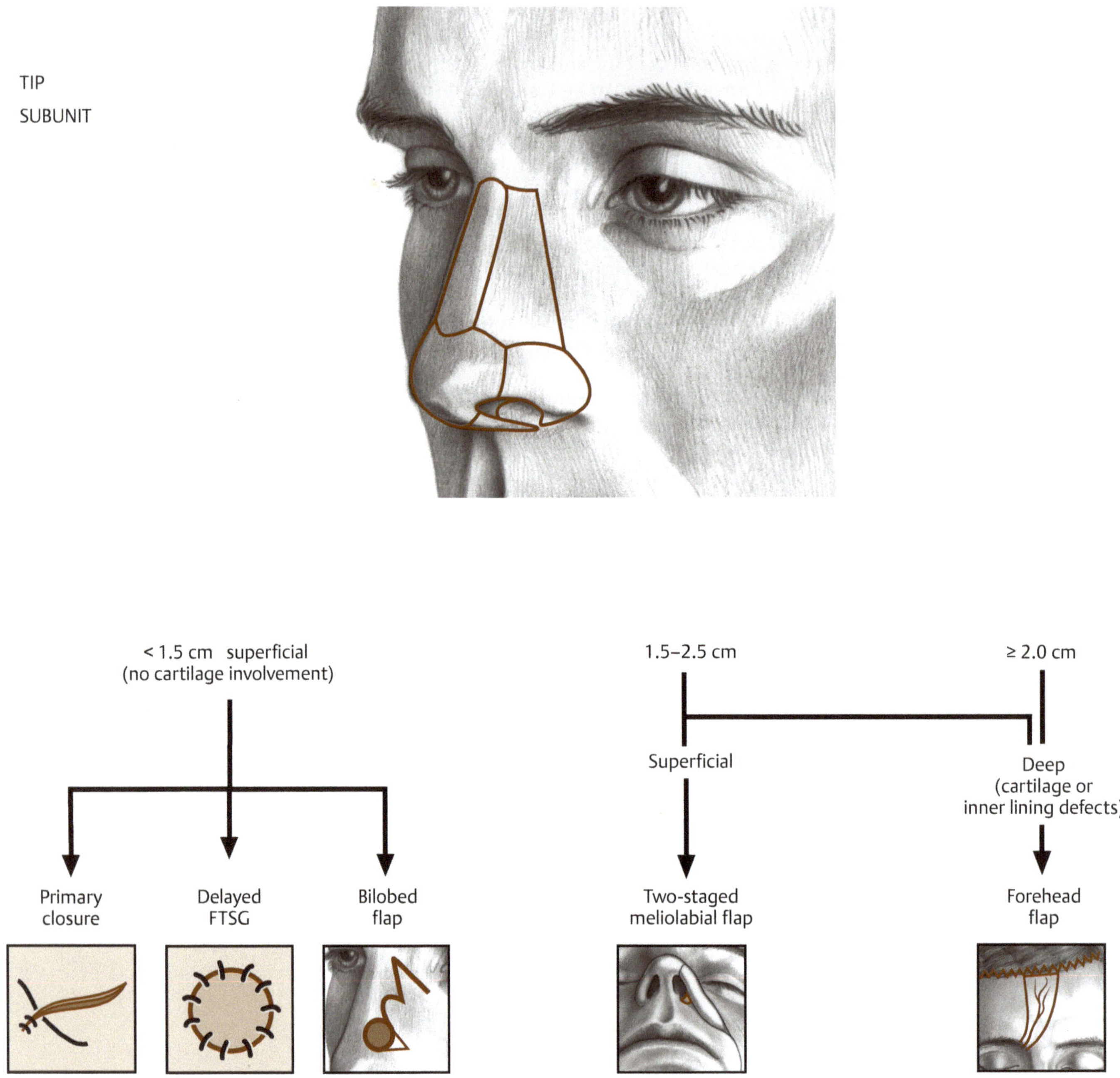

Fig. 6.13 Tip subunit. FTSG, full-thickness skin graft.

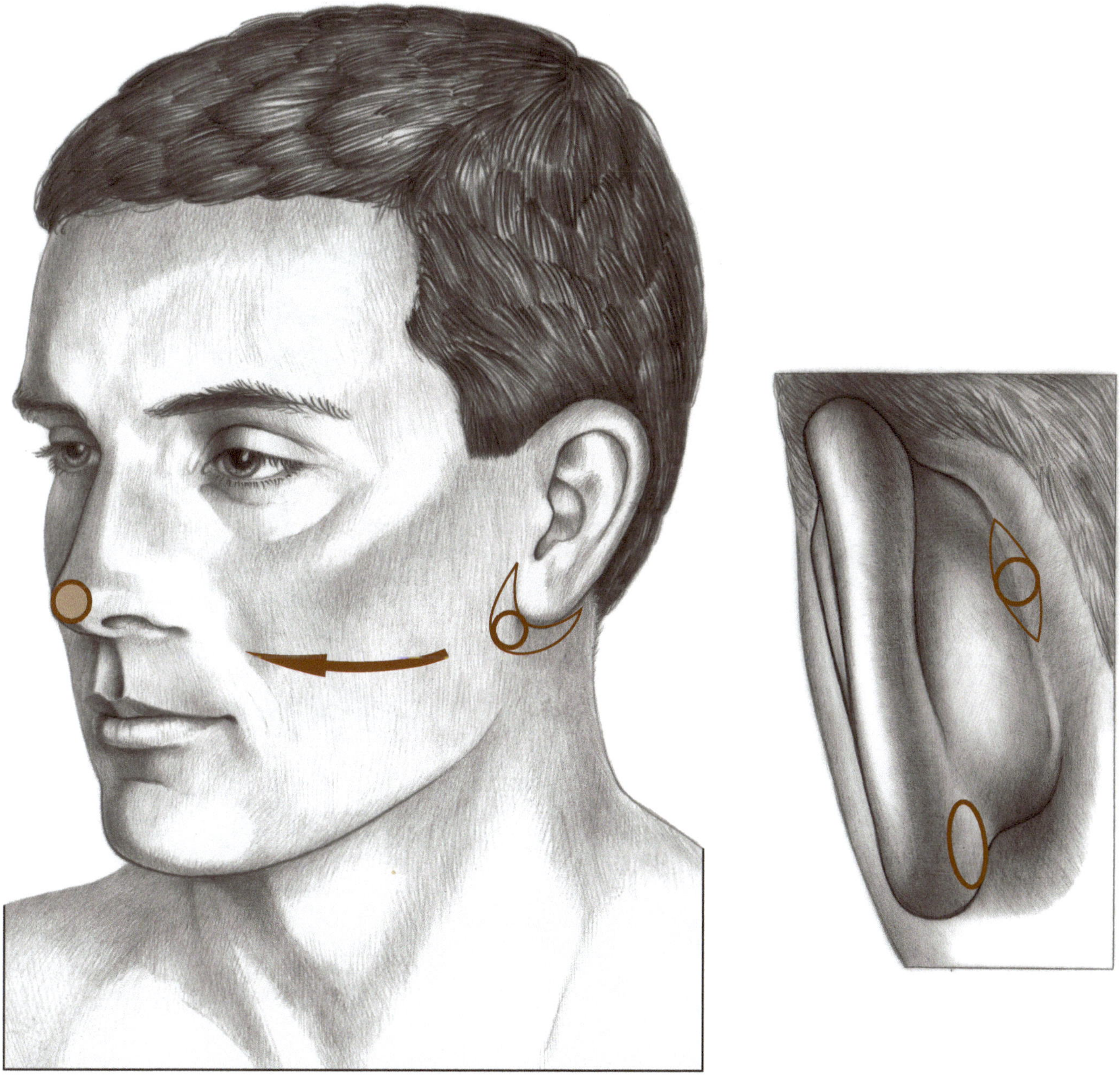

Fig. 6.14 Skin graft to the nasal tip.

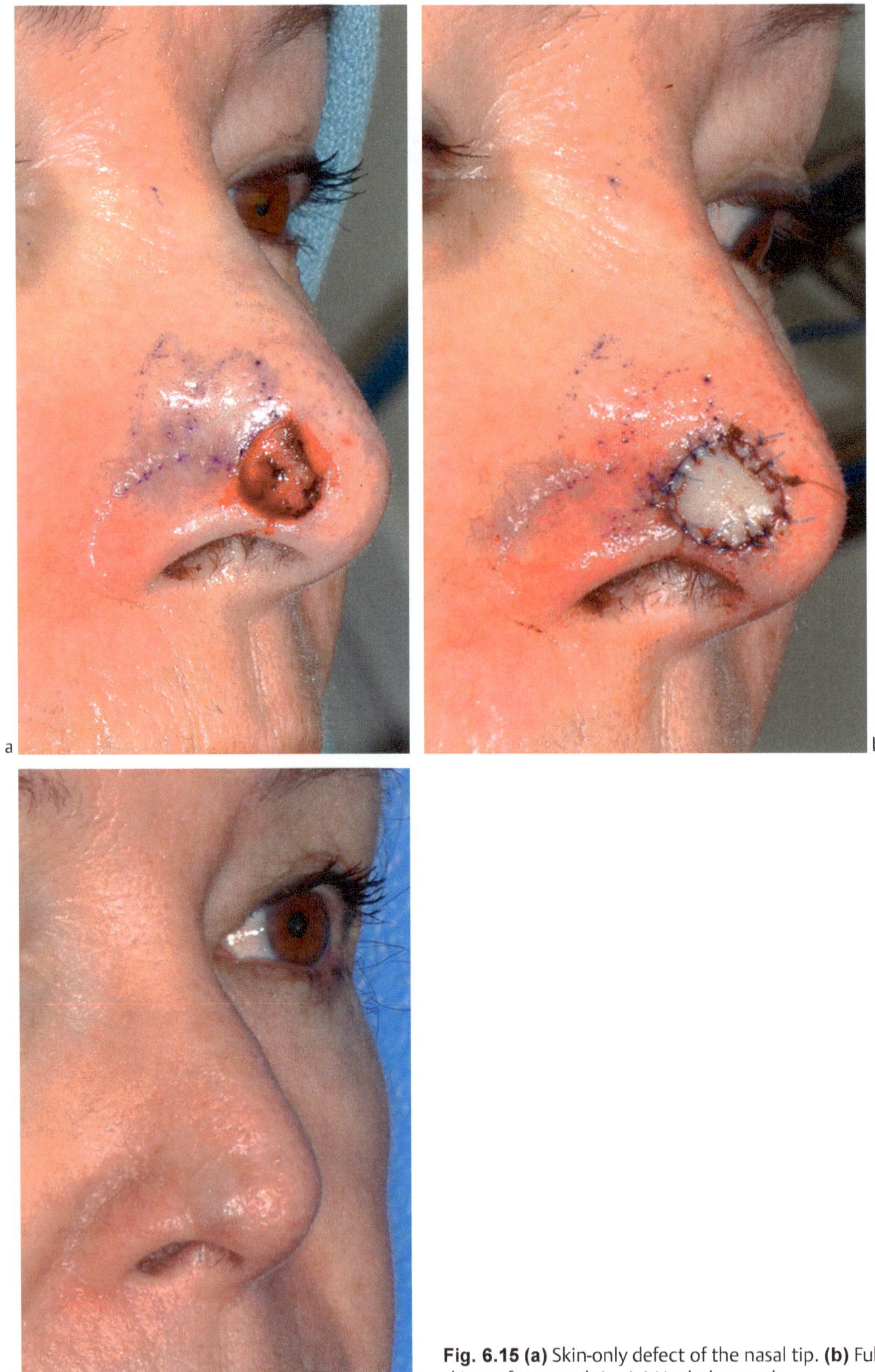

Fig. 6.15 (a) Skin-only defect of the nasal tip. (b) Full thickness skin graft to nasal tip. (c) Healed wound.

♦ Columella and Soft Tissue Subunits

The soft tissue triangles are natural webbed regions that are difficult to re-create. If they are present prior to reconstruction, then the natural soft tissue triangles are carefully preserved. A defect that involves the soft tissue triangle almost always involves the tip also and/or the columella. The best way to re-create the natural webbed appearance of the soft tissue triangles is to reconstruct the other involved subunit as planned but to leave the triangles open to granulate. Notching of the region frequently occurs if sutures are placed into the soft tissue triangles for exact tissue reapproximation.

The columella can be reconstructed with either grafts or flaps (**Fig. 6.16**). Skin-only defects are best repaired with either secondary intention healing or an FTSG (**Fig. 6.17**). The skin of the ear lobule is particularly well suited in shape and elasticity for this purpose. Larger columellar defects that include the cartilage of the medial crura can be repaired with a composite graft from the ear. A technique that works particularly well is to take the lobule of the ear and bury a cartilage graft in it through a stab incision. The cartilage graft can be taken from either the septum or concha of the ear. In larger defects, especially combined with tip defects, or in cases of impaired tissue perfusion, such as in postradiation patients, a staged, superiorly based melolabial flap or a forehead flap is chosen preferentially over a composite graft (**Fig. 6.18**). A nasolabial sulcus flap is also useful for full-thickness columellar defects (**Fig. 6.19**). This flap is an island pedicled flap from the nasofacial sulcus, which is tunneled under the nostril sill and put into place. Typically, the flap is wrapped around an autogenous cartilage columellar strut for tip support. Finally, for large columellar and upper lip defects, the extended Abbe flap is an excellent alternative (see Chapter 9 of this book).

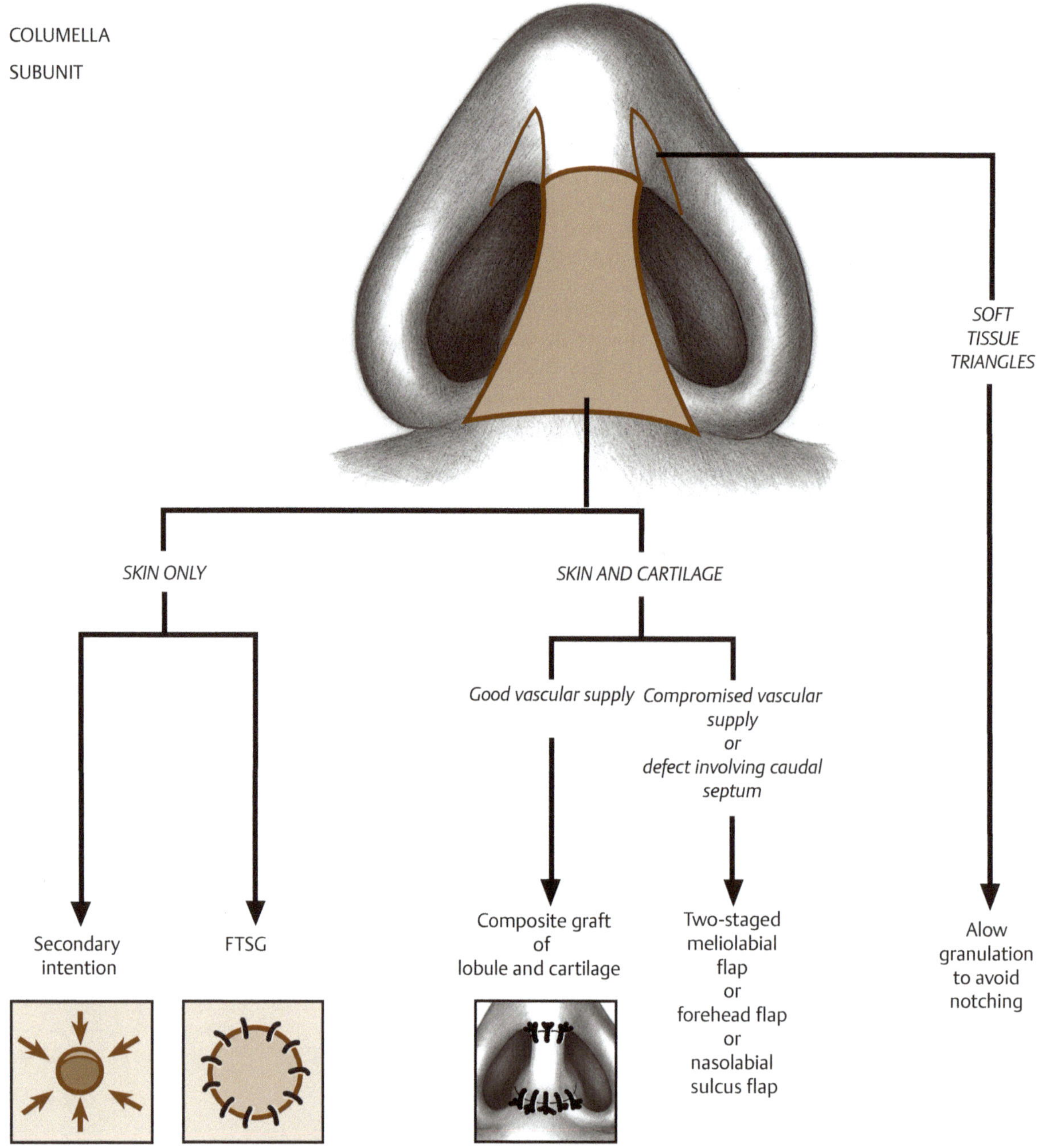

Fig. 6.16 Columella subunit. FTSG, full-thickness skin graft.

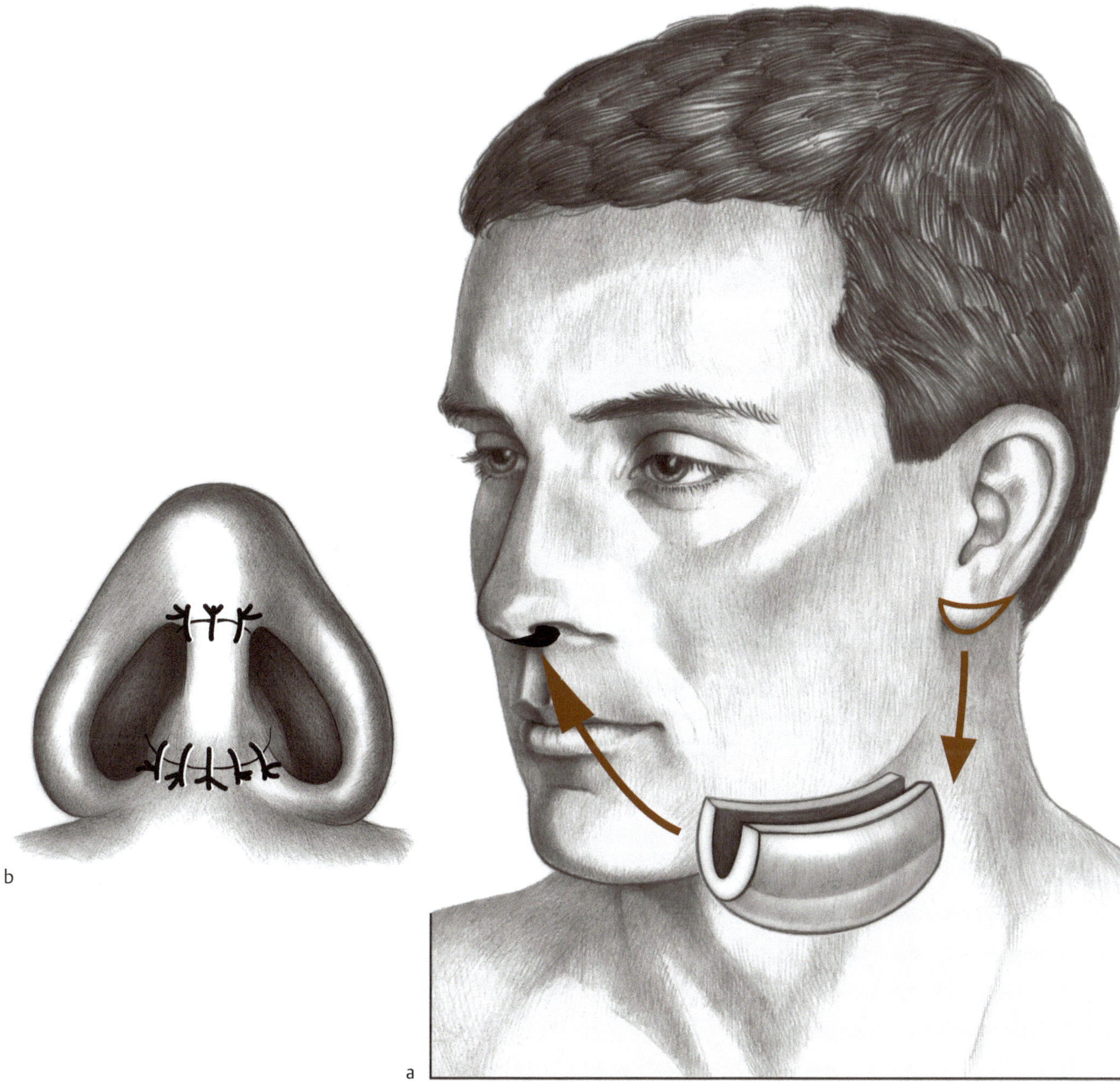

Fig. 6.17 (a, b) Full-thickness skin graft to the columella.

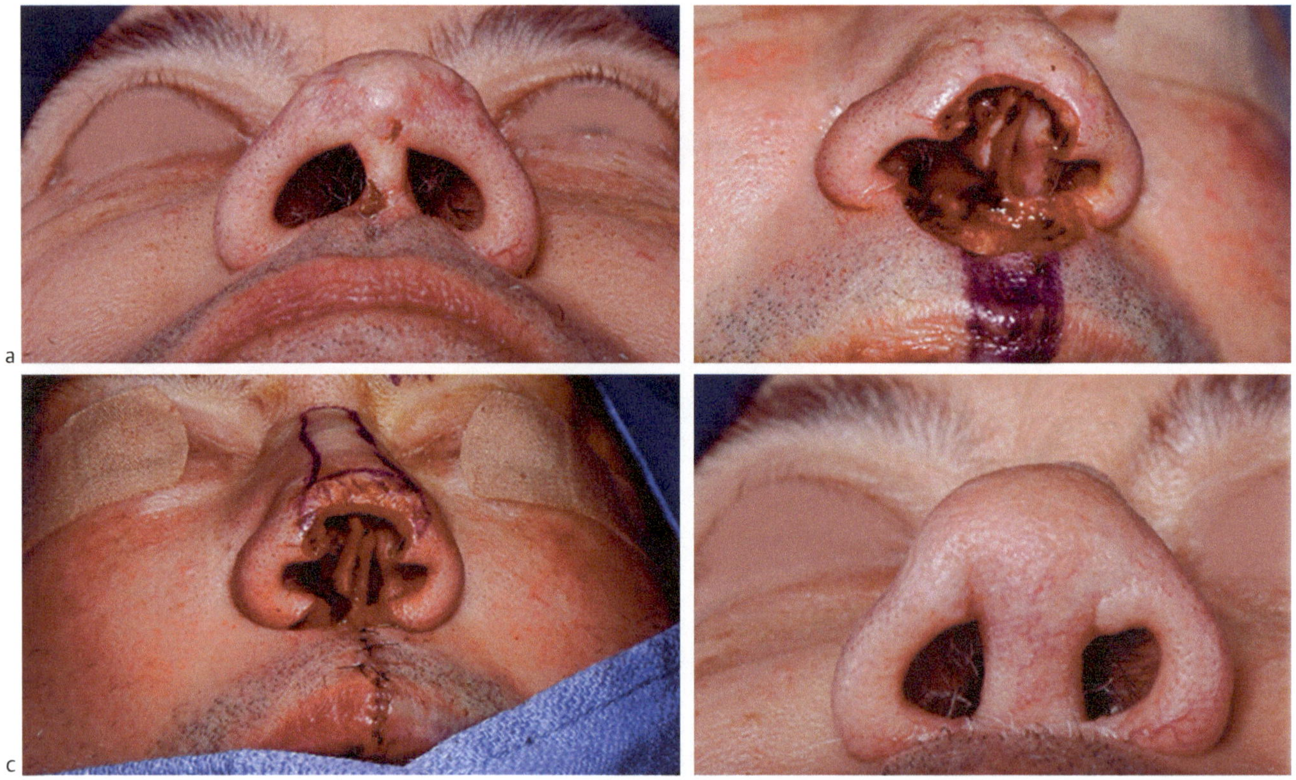

Fig. 6.18 (a) Malignancy of the columella, tip, and upper lip. **(b)** Planned full-thickness upper lip excision with primary closure. **(c)** The lip is closed. A paramedian forehead flap is planned to replace the columella, tip, and dorsum, as well as the caudal septal mucosa. **(d)** Postoperative result.

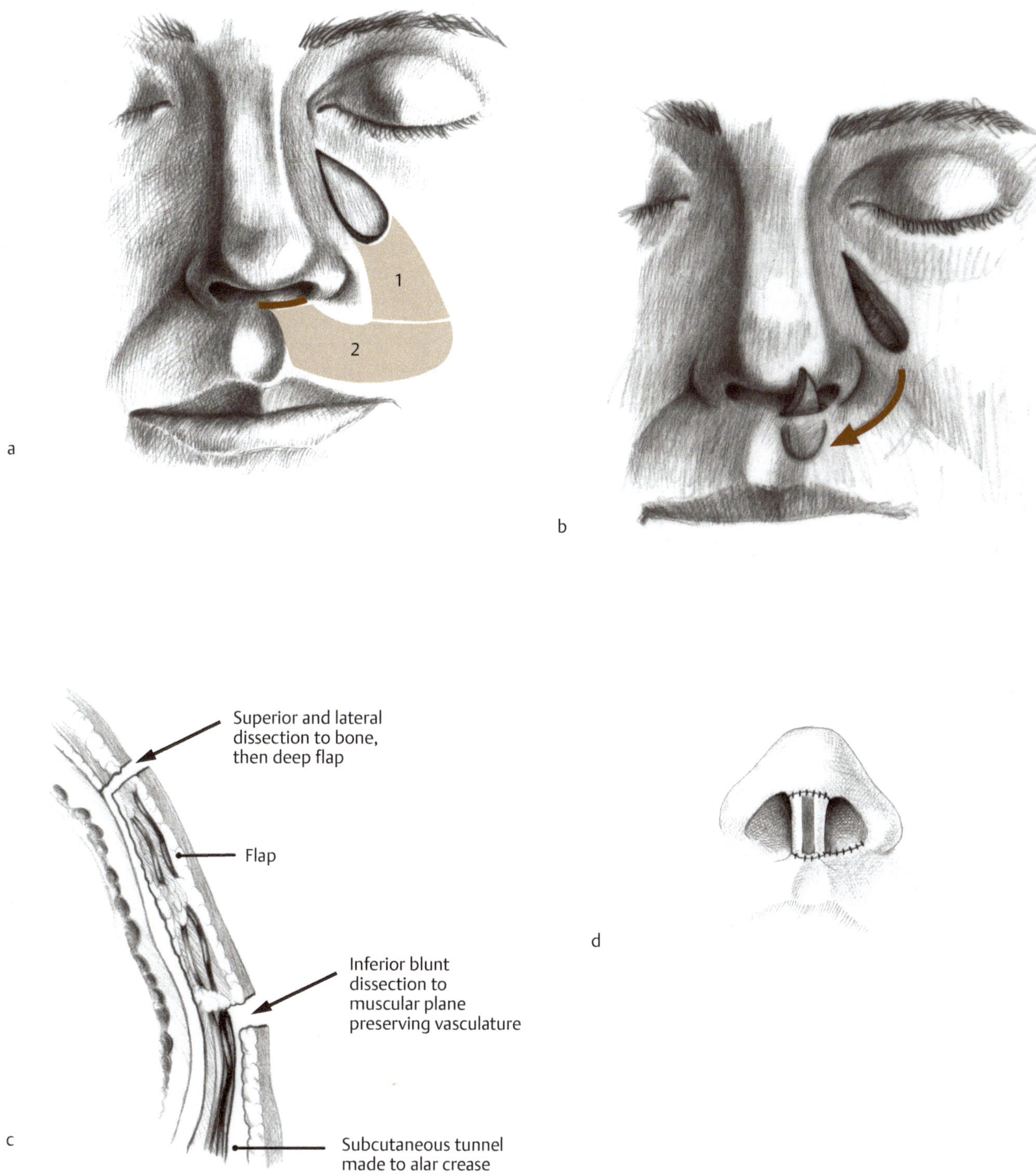

Fig. 6.19 (a, b) Nasofacial sulcus flap (after Hilger). **(c)** Explanation of tissue planes for nasofacial sulcus flap elevation. **(d)** Flap in place.

♦ Alar Subunit

Partial-thickness defects that are centered on the concave alar nasal groove and that do not approach the alar margin can be allowed to heal by secondary intention with satisfactory results (**Fig. 6.20**). These areas will close in ~3 to 4 weeks, with conservative local wounds treated with gentle cleansing and antibiotic ointment. Other partial-thickness defects of the ala are commonly repaired with a modified bilobed flap, a two-stage melolabial flap, or a nasofacial groove flap.

The nasofacial groove flap is a two-stage procedure (**Figs. 6.21** and **Fig. 6.22**). The small remainder of skin at the lower lateral nasofacial groove is left intact at the first stage (**Fig. 6.21** and **Fig. 6.22a, b**). At the second stage, the lateral aspect is inset 2 to 3 weeks later (**Fig. 6.21c** and **Fig. 6.22c, d**).

Full-thickness defects of the alar margins that are ~1.5 cm or less can be reconstructed with a composite graft of skin and cartilage from the ear (**Fig. 6.23**). A defect involving primarily the alar margin is repaired with the cartilage of the crus helices and associated preauricular skin. This particular composite is also ideal for a small "cookie bite" deformity of the alar margin and a larger associated skin deficiency over the lateral nasal wall; a large paddle of skin can be harvested with the small amount of cartilage and the donor defect closed cosmetically as in a facelift. One can create a more favorable recipient site for a large "cookie bite" deformity by using either a melolabial or an adjacent nasal skin turn-in flap to create an inner lining, then using this same crus helices composite. The nasal skin turn-in flap is used primarily for healed defects that are being reconstructed secondarily. Full-thickness defects, 1.5 cm or less, that involve more than the alar margin, can be repaired with a composite graft harvested as a wedge (or star) excision from the helix; these composites receive blood supply only on the margins and heal less predictably than the crus helices composite.

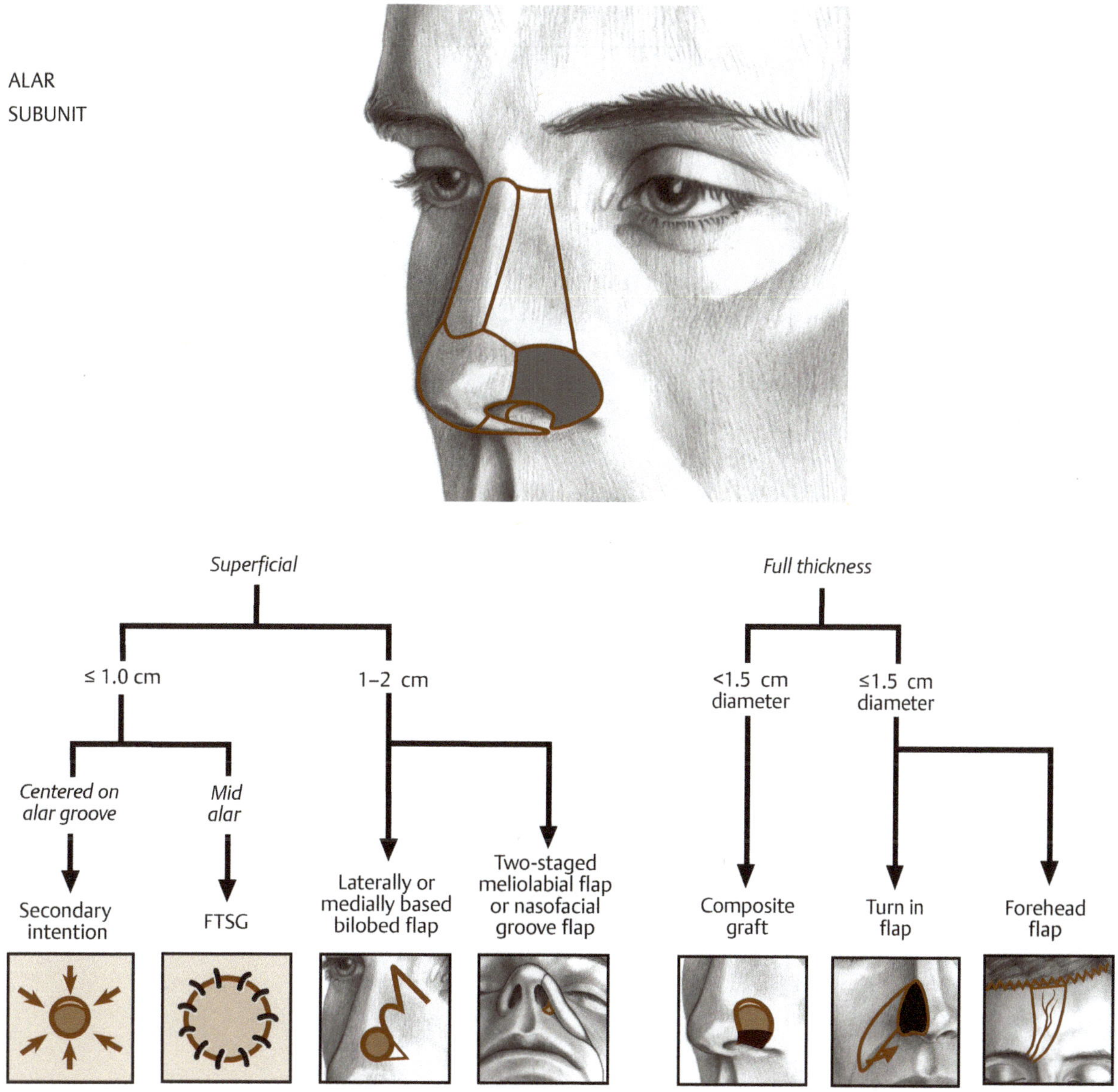

Fig. 6.20 Alar subunit. FTSG, full-thickness skin graft.

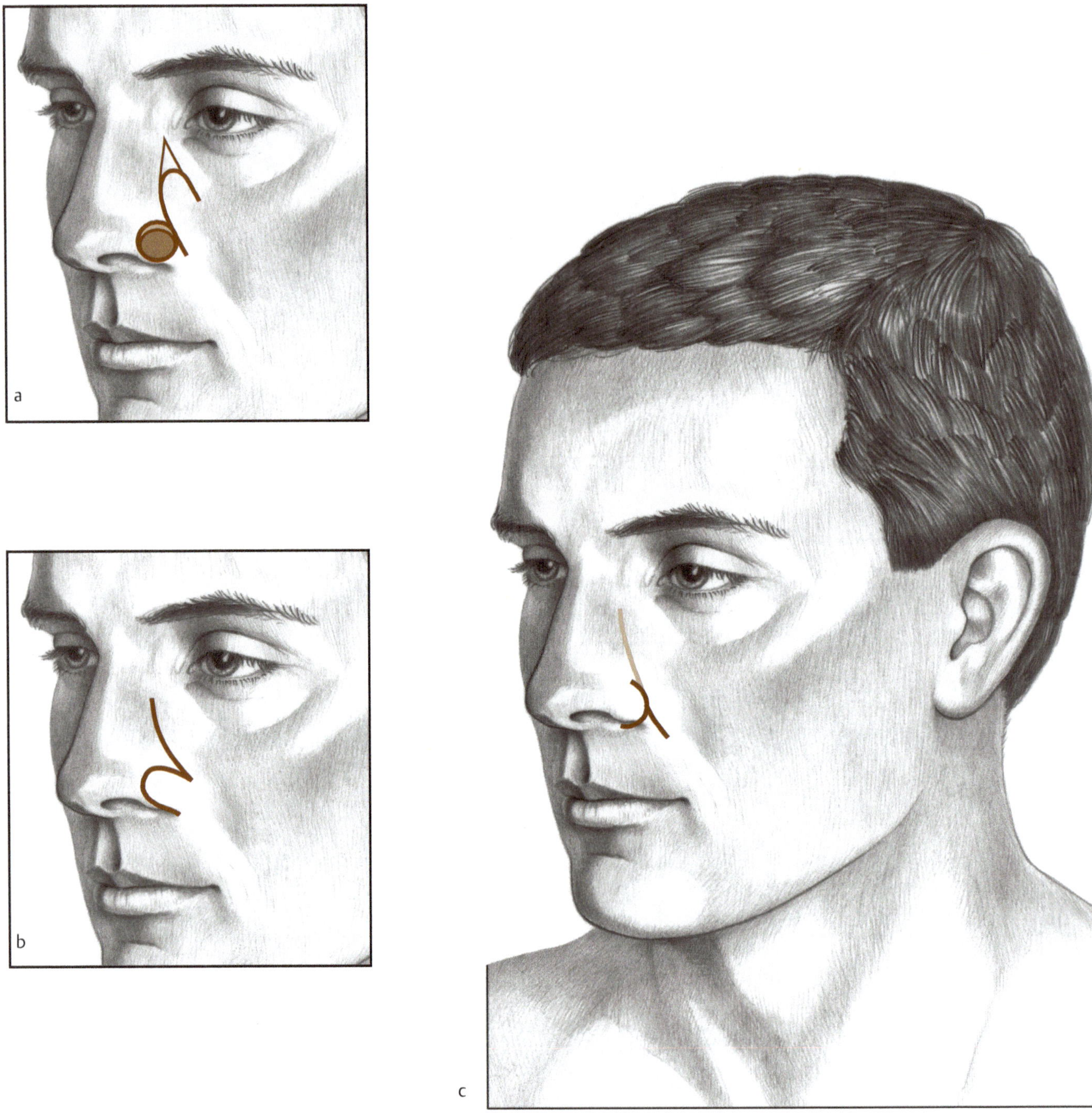

Fig. 6.21 (a–c) The nasofacial groove flap.

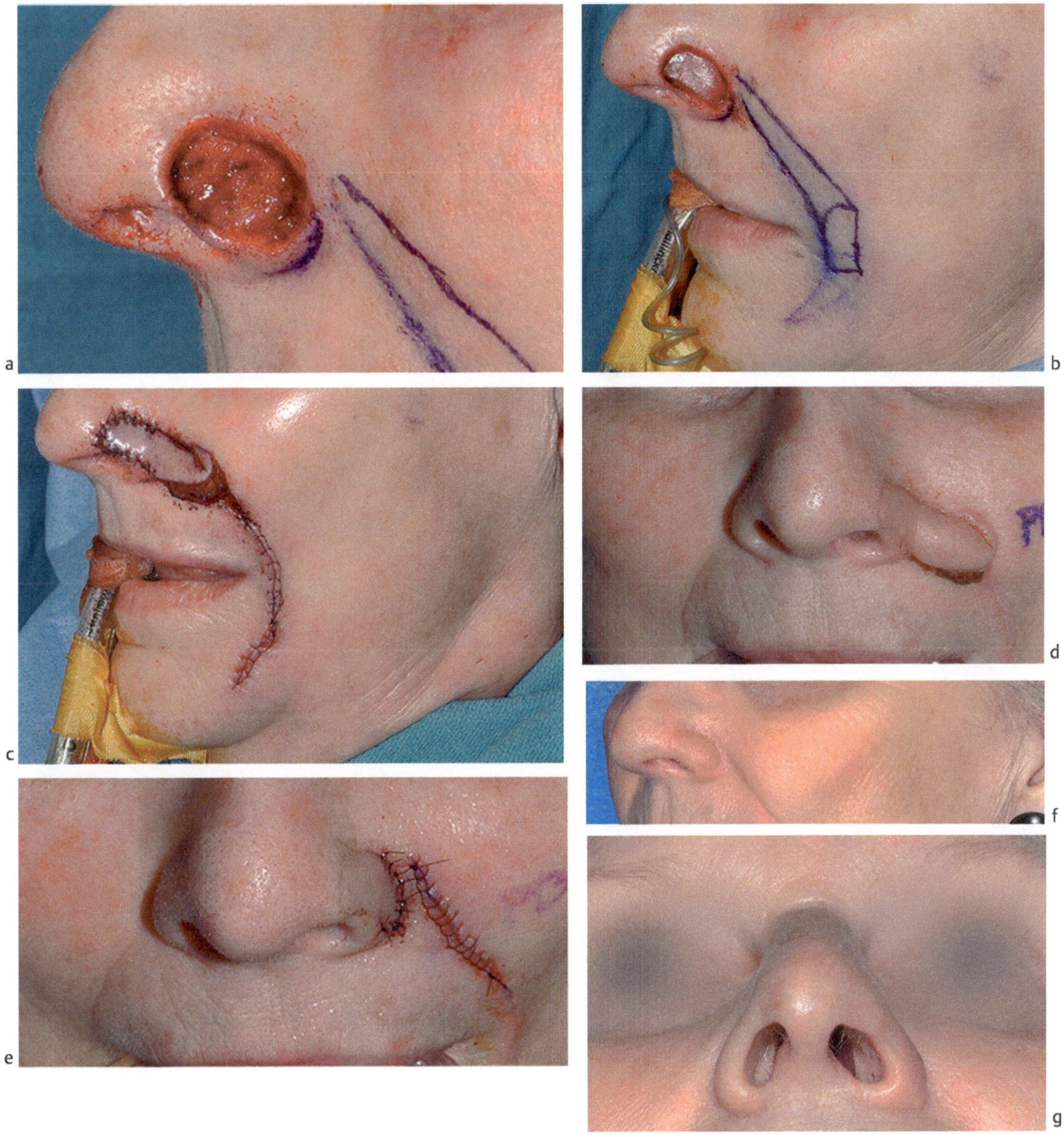

Fig. 6.22 (a) Nasal ala defect. **(b)** Cartilage graft and melolabial flap template. **(c)** Melolabial flap in place at the end of stage 1. **(d)** Melolabial flap healing prior to stage 2. **(e)** Melolabial flap divided and closed. **(f)** healed wound sideview. **(g)** Healed wound base view.

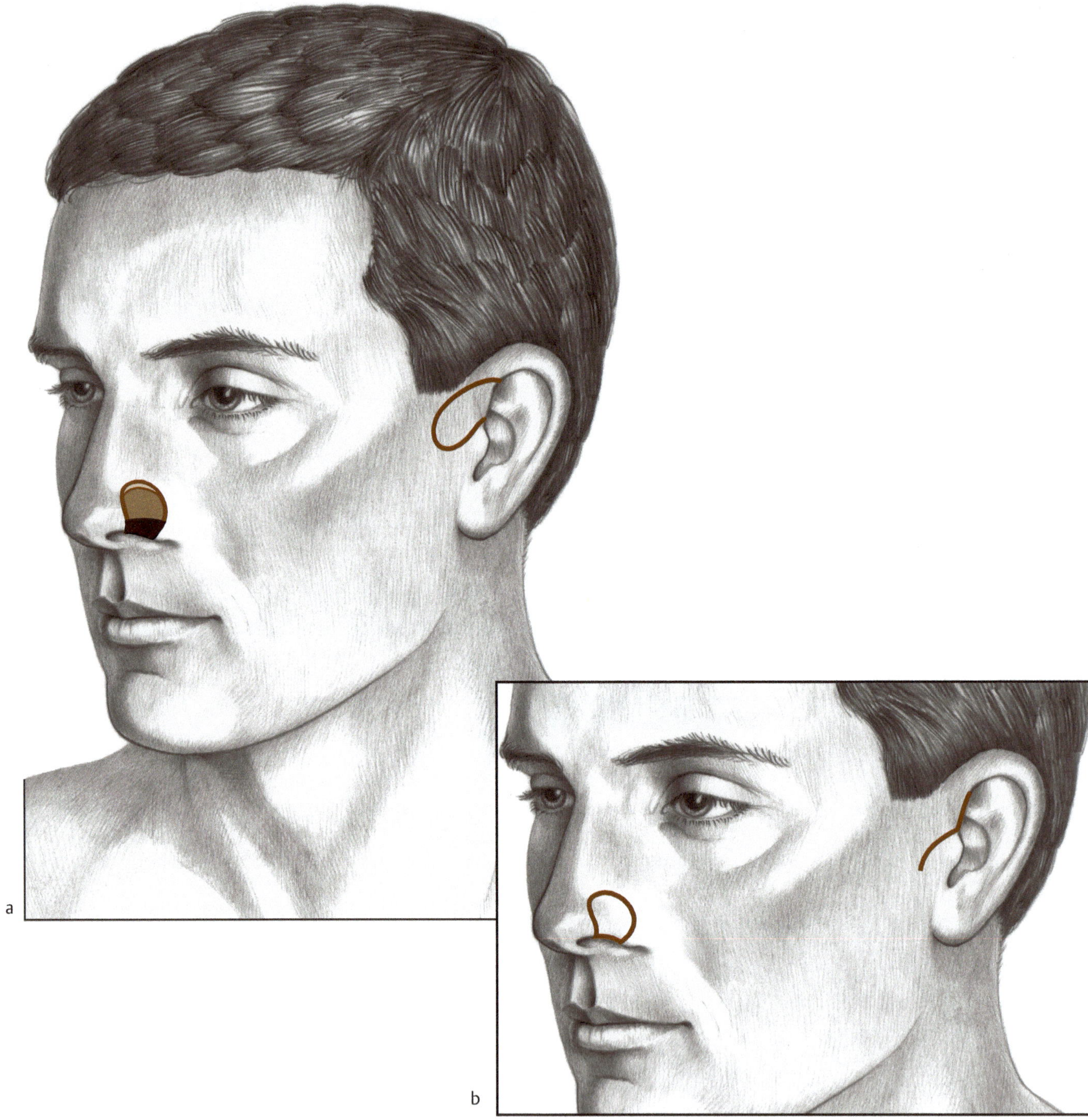

Fig. 6.23 (a, b) Composite graft reconstruction of the alar rim.

c 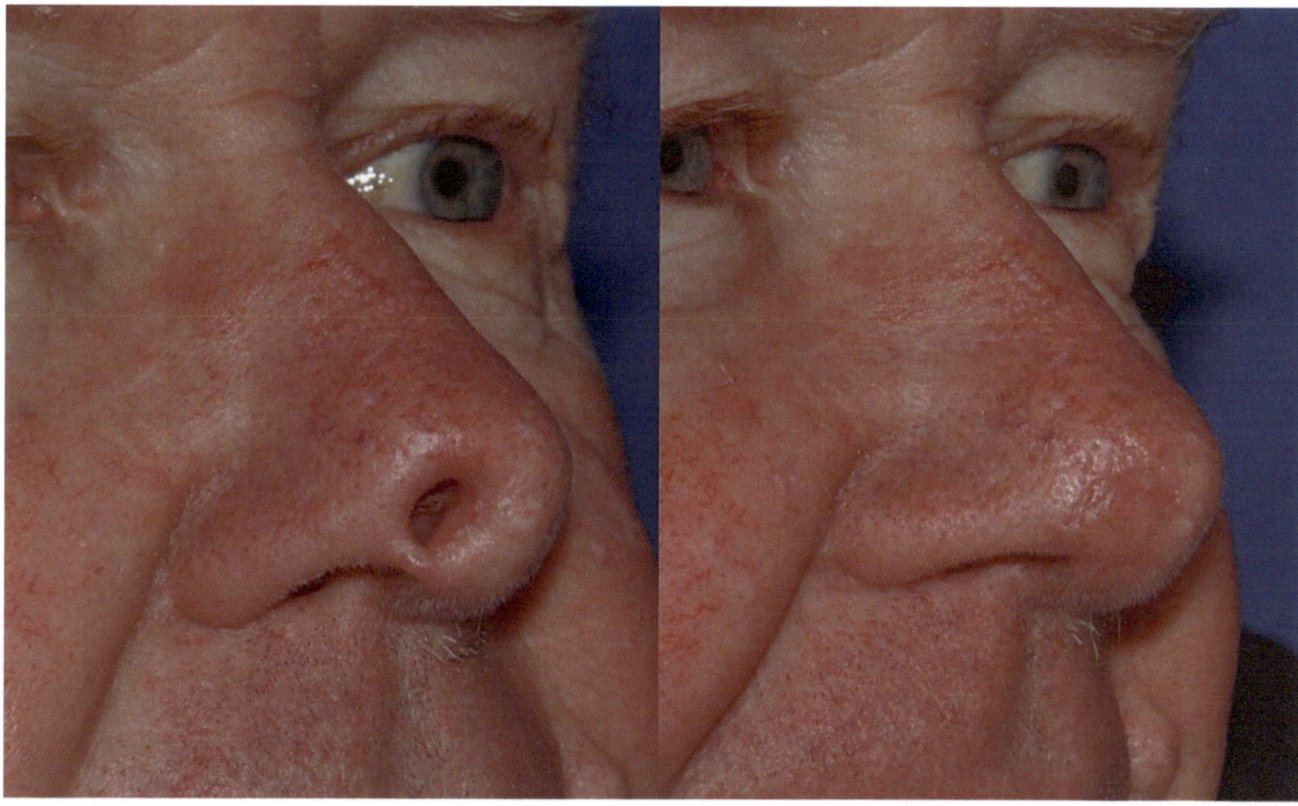

Fig. 6.23 (c) Before and after composite graft reconstruction.

Large full-thickness alar defects (>1.5 cm) are repaired using a melolabial flap, executed as described by Burget and Menick (**Fig. 6.24**). The melolabial flap is planned using a template created from the contralateral, intact ala. The flap is then drawn with tapered ends over the melolabial crease and is planned 1 to 2 mm wider than anticipated to allow for the scar contracture that inevitably accompanies this flap. In general, the flap should also be carried somewhat further in an inferior direction than seems necessary, because this incision heals very well, and the extra tissue is sometimes necessary to obtain defect closure without tension or distortion.

The triangular tip necessary for closure of the donor site without a standing cone formation is never trimmed until the final contouring of the flap at the defect site. The flap is incised through skin, and the distal end is elevated in a subcutaneous plane above the facial musculature. The proximal superior skin is left attached to a subcutaneous pedicle that allows for thinning of the distal flap to the level just deep to the dermis. The pedicle can be mobilized with blunt dissection. It is very difficult to re-create an anatomical alar base; therefore, if any of the alar base remains, it is preserved, and the melolabial flap is transposed over it and sutured into position. The donor site is closed by advancing the cheek flap to the melolabial groove.

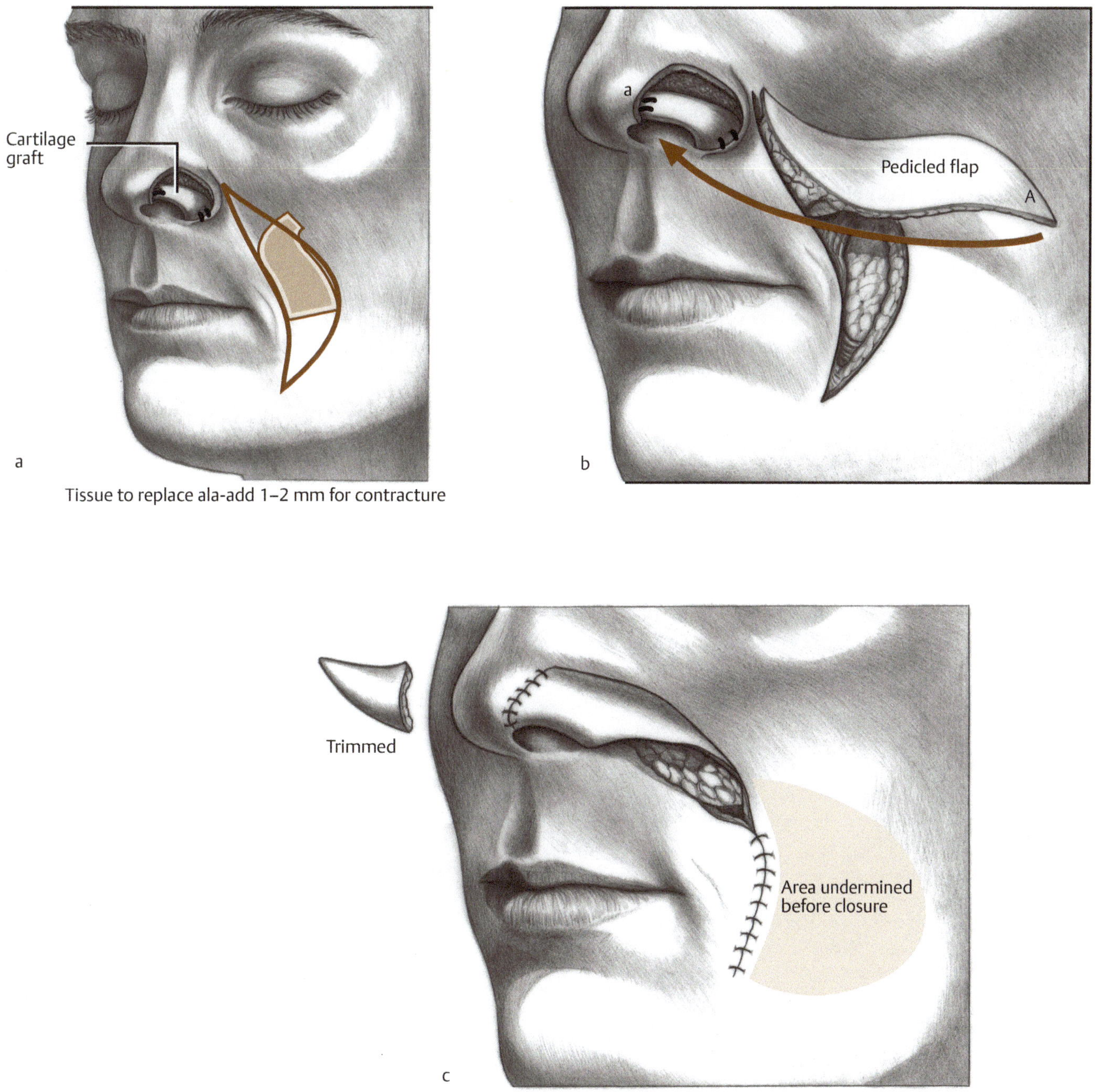

Fig. 6.24 (a–c) Melolabial flap repair of complete alar defect (after Burget and Menick).

When the melolabial flap is used for a large full-thickness alar defect, the flap can be rolled on itself to reconstruct both internal and external nasal lining if no local intranasal tissue is available to recruit for lining reconstruction (**Fig. 6.25**). If local intranasal tissue is available to re-create the lining, then this is the preferred technique of lining reconstruction (**Fig. 6.26a**). A suture-fixated graft of auricular or septal cartilage is placed precisely at the most inferior aspect of the planned alar margin to help prevent alar retraction (**Fig. 6.26b, c**). This site is lower than the inferior border of the lower lateral cartilage. The flap is inset with minimal tension over the alar batten (**Fig. 6.26d, e**). The supra-alar hollow is re-created with either triangular fixation sutures or transnasal sutures tied over external bolsters. After this first stage of the operation, the alar margin should appear 1 to 3 mm lower than the rim on the contralateral side.

About 3 weeks after the initial surgery, pedicle division may be undertaken (**Fig. 6.27a, b**). At this time, the alar base remnant may be either resected and carefully replaced with the flap remnant, or else left in place and the flap inset into it. Either way, the flap is further thinned prior to inset and is then inset with minimal tension (**Fig. 6.27c**). The flap pedicle is excised and is closed in the melolabial crease (**Fig. 6.27d–f**).

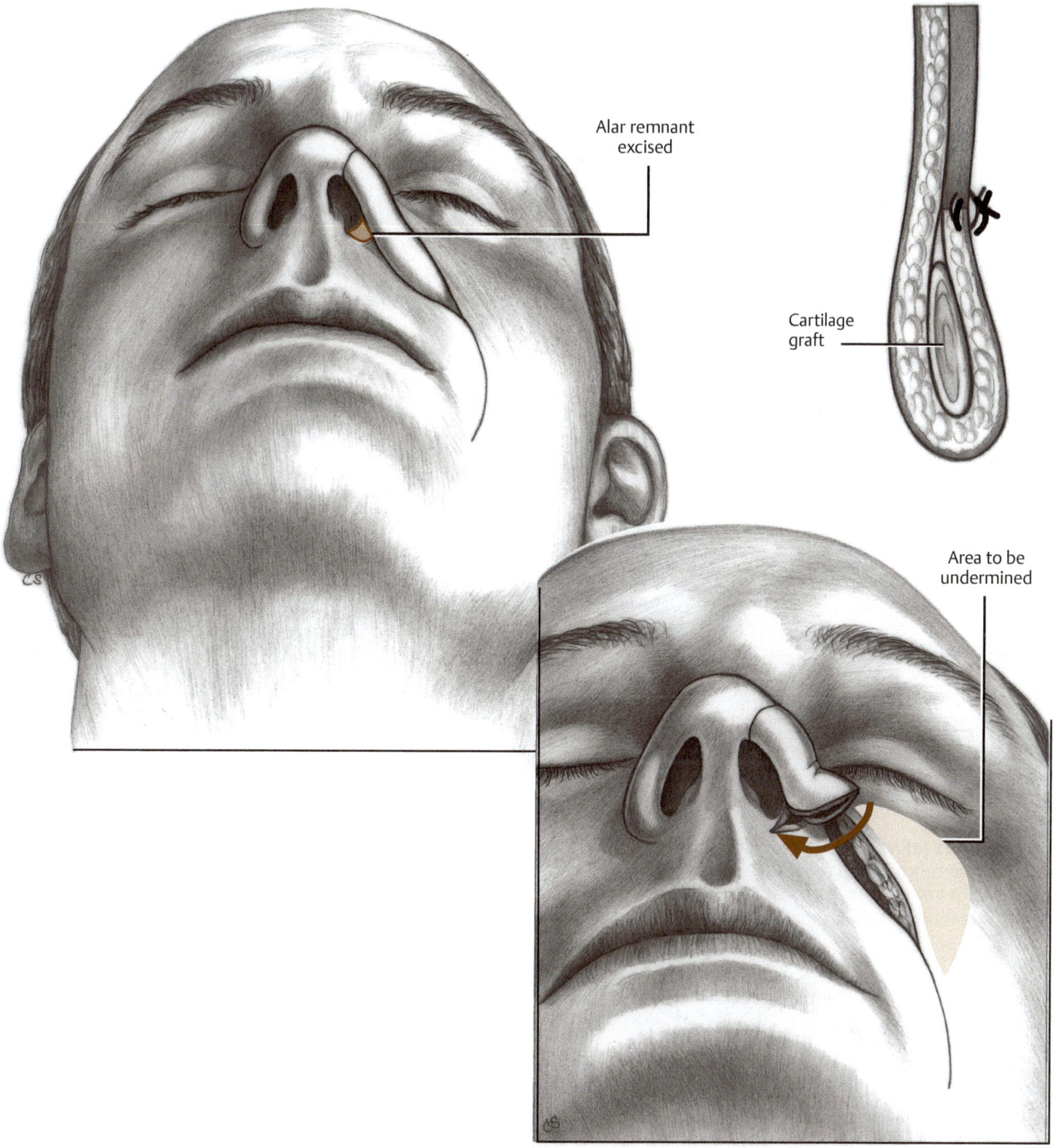

Fig. 6.25 Rolling the melolabial flap internally to reconstruct larger lining defects.

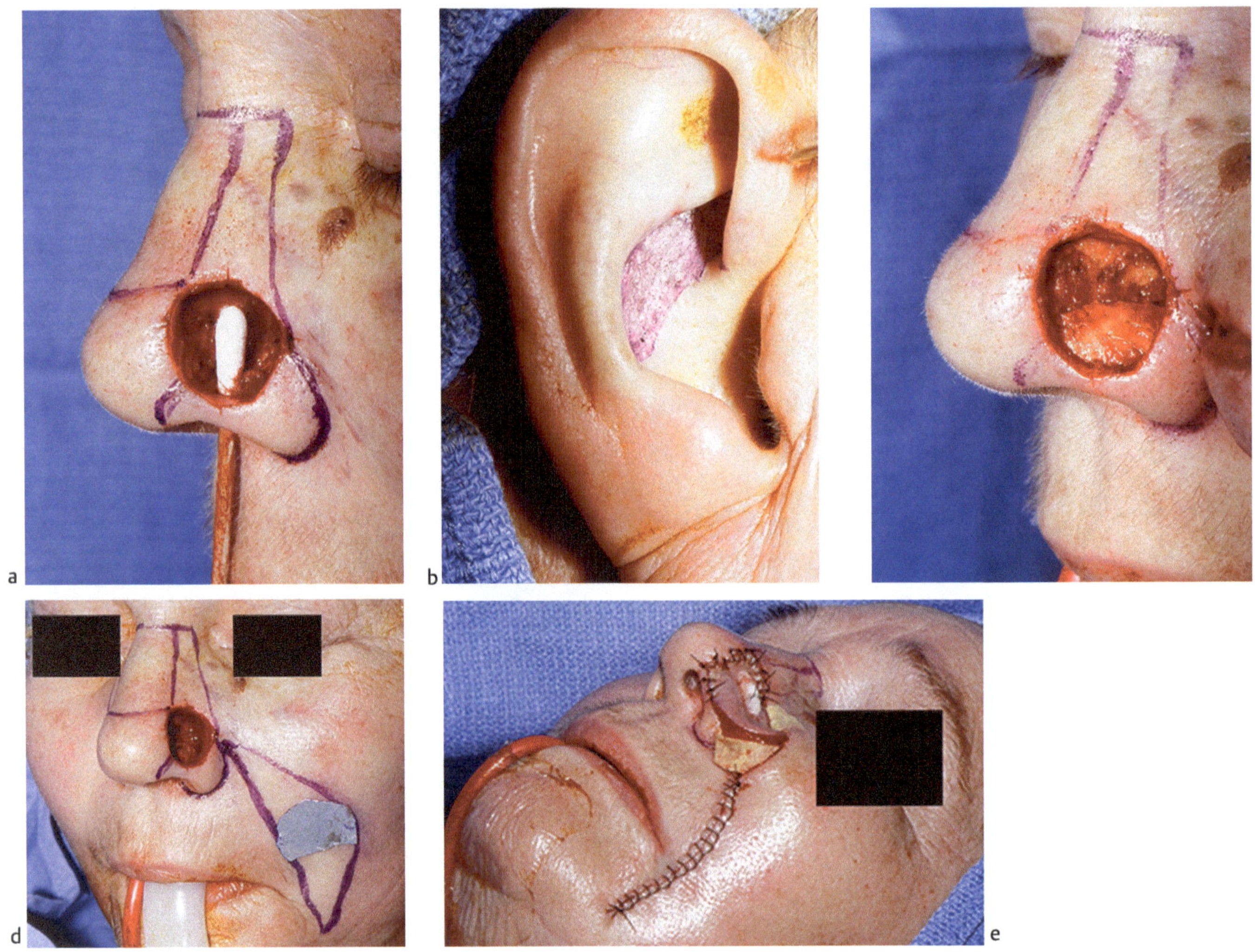

Fig. 6.26 (a) A near complete alar defect with a small lining defect amenable to local tissue closure for the lining defect. **(b)** The concha cymba cartilage graft is excellent for re-creating the alar rim. **(c)** The cartilage graft is fixated into place with its lower border precisely at the site where the planned alar rim will sit. **(d)** The flap is planned with a template from the opposite, intact alar subunit. **(e)** The melolabial flap at completion of stage 1.

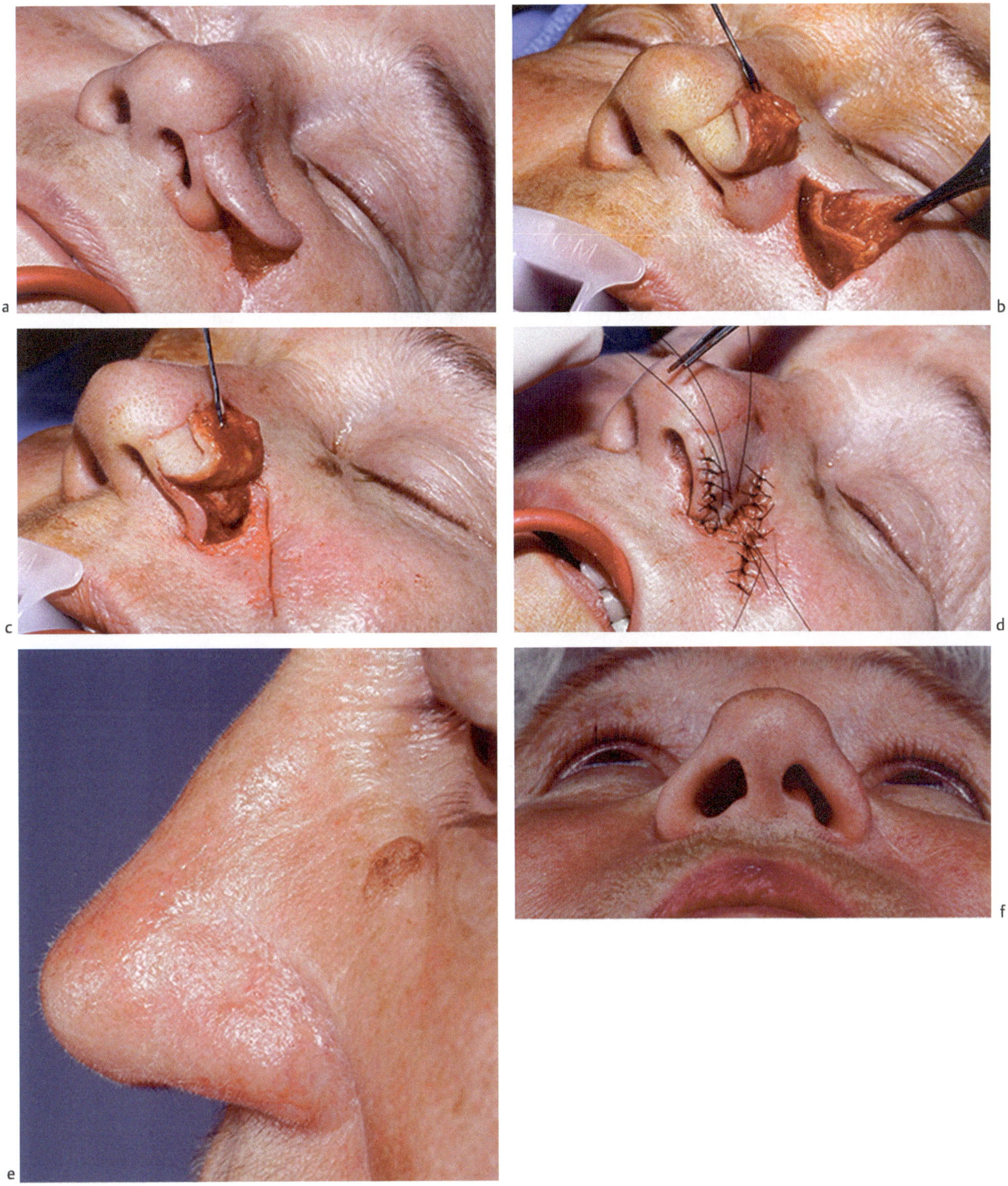

Fig. 6.27 (a) The pedicle 3 weeks later. **(b)** The pedicle is divided. **(c)** The flap is thinned. Note the 1- to 2-mm cuff of tissue of the alar–facial groove left intact. **(d)** The flap is inset. Bolster sutures are in place to affix a cotton bolster in the alar–facial groove to re-create the inversion. **(e)** Late postoperative result of alar reconstruction. **(f)** The reconstructed left alar rim re-creates the intact right alar rim well.

♦ Forehead Flap

The forehead flap is the reconstructive method of choice for significant nasal defects. This versatile, reliable flap can be used for a spectrum of defects, up to and including total nasal reconstruction. Both the midline and the paramedian forehead flaps carry with them a robust vertically oriented blood supply that readily nourishes skin, subcutaneous tissue, and cartilage grafts applied at the time of reconstruction. By using the paramedian forehead flap design, in the rare case the need arises, the opposite supratrochlear vascular pedicle can be used to harvest a second flap at a later date (**Fig. 6.28**). Forehead flaps are supplied primarily by the supratrochlear vessels, and secondarily by the angular and supraorbital vessels. The supratrochlear vessels exit the orbital septum between 1.7 to 2.2 cm lateral to the midline, then pass beneath the orbicularis oculi muscle over the corrugator muscle. Flap design begins with precise Doppler identification and marking of the supratrochlear pedicle contralateral to the nasal defect to be reconstructed.

The shape of the flap to be harvested is planned with a foil template made from the corresponding undisturbed subunits. The length of the flap is determined using a suture or gauze to measure from the pedicle base to the most distal reconstruction site. The flap is then drawn as close to the midline as the hairline and pedicle allow. Precise Doppler identification of supratrochlear vessels allows safe thinning of the pedicle base to 1 cm, which facilitates ease of rotation and provides maximal flap length. The flap is then elevated in the subgaleal plane. Beginning 1 to 2 cm superior to the pedicle base, blunt dissection is used to prevent inadvertent damage to the vascular supply.

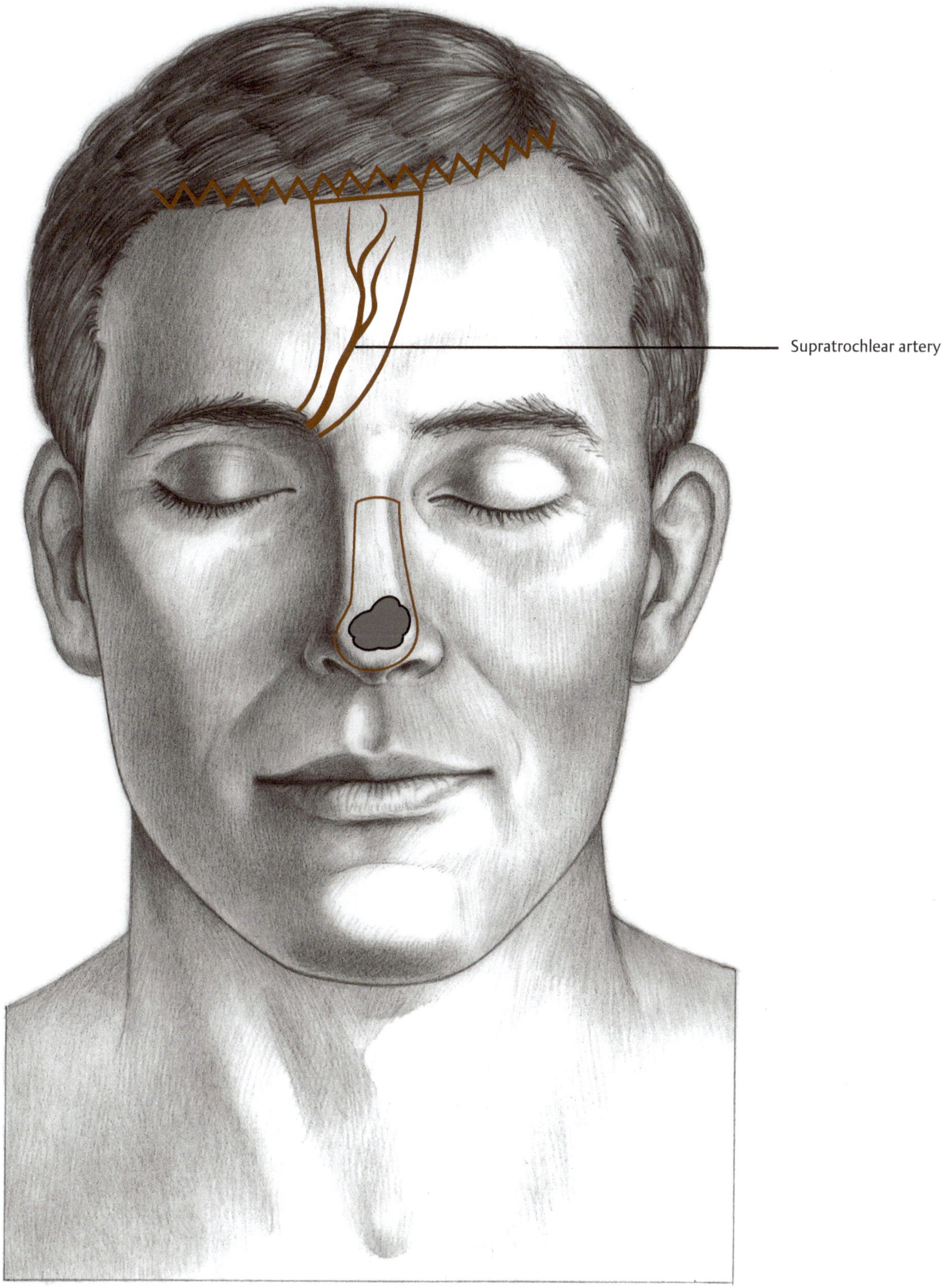

Fig. 6.28 Paramedian forehead flap planned on one supratrochlear vascular pedicle.

One-half to three-fourths of the tissue that is planned to be excised to complete subunit reconstruction is removed at the first stage to provide a large base for flap insertion. The rest of the subunit excision is performed at the secondary flap inset.

Prior to initial flap inset, any nasal lining defect must be reconstructed. Many times the nasal lining reconstruction proves the most challenging aspect of nasal reconstruction. Epidermal turn-in flaps are an excellent option (**Fig. 6.29**). The intact skin of the subunit being reconstructed adjacent to the defect provides the lining tissue. The 3 to 4 mm of skin adjacent to the defect is de-epithelialized prior to turning the flap in to prevent cyst formation. The flap is elevated in the plane just superficial to the periosteum and perichondrium of the nasal dorsum. It is left intact ~3 to 4 mm superior to the defect to provide a subcutaneous pedicle. For lateral nasal defects, a one-stage melolabial or cheek flap can be used as a turn-in flap in the same way (**Fig. 6.30**).

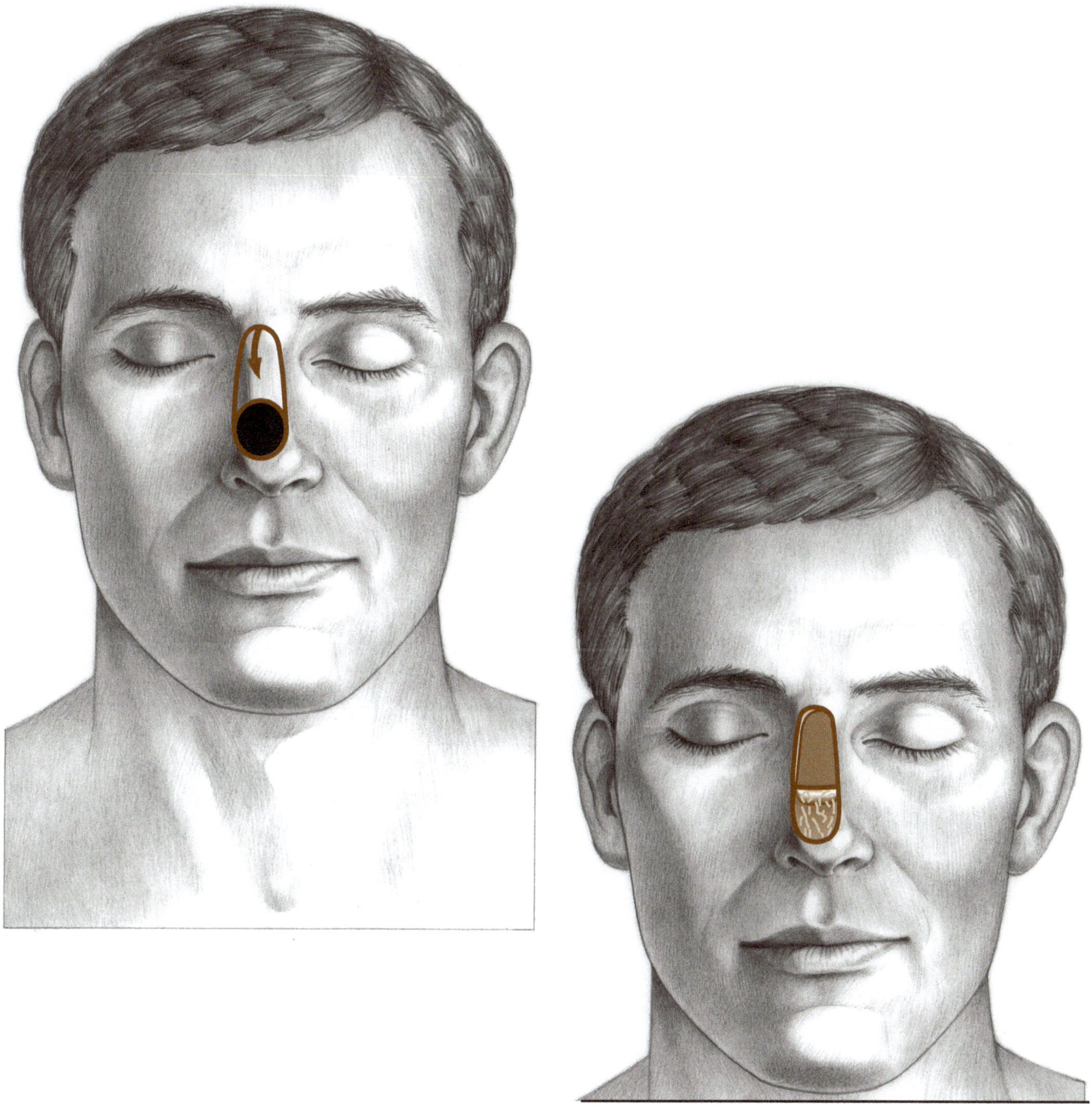

Fig. 6.29 Epidermal turn-in flap planned on the intact dorsal subunit skin that would be removed at pedicle inset. At the border of the turn-in, the skin is de-epithelialized to prevent cyst formation.

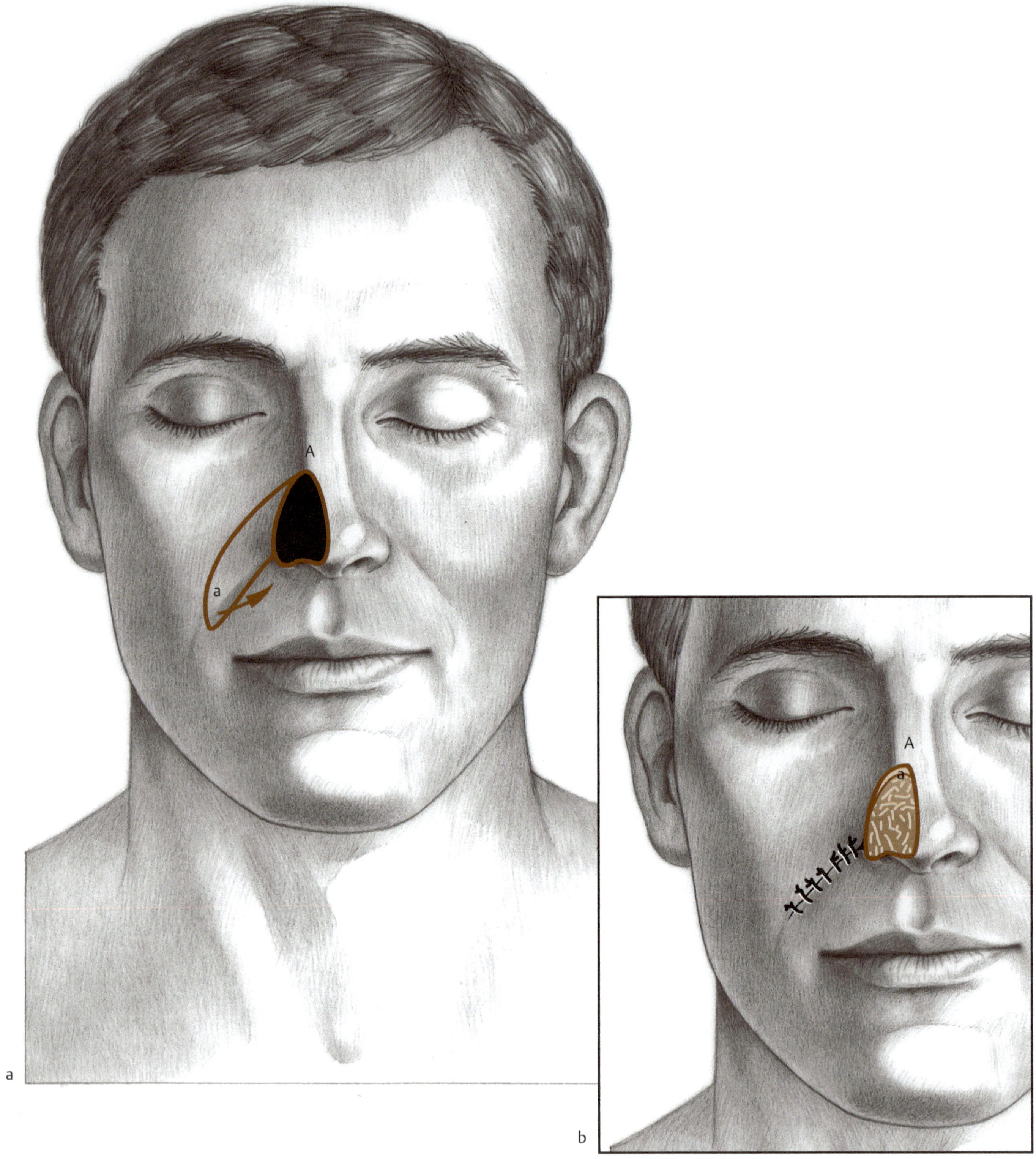

Fig. 6.30 (a, b) A one-stage melolabial flap for internal nasal lining reconstruction.

For very small lining defects, local nasal mucosa may be advanced for closure. The bipedicled advancement flap works well for defects close to the alar margin. The mucosal is incised superiorly at the defect boundary and left pedicled medially and laterally. This flap is advanced to the alar margin, and the resultant defect is closed with either an epidermal turn-in flap or a septal flap.

When possible with septal flaps, the mucosa is "rolled down" through caudal and dorsal mucosal perichondrial incisions, and the flap is then reattached to prevent or minimize any septal perforation.

In cases of large lining tissue losses, septal flaps that result in major nasal septal perforations may be necessary (**Fig. 6.31**). Alternatively, two-stage melolabial flaps placed through a nostril or free flaps are viable alternatives. For caudal septal mucosal reconstruction with a columellar defect, the forehead flap and the extended Abbe flap are good choices for mucosal and defect reconstruction.

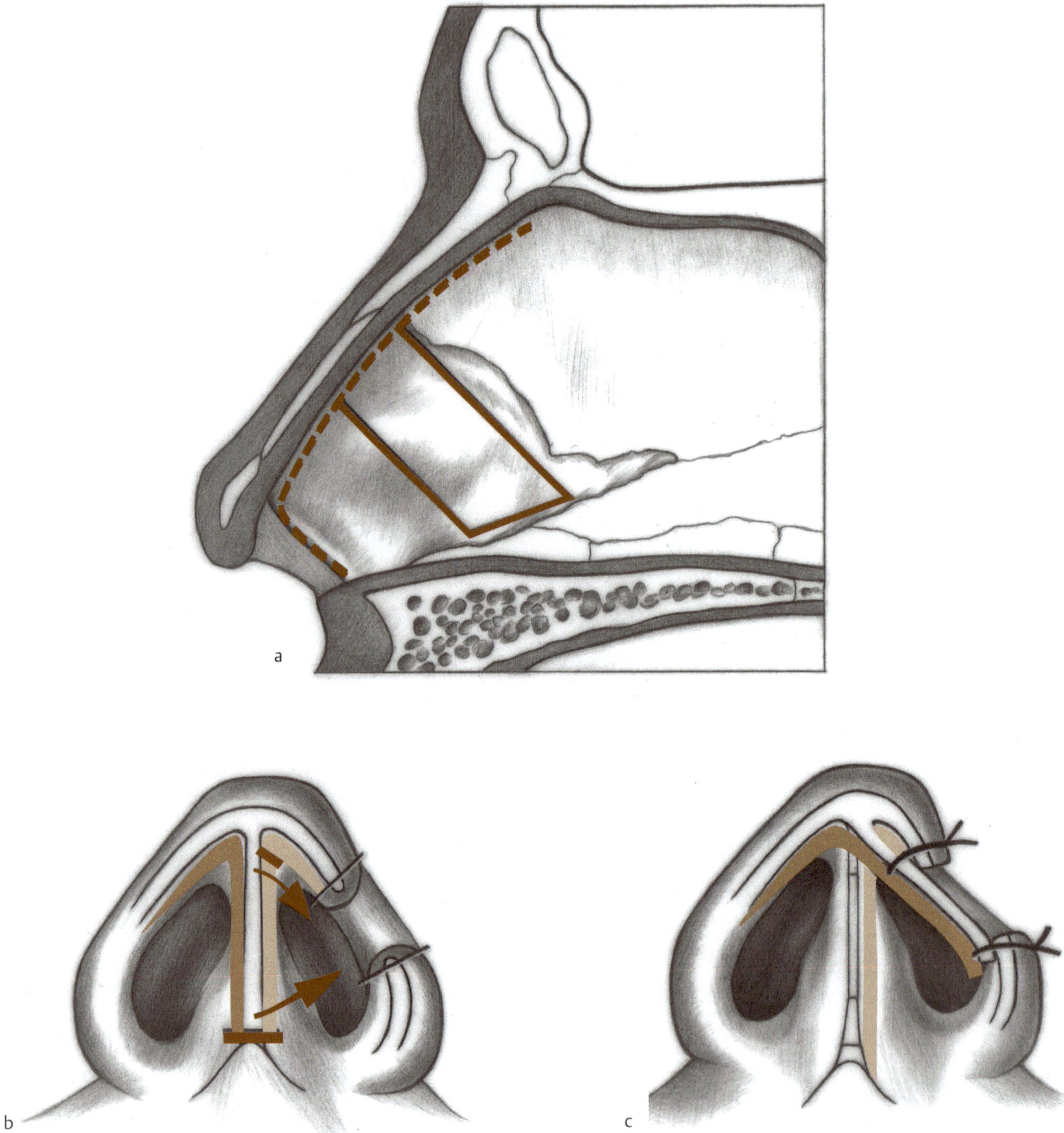

a b c

Fig. 6.31 (a–c) Large septal mucosal and cartilage flap for a large lining defect. A disadvantage of this flap is the resultant septal perforation.

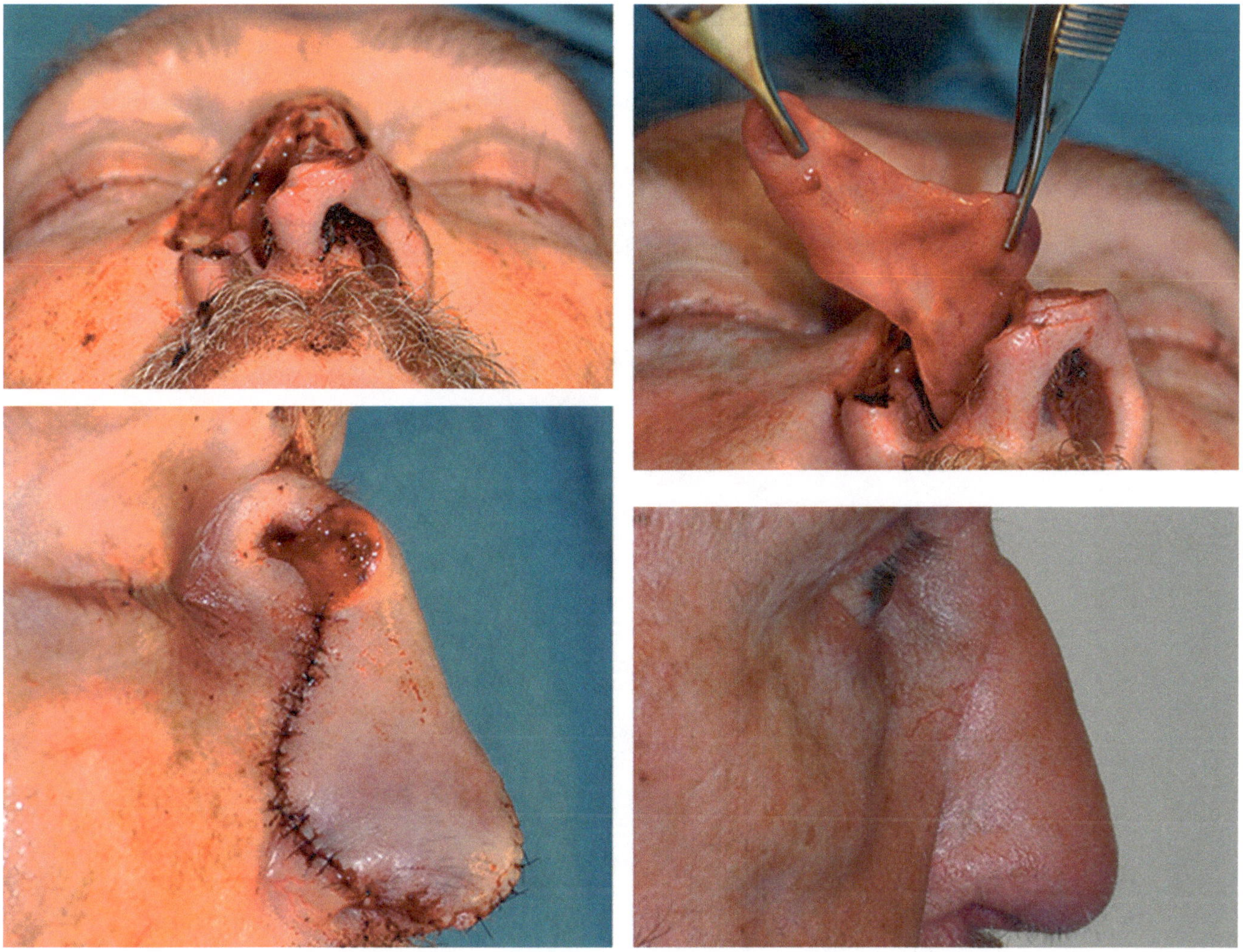

d e f g

Fig. 6.31 (d) Large lining defect. **(e)** Septal lining flap. **(f)** Paramedian forehead flap in place. **(g)** Healed wound.

A running W-plasty closure in the pretrichal region, combined with bilateral forehead advancement flaps, is used for flap donor site closure in women and in men at low risk for alopecia (**Fig. 6.32**). The edges of each unit of the W-plasty measure ~1 cm and are beveled opposite to the direction of hair follicles to facilitate hair growth through the incision. Subgaleal advancement flaps are elevated over both sides of the forehead. The galea is then closed in the midline with 2–0 or 3–0 long-lasting absorbable sutures. The lateralmost cephalic limbs of the W-plasty are each closed upon themselves to prevent standing cone formation. In men at high risk for alopecia, the bilateral advancement flaps can be bluntly elevated from the flap site without the W-plasty incisions. The resultant "dog-ear" formation is excised appropriately. If the superiormost region of the donor site does not close primarily, this region will heal well by secondary intention.

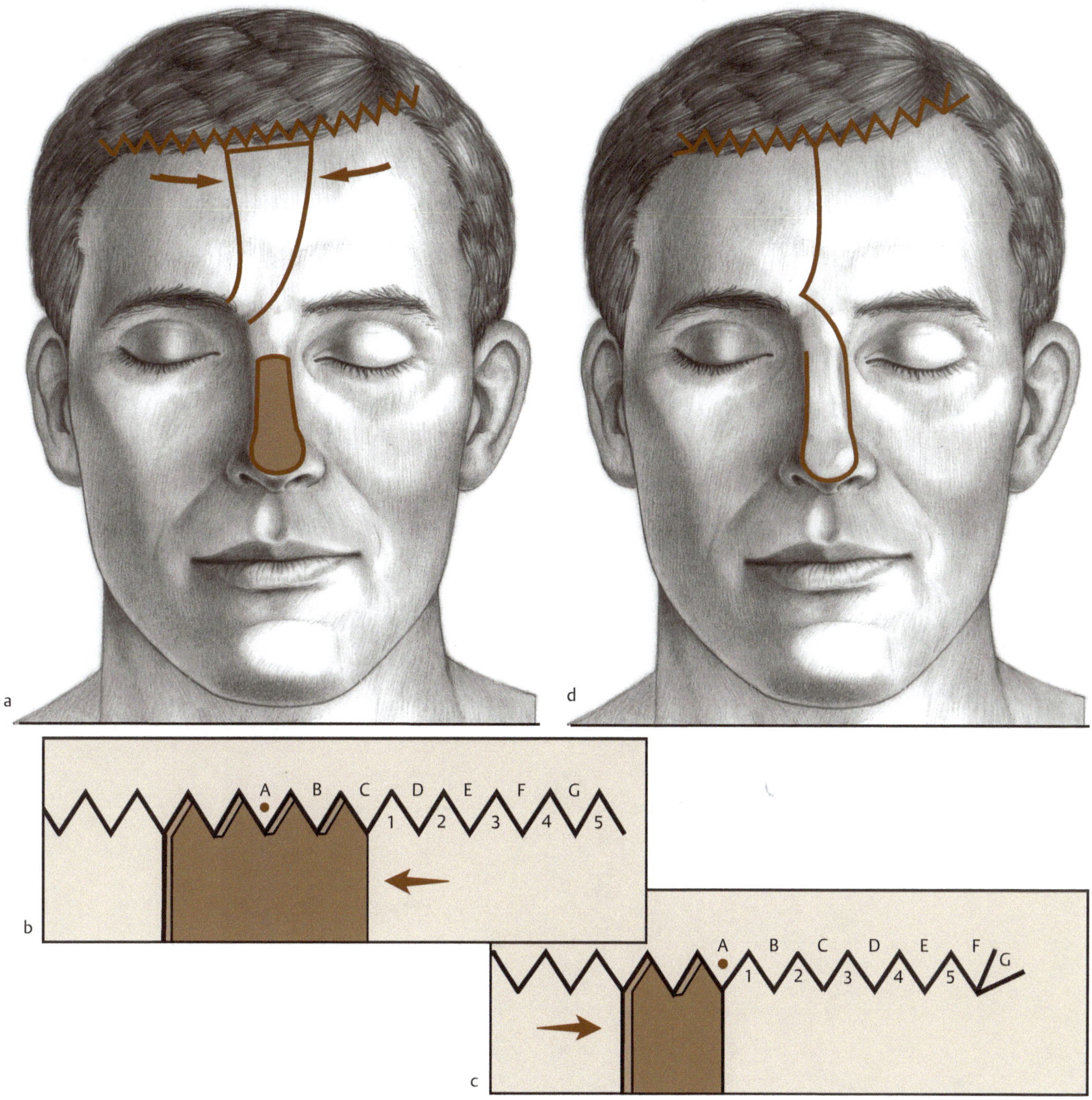

Fig. 6.32 (a-d) A running W-plasty closure of large forehead flap donor sites is useful in patients with intact stable hairlines. The closure re-creates a pretrichal forehead lift closure.

The cartilaginous structure of the nose is reconstructed with suture-fixated septal or auricular cartilage grafts. The reconstructed cartilaginous structure must be stronger than the pre-existing structure of the nose to avoid the inevitable contraction of the skin–soft tissue envelope formed by the forehead flap. The distal one-third of the forehead flap is thinned to the subdermal layer, prior to flap inset. The flap is inset with subdermal absorbable 5–0 sutures and monofilament nonabsorbable 5–0 and 6–0 skin sutures. Triangular fixation sutures or external cotton bolsters are placed in the supra-alar region to better re-create this hollow if there is no concern with flap viability (**Fig. 6.33**). A case of complex full-thickness nasal tip defect is presented through initial flap inset (**Fig. 6.34**).

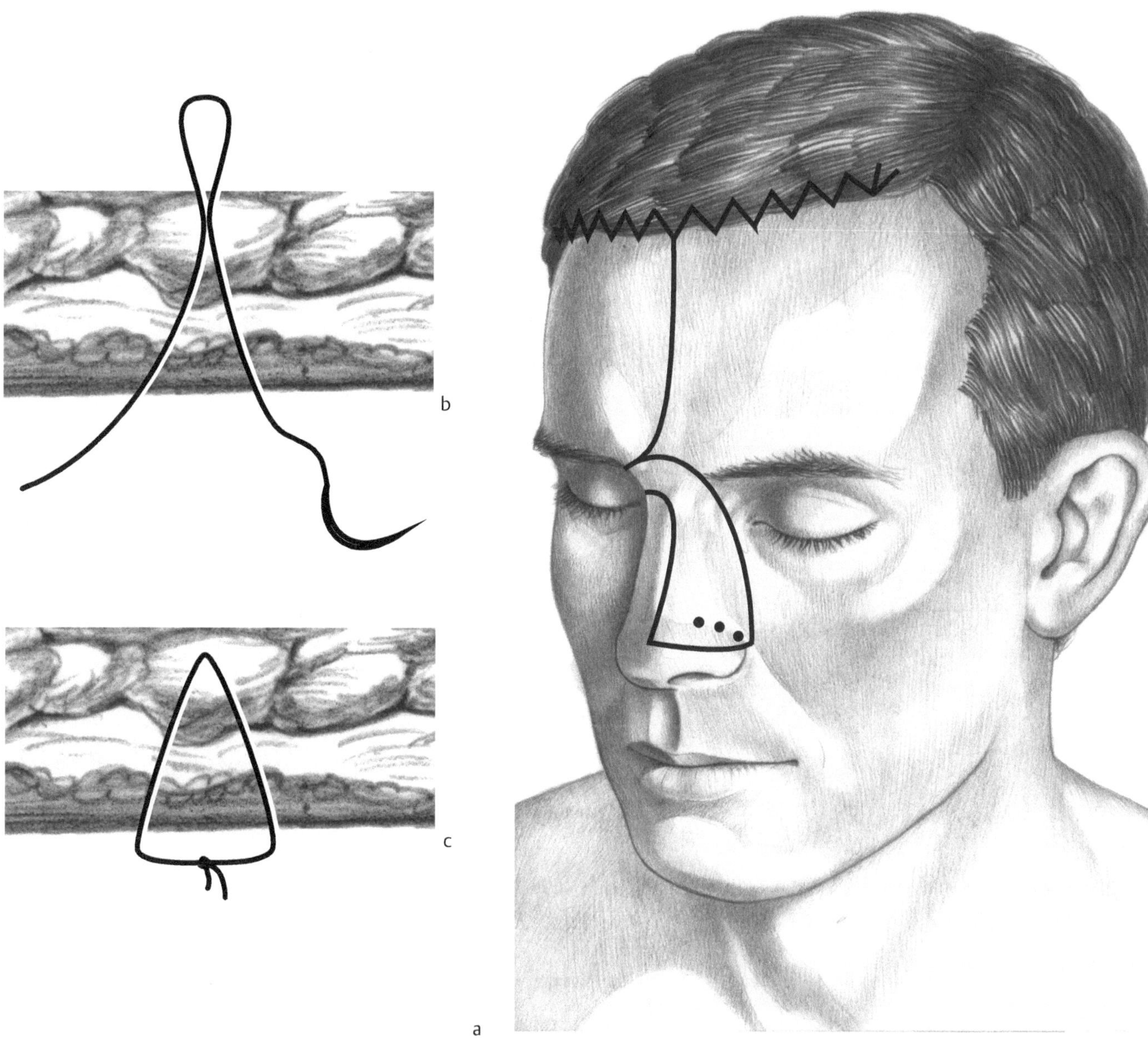

Fig. 6.33 (a-c) Triangular fixation sutures can be used to re-create the sparkler groove.

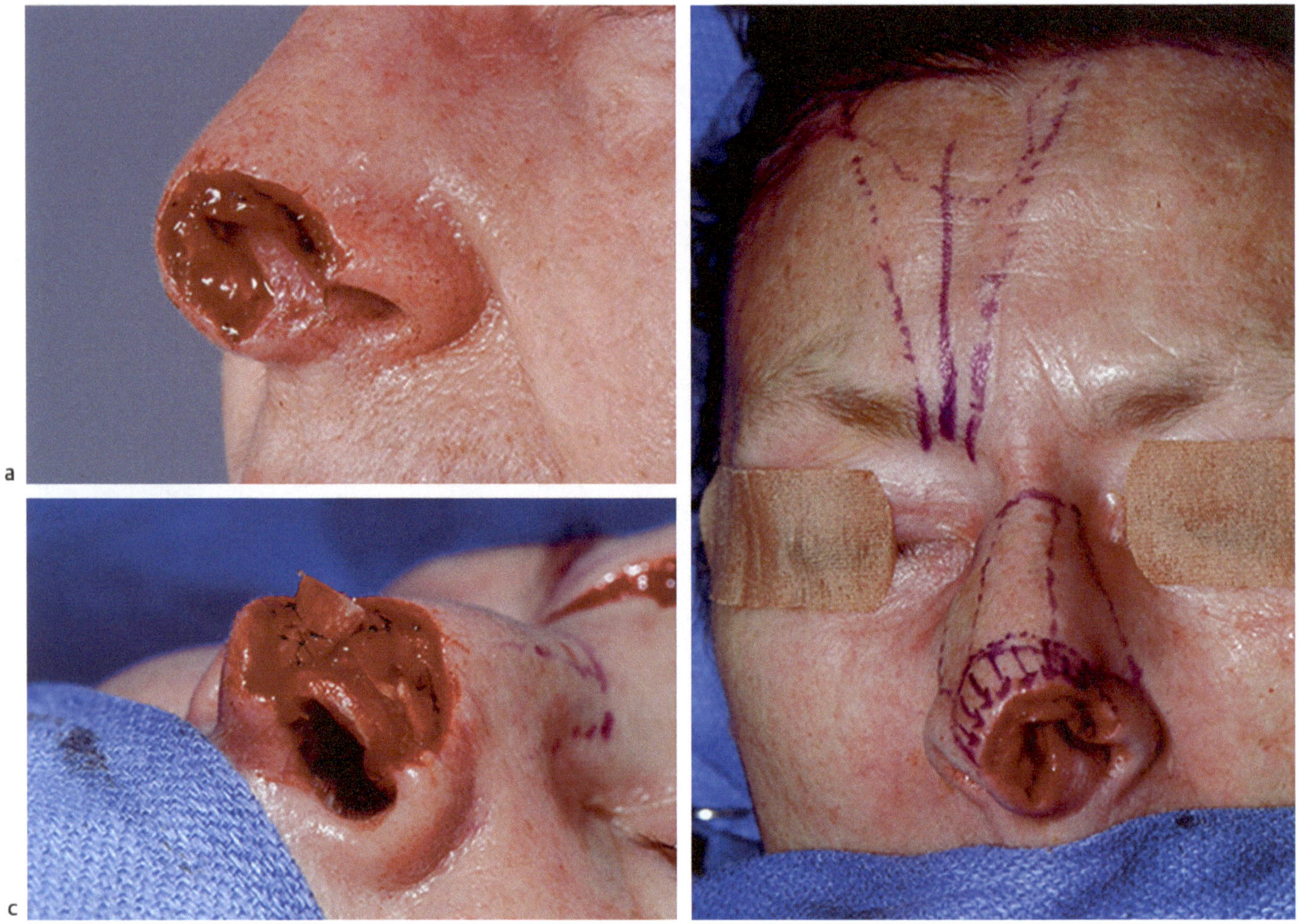

Fig. 6.34 (a) Complex full-thickness nasal tip defect. **(b)** The skin marked with arrows is planned as an epidermal turn-in flap. The paramedian forehead flap is drawn on the right supratrochlear vascular pedicle. **(c)** The epidermal turn-in flap is in place, along with a septal cartilage tip graft and partial left lower lateral cartilage reconstruction graft.

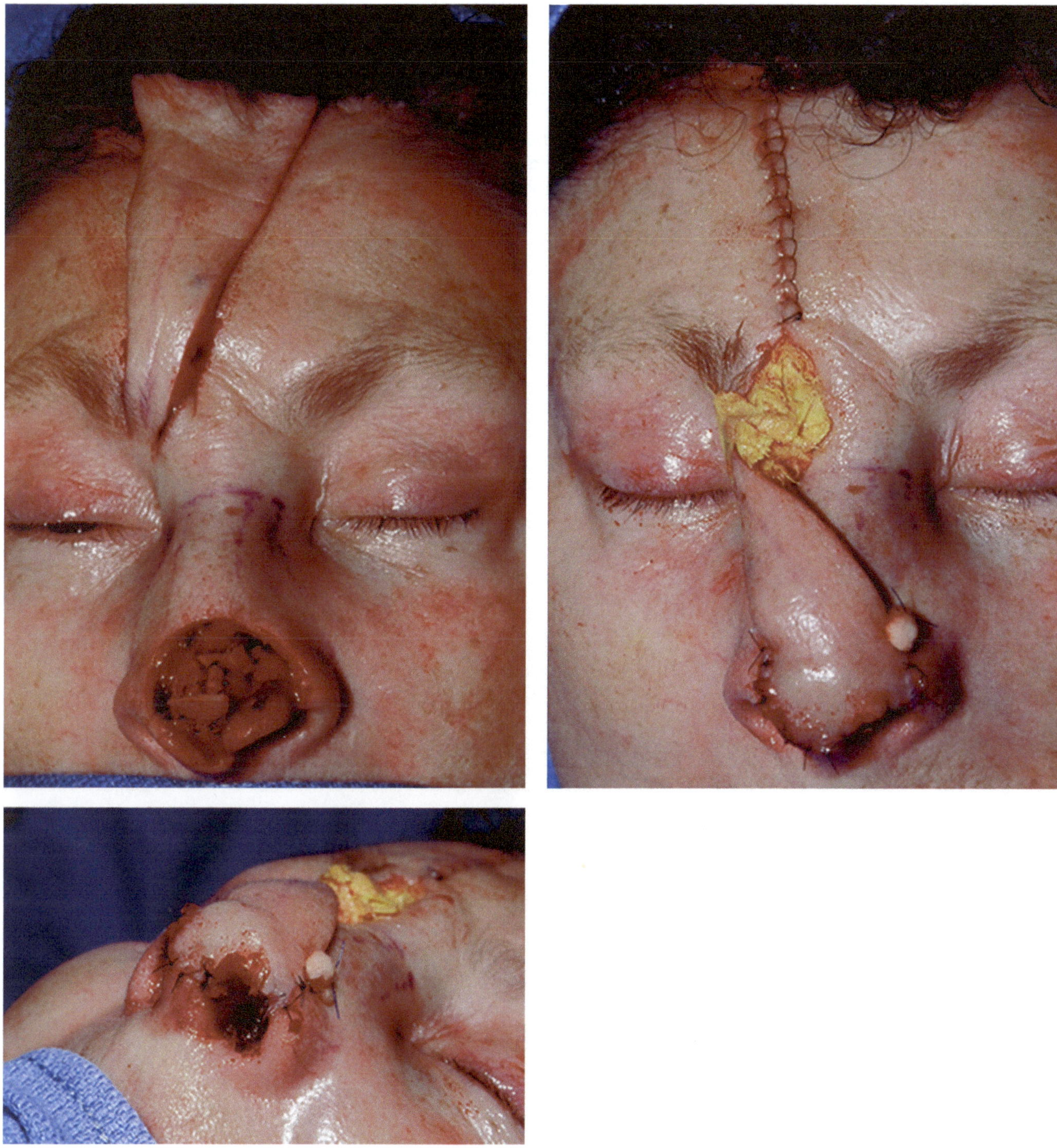

Fig. 6.34 (d) The forehead flap is incised. **(e)** The forehead flap is in place with running W-plasty forehead closure. **(f)** Note the notches left to re-epithelialize for soft triangle reconstruction.

The final pedicle division, flap inset, and trimming are performed 3 weeks later. The previously inset distal flap is not disturbed, as the new blood supply is via the subdermal plexus from the distal flap. The vascular pedicle is divided, and the remaining subunit skin is excised to the depth of the perichondrium. The region is then replaced with the flap after appropriate thinning and trimming. Minimal skin is returned to the forehead to obtain the best cosmetic result in the glabellar area. In general, do not return any tissue beyond the extension of the glabellar frown lines (**Fig. 6.35**). If appropriate, thinning is done prior to flap inset (**Fig. 6.36** and **Fig. 6.37**). Further revisions, though rarely needed, are done at 3 to 6 months. The entire nasal unit is dermabraded at 4 to 6 weeks for skin color blending if there is a discrepancy. Another case where both epidermal turn-in flaps and rib bone and cartilage graft are necessary for a full-thickness nasal dorsal defect is illustrated in **Fig. 6.38**.

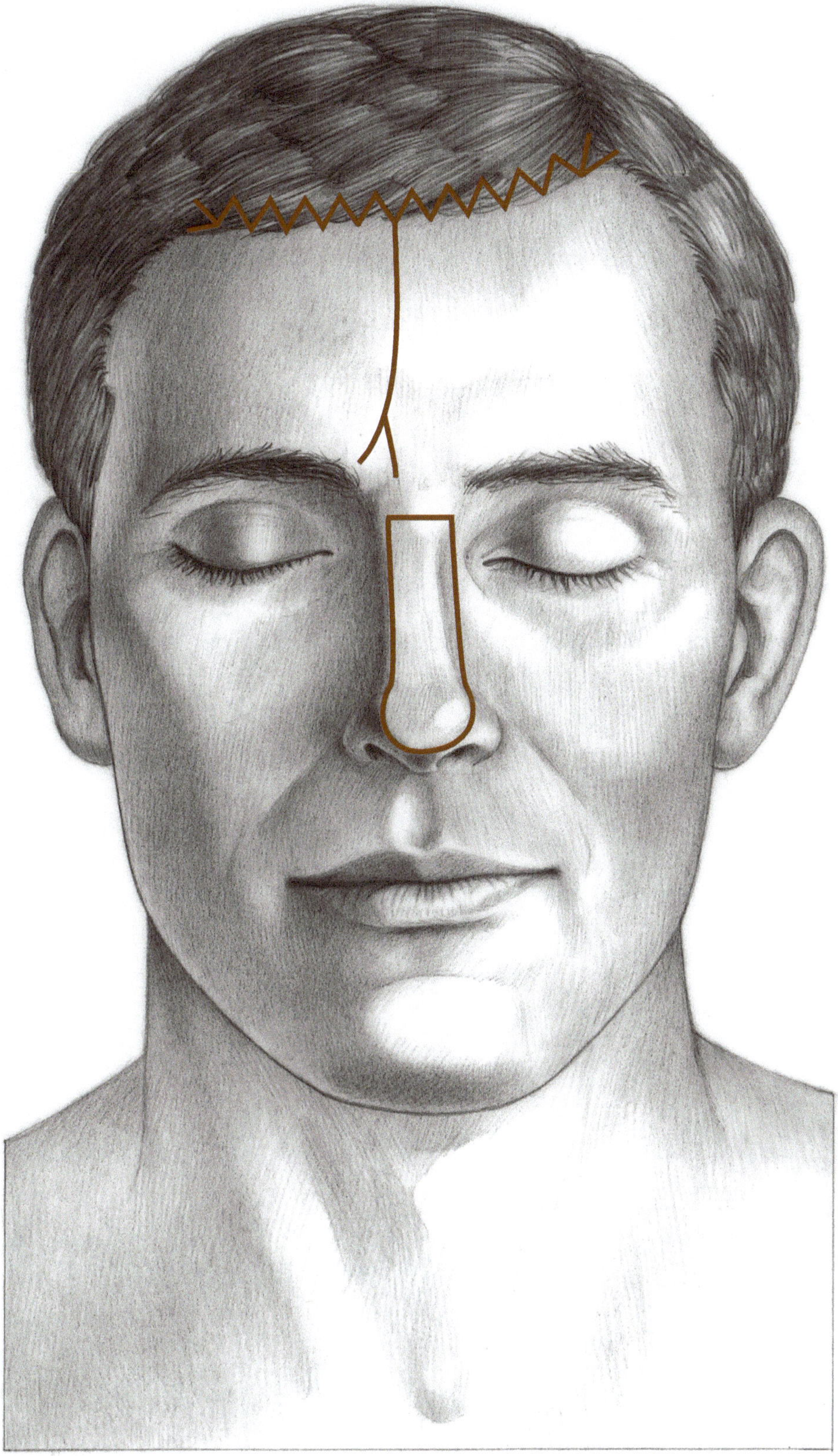

Fig. 6.35 Appearance at the pedicle inset.

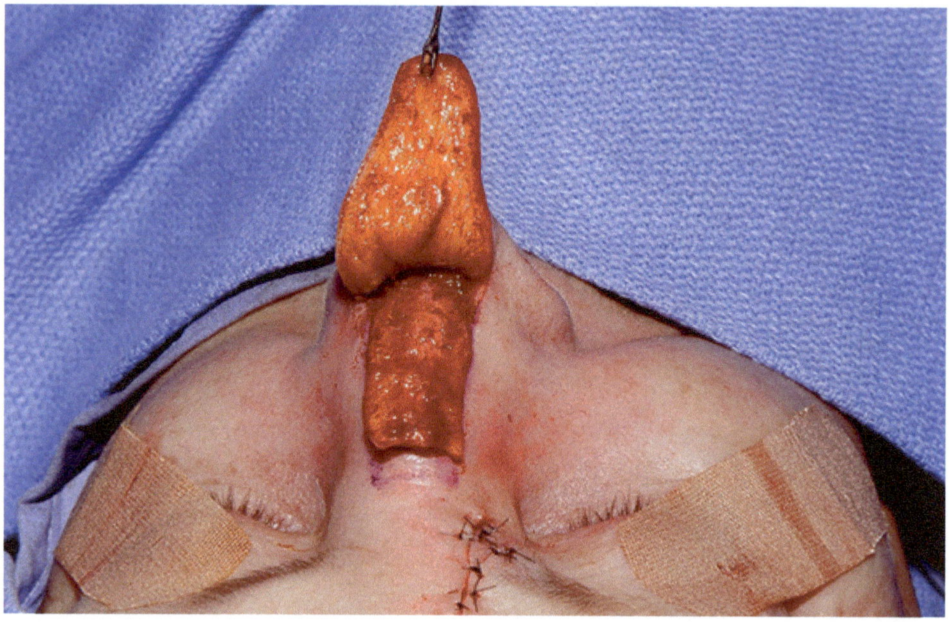

Fig. 6.36 Pedicle inset in the same case from **Fig. 6.34**. In most instances, it is best to replace both the tip and the nasal dorsal subunit skin in total tip defect reconstruction. The skin of the flap has been thinned, and the nasal dorsal skin has been excised to the layer of the perichondrium.

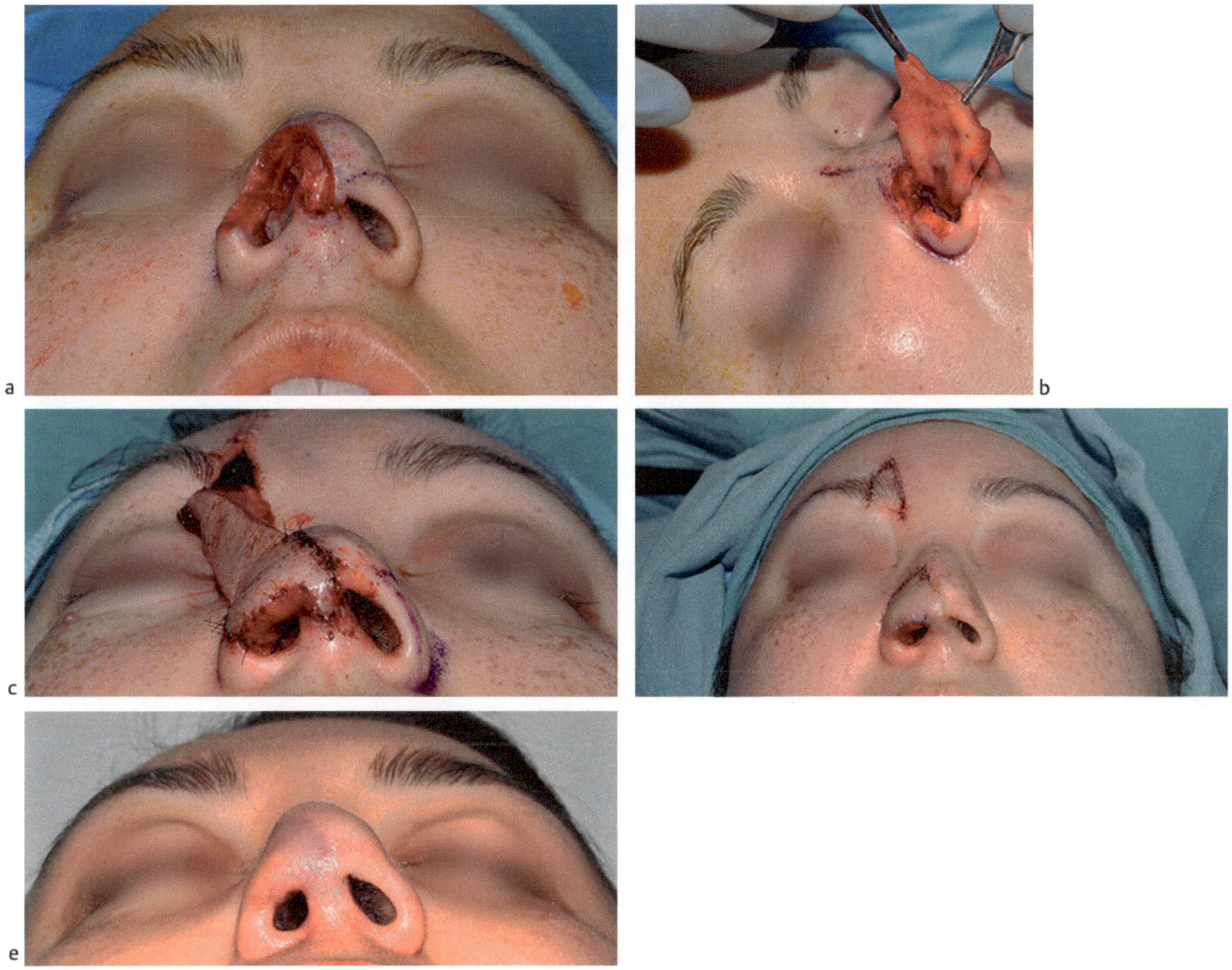

Fig. 6.37 (a) Nasal tip and ala defect. **(b)** Septal mucosal flap for lining defect. **(c)** Paramedian flap in place. **(d)** Second stage after takedown. **(e)** Healed wound.

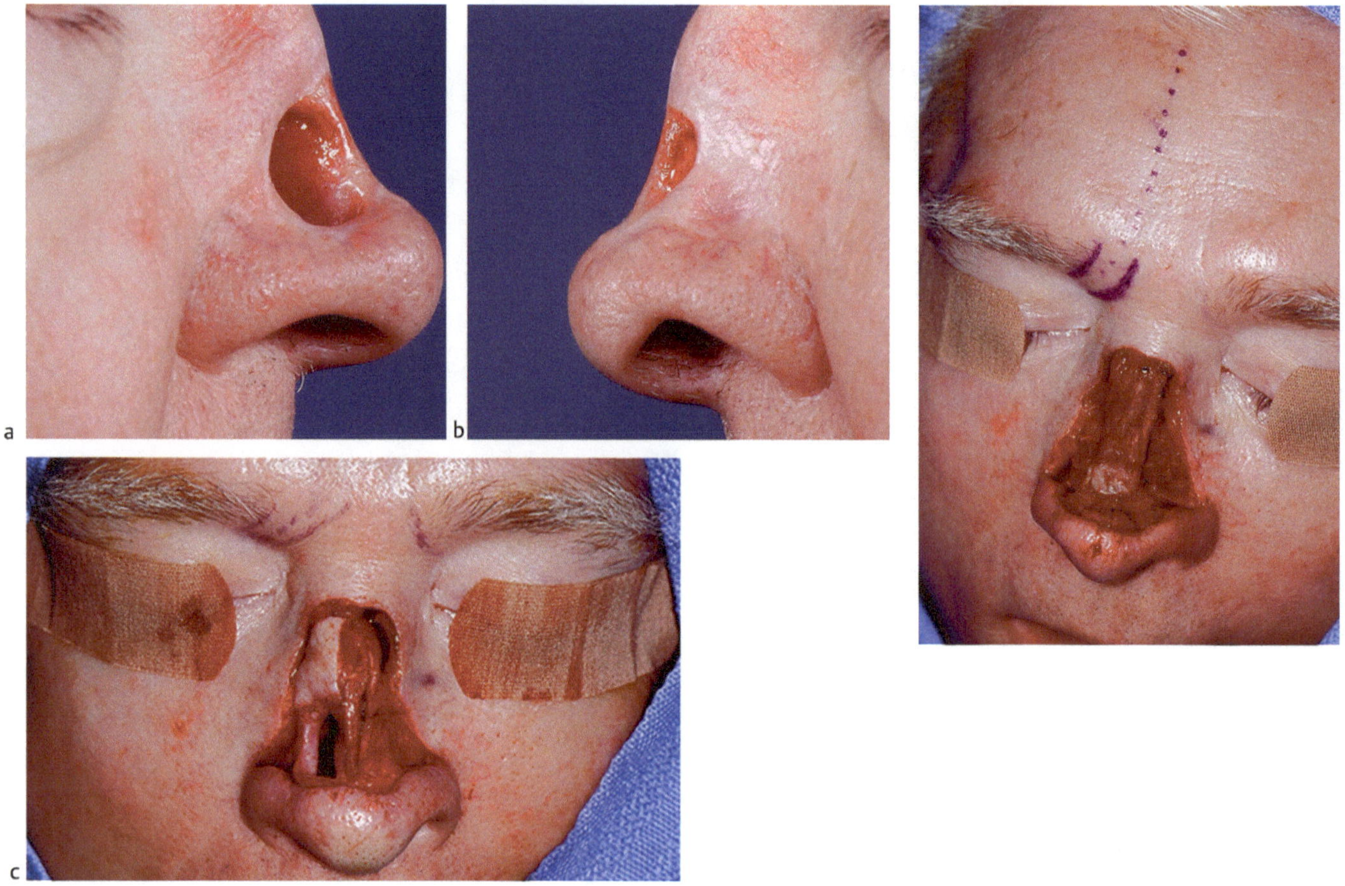

Fig. 6.38 (a) Full-thickness nasal dorsal defect, right side. **(b)** Left side of the same defect. **(c)** Epidermal turn-in flap incised and planned for the right side and inset on the left side of the lining defects. **(d)** Rib bone and costal cartilage graft in place for structural reconstruction. The right supratrochlear vascular pedicle is marked by Doppler for the forehead flap.

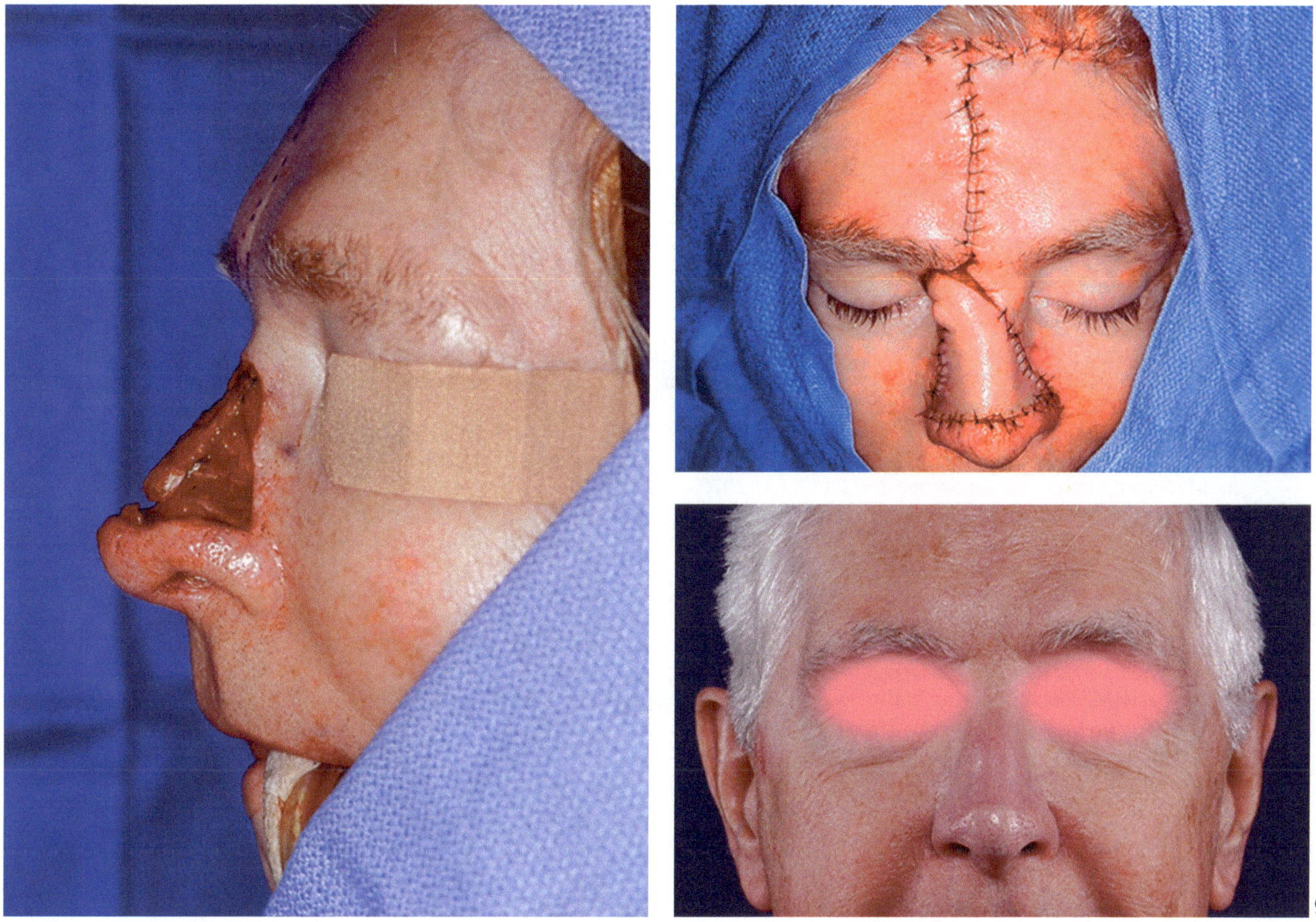

e f g

Fig. 6.38 (e) Lateral view of the dorsal reconstruction. **(f)** Paramedian forehead flap in place, with running W-plasty closure of the forehead donor site. **(g)** Late postoperative result. Note the result of the donor site closure.

Suggested Reading

Becker GD, Adams LA, Levin BC. Nonsurgical repair of perinasal skin defects. Plast Reconstr Surg 1991;88(5):768–776, discussion 777–778

Branham GH, Thomas JR. Skin grafts. Otolaryngol Clin North Am 1990;23(5):889–897

Burget GC. Aesthetic restoration of the nose. Clin Plast Surg 1985;12(3):463–480

Burget GC, Menick FJ. The subunit principle in nasal reconstruction. Plast Reconstr Surg 1985;76(2):239–247

Burget GC, Menick FJ. Aesthetic reconstruction of the nose. St. Louis: CV Mosby; 1994

Burget GC, Menick FJ. Nasal reconstruction: seeking a fourth dimension. Plast Reconstr Surg 1986;78(2):145–157

Burget GC, Menick FJ. Nasal support and lining: the marriage of beauty and blood supply. Plast Reconstr Surg 1989;84(2):189–202

Giberson WG, Freeman JL. Use of free auricular composite graft in nasal alar/vestibular reconstruction. J Otolaryngol 1992;21(2):153–155

Koranda FC, Webster RC. Trapdoor effect in nasolabial flaps: causes and corrections. Arch Otolaryngol 1985;111(7):421–424

Maves MD, Yessenow RS. The use of composite auricular grafts in nasal reconstruction. J Dermatol Surg Oncol 1988;14(9):994–999

McGregor JC, Soutar DS. A critical assessment of the bilobed flap. Br J Plast Surg 1981;34(2):197–205

Moore EJ, Strome SA, Kasperbauer JL, Sherris DA, Manning LA. Vascularized radial forearm free tissue transfer for lining in nasal reconstruction. Laryngoscope 2003;113(12):2078–2085

Quatela VC, Sherris DA, Rounds MMMF. Aesthetic refinements in forehead flap nasal reconstruction. Arch Otol HNS 1995

Sherris DA, Fuerstenberg J, Danahey D, Hilger PA. Reconstruction of the nasal columella. Arch Facial Plast Surg 2002;4(1):42–46

Shumrick KA, Smith TL. The anatomic basis for the design of forehead flaps in nasal reconstruction. Arch Otolaryngol Head Neck Surg 1992;118(4):373–379

Younger RA. The versatile melolabial flap. Otolaryngol Head Neck Surg 1992;107(6 Pt 1):721–726

Zitelli JA. The bilobed flap for nasal reconstruction. Arch Dermatol 1989;125(7):957–959

Zitelli JA, Fazio MJ. Reconstruction of the nose with local flaps. J Dermatol Surg Oncol 1991;17(2):184–189

7 Cheek

Summary

This chapter focuses on the reconstructive principles with respect to the cheek. The cheek is broken up into several subunits including lateral cheek, medial cheek, zygomatic area, and buccal area. Flap design is guided based on location, and special attention must be paid to medial and zygomatic defects that also involve the lower eyelid in order to avoid ectropion. Cheek defects classically involved extensive back cuts and undermining in order to provide tension-free closure.

Keywords: medial cheek, lateral cheek, cervicofacial advancement flap, rhombic flap, transposition flap, undermining, zygomatic

♦ Introduction

The boundaries of the cheek unit are the preauricular crease, the superior border of the malar eminence and zygomatic arch, the inferior orbital rim, the nasofacial groove, the melolabial crease, and the inferior border of the mandible. The cheek is divided into the medial, zygomatic, buccal, and lateral subunits (**Fig. 7.1**). The medial and buccal cheek subunits consist of thicker skin that is freely mobile over the underlying fat. The skin of the lateral subunit, over the parotid, is somewhat more attached to the underlying fat and fascia. The skin of the zygomatic subunit (sometimes referred to as the "McGregor's patch") has firm fibrous attachments to the underlying fascia.

Because of the broad, relatively flat contour of the cheek, incisions are best placed at the boundaries of this aesthetic unit; rotation and advancement flaps are thus used when possible. For a defect whose position away from the boundaries of the aesthetic unit does not permit use of rotation or advancement flaps, transposition flaps are selected. In the design of local cheek flaps, tension is placed where it will not distort landmarks, such as the eyelid, lip, and ala. Island pedicle flaps are occasionally useful in the medial and central cheek, where the subcutaneous fat allows easy mobility of the attached skin. The flaps are especially valuable if the closure can be camouflaged in the melolabial fold.

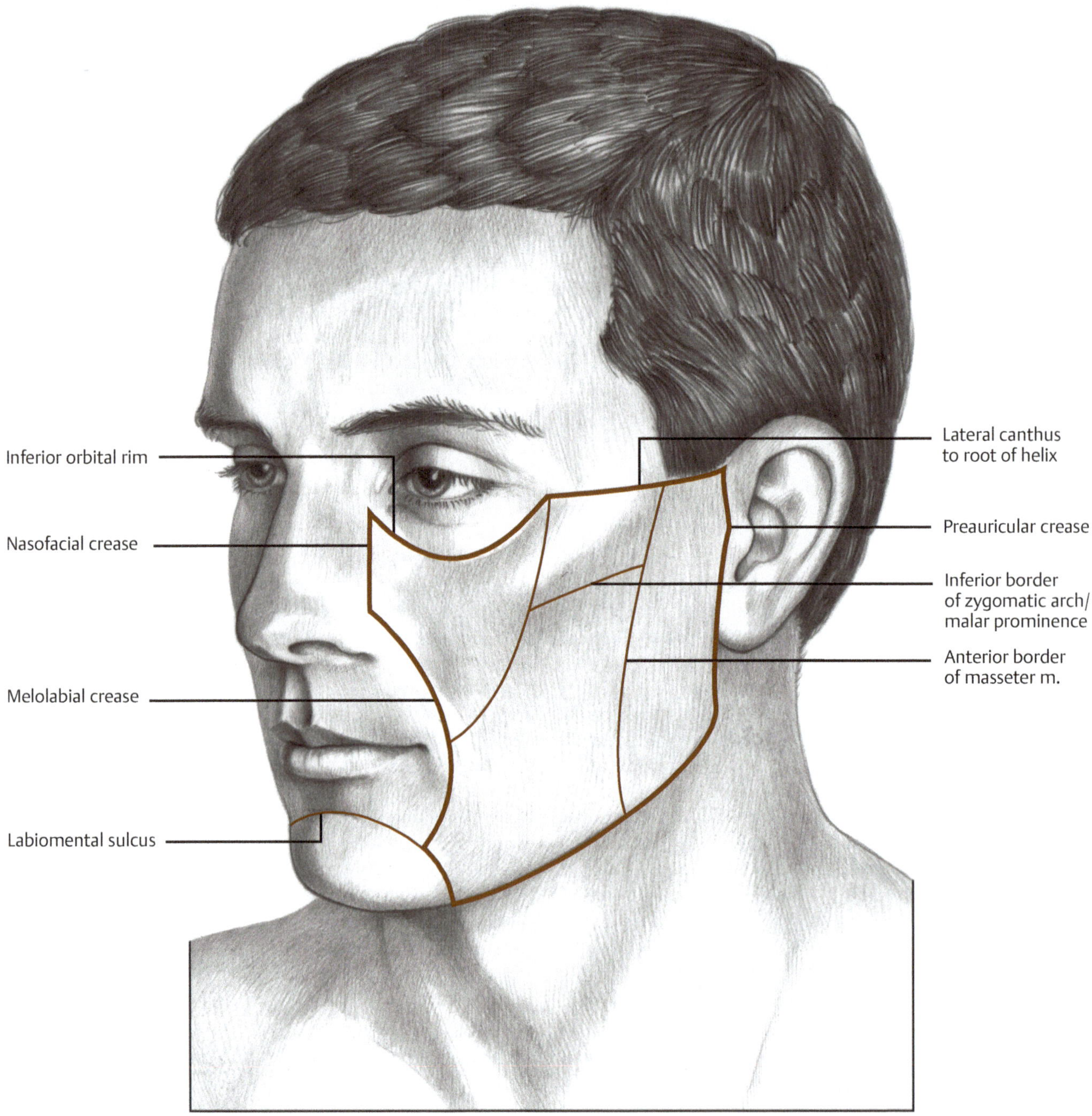

Fig. 7.1 Aesthetic subunits of the cheek.

♦ Medial Cheek Subunit

Medial cheek lesions are closed directly in the cheek–nose junction and melolabial fold, when possible (**Fig. 7.2**). For lesions adjacent to the nose–cheek junction, this closure simply involves undermining the cheek and advancing it (**Fig. 7.3**). To avoid distortion of the junction of the cheek with the nose, deep sutures from the dermis of the flap are fixed to the periosteum of the nasal bone or pyriform aperture with 3–0 or 4–0 permanent or long-lasting absorbable sutures.

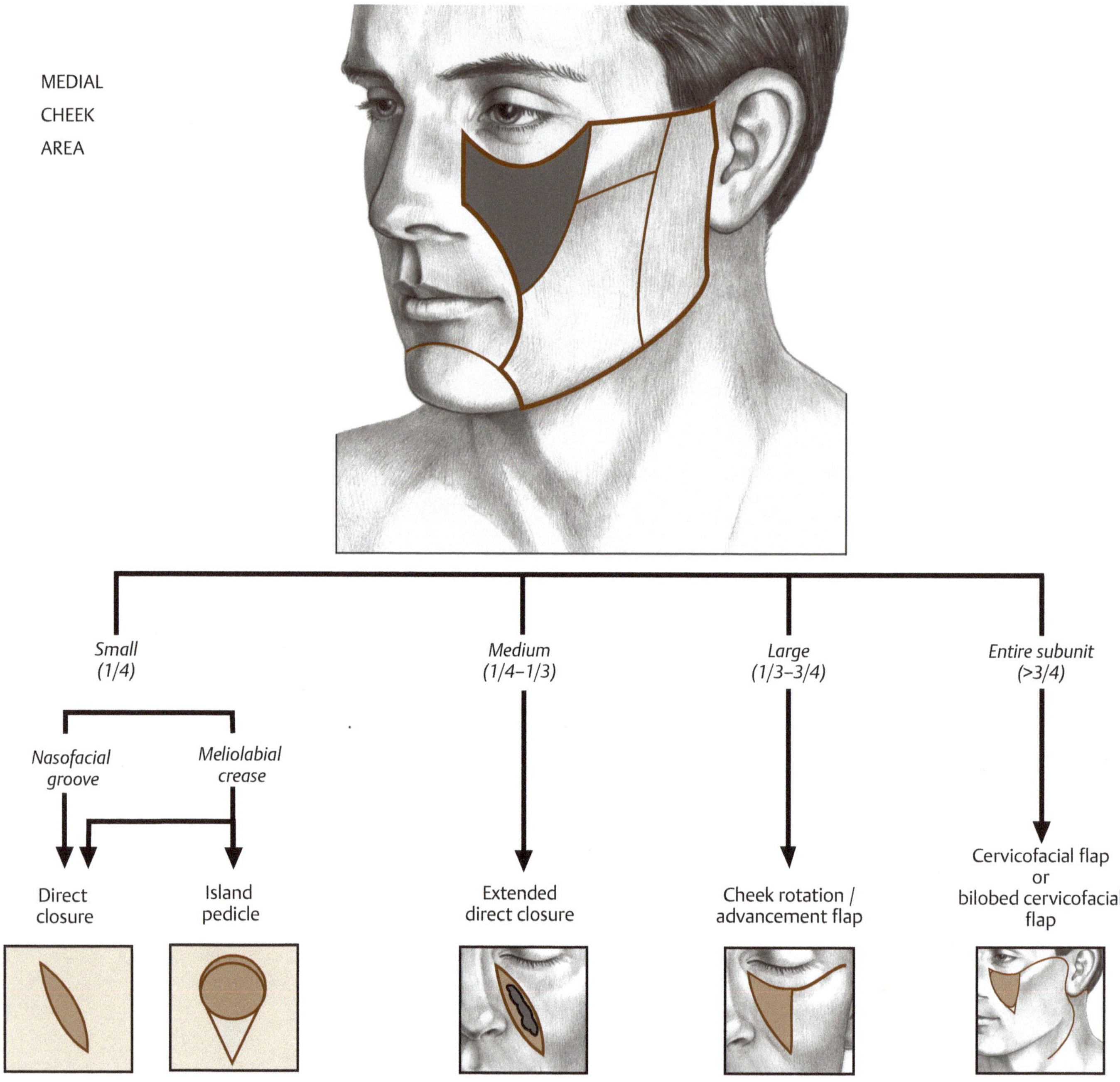

Fig. 7.2 Medial cheek area.

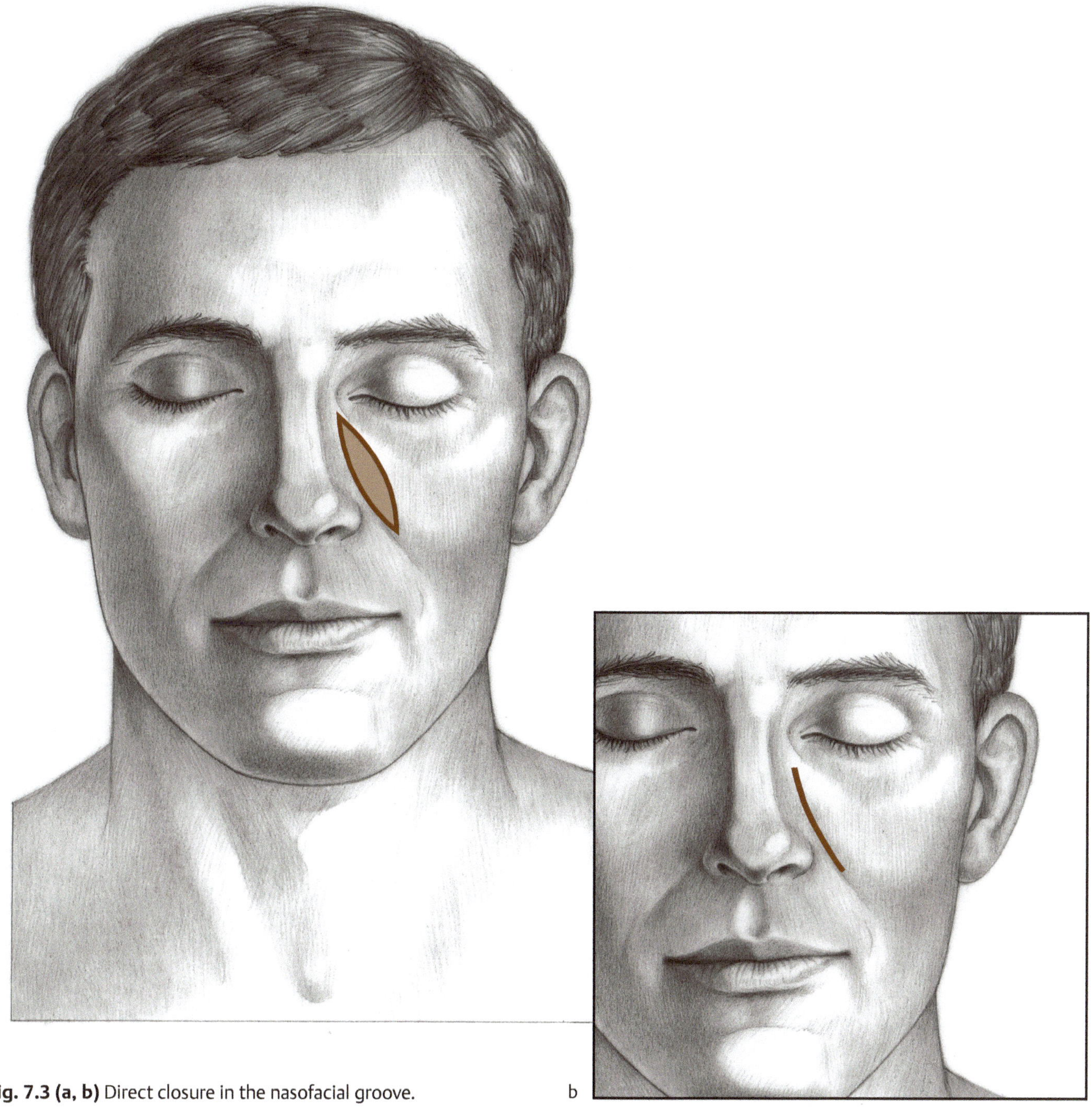

a

b

Fig. 7.3 (a, b) Direct closure in the nasofacial groove.

In patients with sufficient cheek laxity, a defect not immediately adjacent to the nose can still be closed in the nasofacial groove by excising intervening skin and creating a simple advancement flap in the plane just deep to the subdermal plexus (**Fig. 7.4** and **Fig. 7.5**). Again, deep sutures must be placed to the pyriform aperture periosteum to prevent distortion of the nasofacial groove.

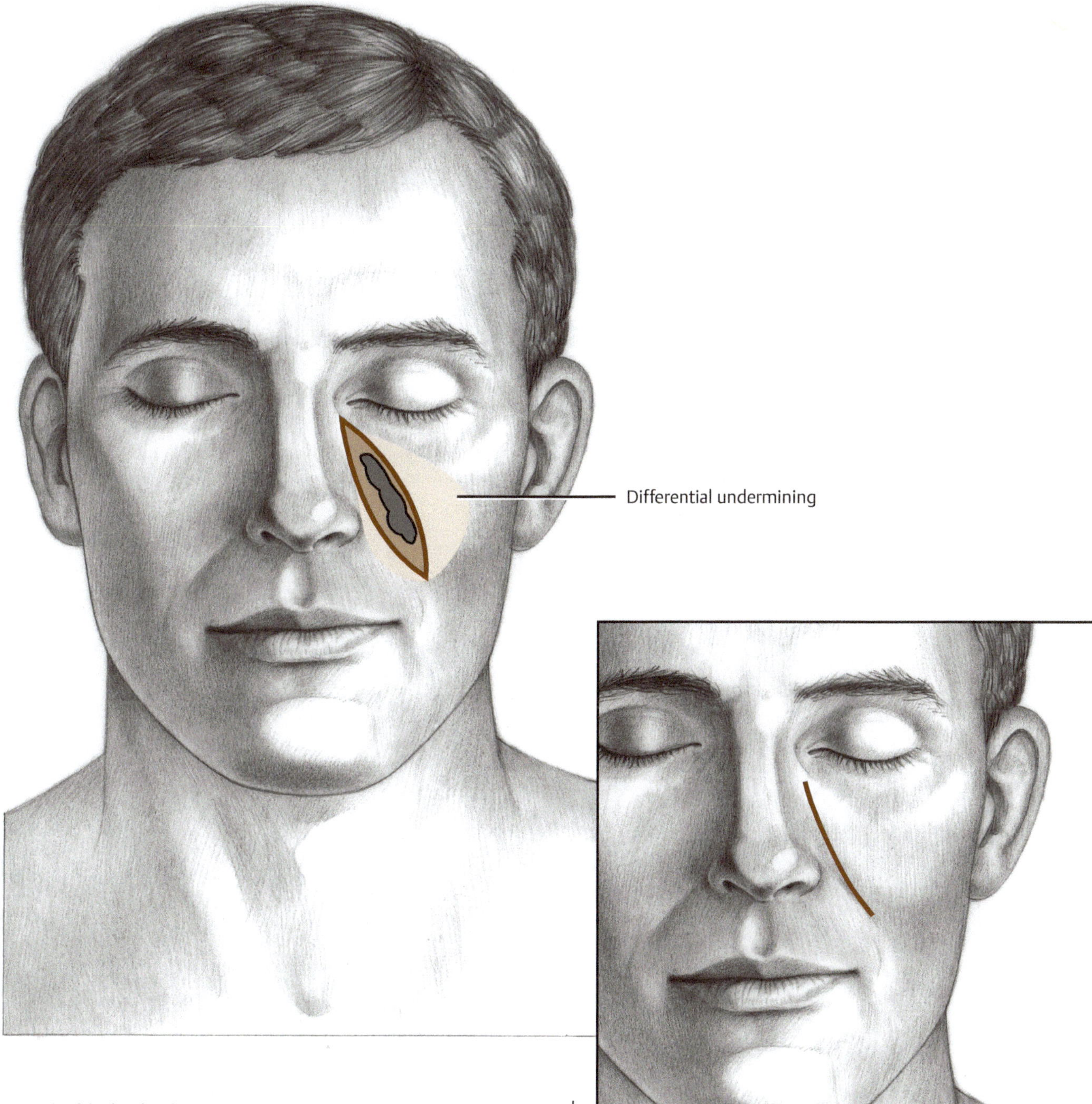

a

b

Fig. 7.4 (a, b) Cheek advancement.

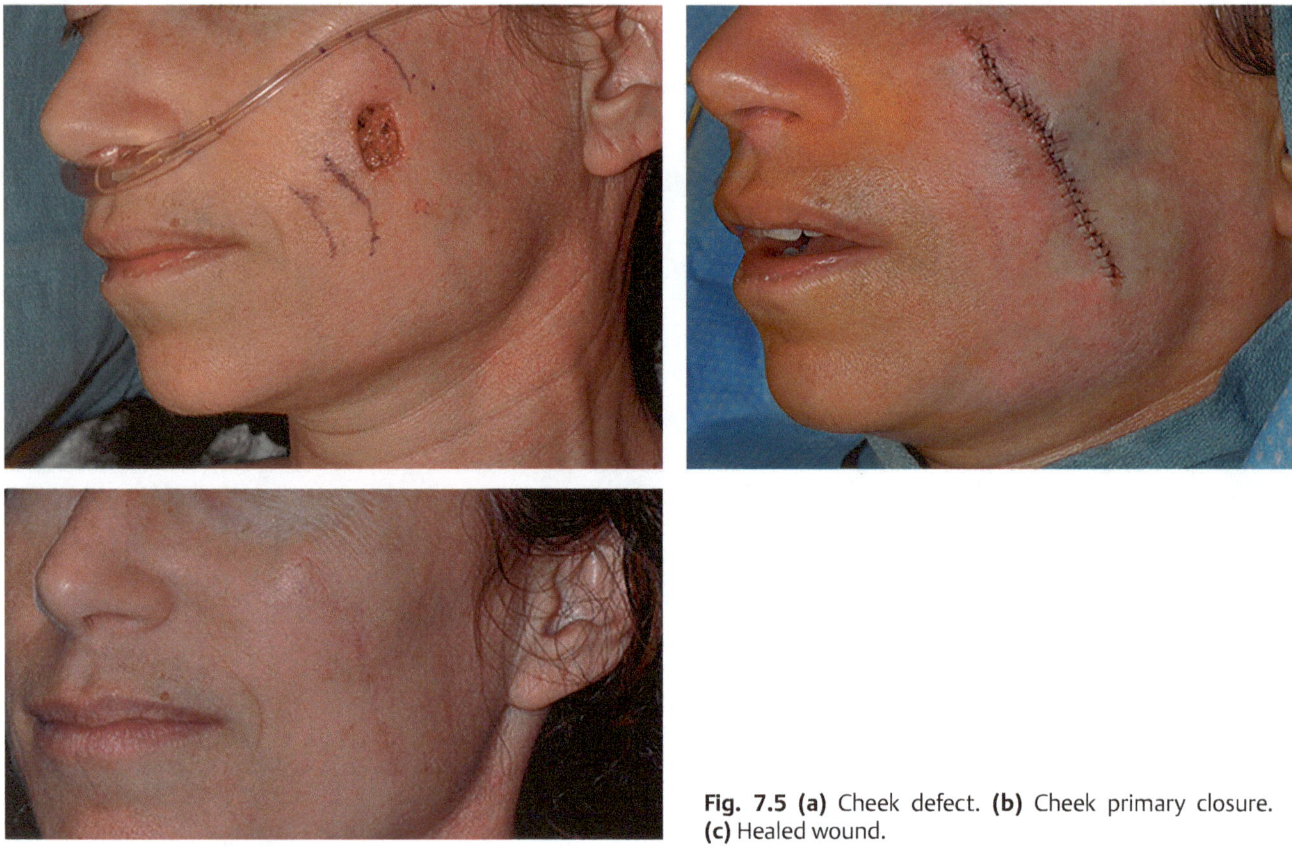

a b c

Fig. 7.5 (a) Cheek defect. **(b)** Cheek primary closure. **(c)** Healed wound.

When a defect becomes too large to close with a simple advancement flap, an incision is made along the orbital rim (the junction of the cheek and lid aesthetic units) to create a cheek rotation flap (**Fig. 7.6** and **Fig. 7.7**). This useful flap is elevated in the same subcutaneous plane. As the defect becomes larger, the releasing incision can be extended to create a cervical facial rotation flap (**Fig. 7.8** and **Fig. 7.9**). In practice, the surgeon can proceed in limited stages by making sequential back cuts in the rotation flap until the defect can be closed with minimal tension and contour distortion. The back cuts allow for recruitment of tissue from the submandibular region and the neck. The dermal layer of this flap should be fixed to the periosteum of the inferior and lateral orbital rim with 4–0 long-lasting absorbable sutures to prevent postoperative ectropion formation. If the depth of the defect is greater than the flap thickness, a local "flip-flop" flap of fat can be rotated into the deep layer of the defect prior to flap inset.

For very large medial cheek defects, a bilobed cervicofacial flap with the bilobe from postauricular skin can be used (**Fig. 7.10** and **Fig. 7.11**). If there is not enough laxity to close the postauricular donor site, a full-thickness skin graft can be used to close the site.

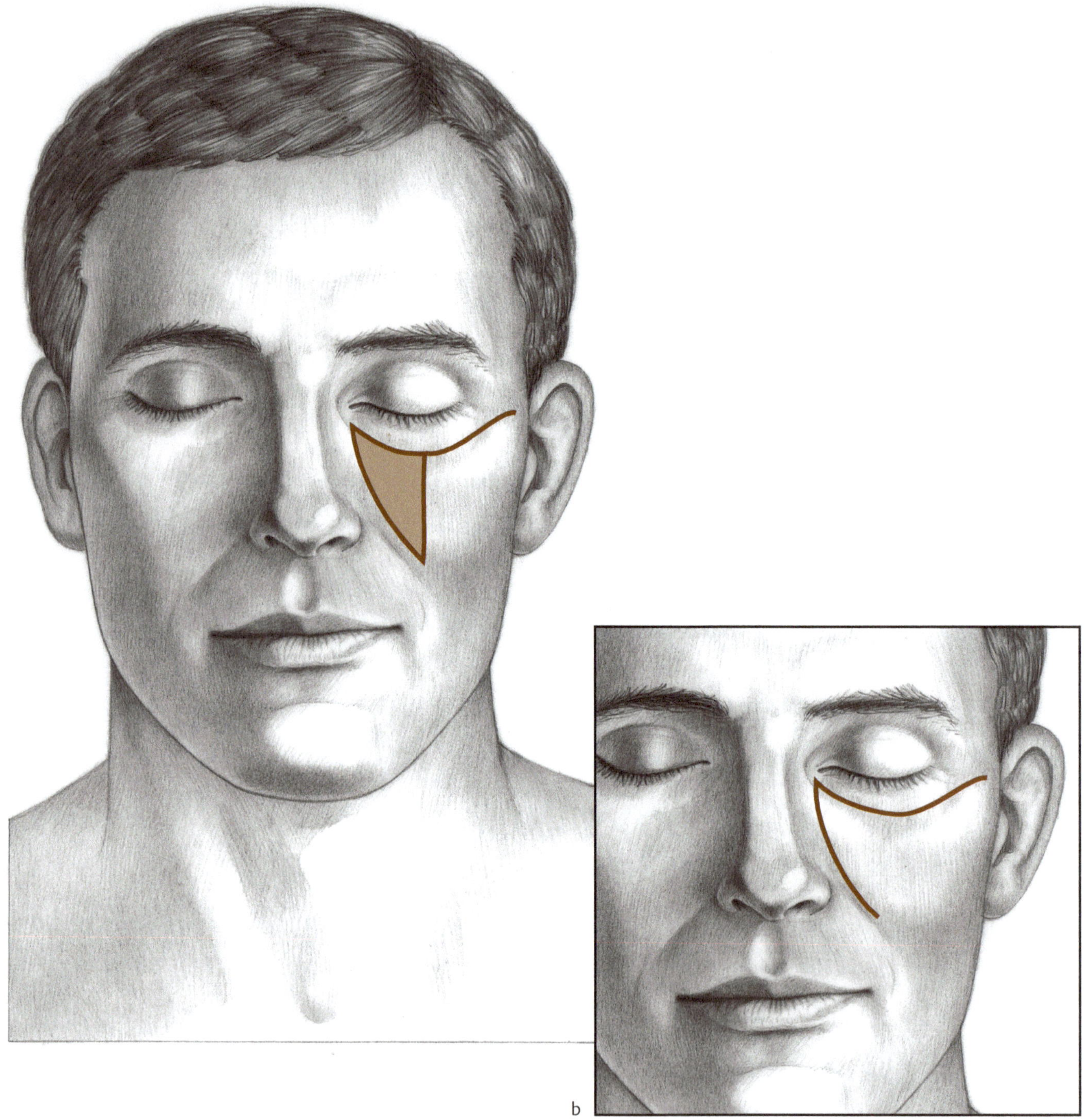

Fig. 7.6 (a, b) Simple cheek rotation flap.

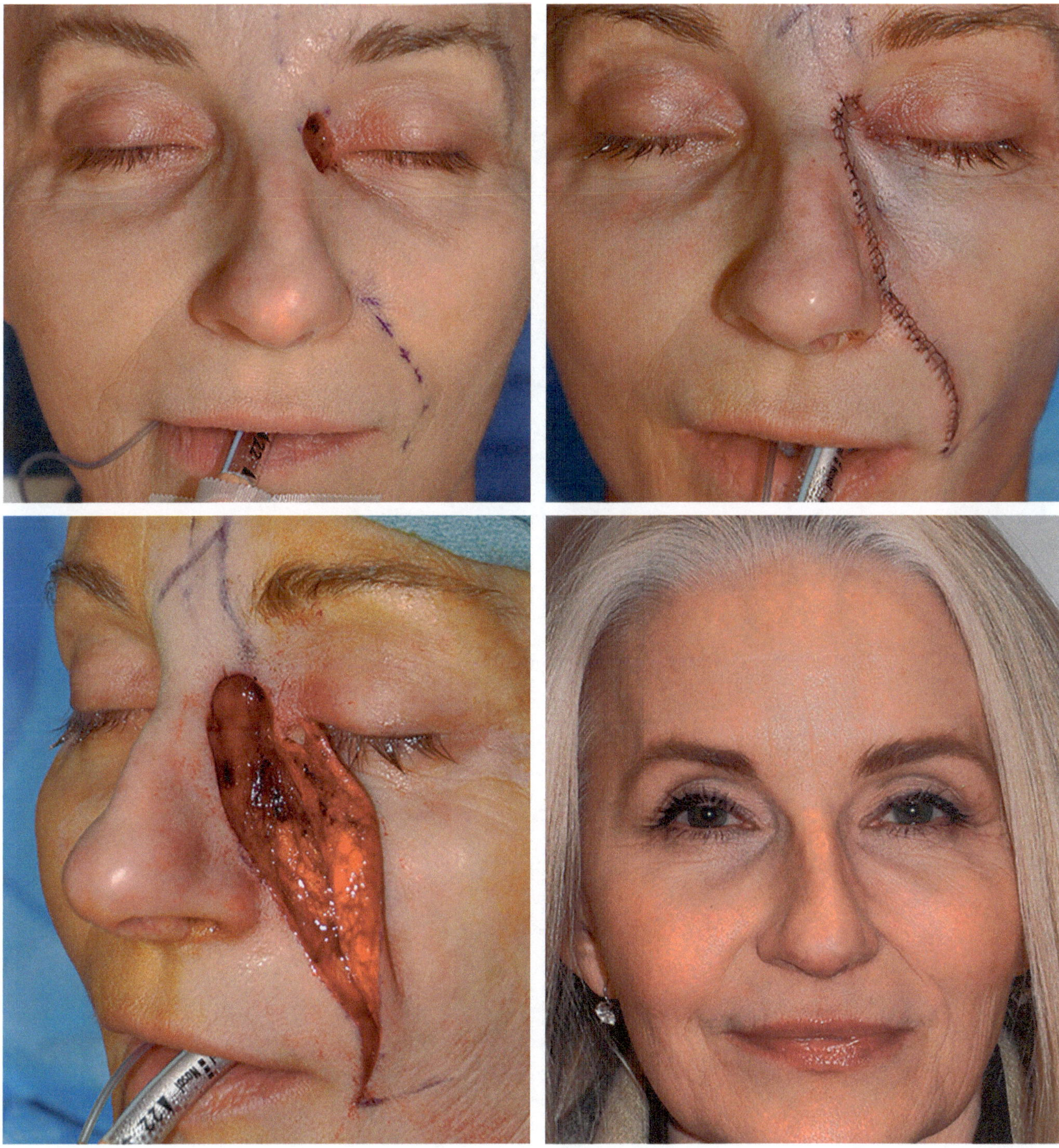

c e d f

Fig. 7.6 **(c)** Medial cheek defect. **(d)** Medial cheek inferiorly based melolabial flap. **(e)** Closure. **(f)** Healed wound.

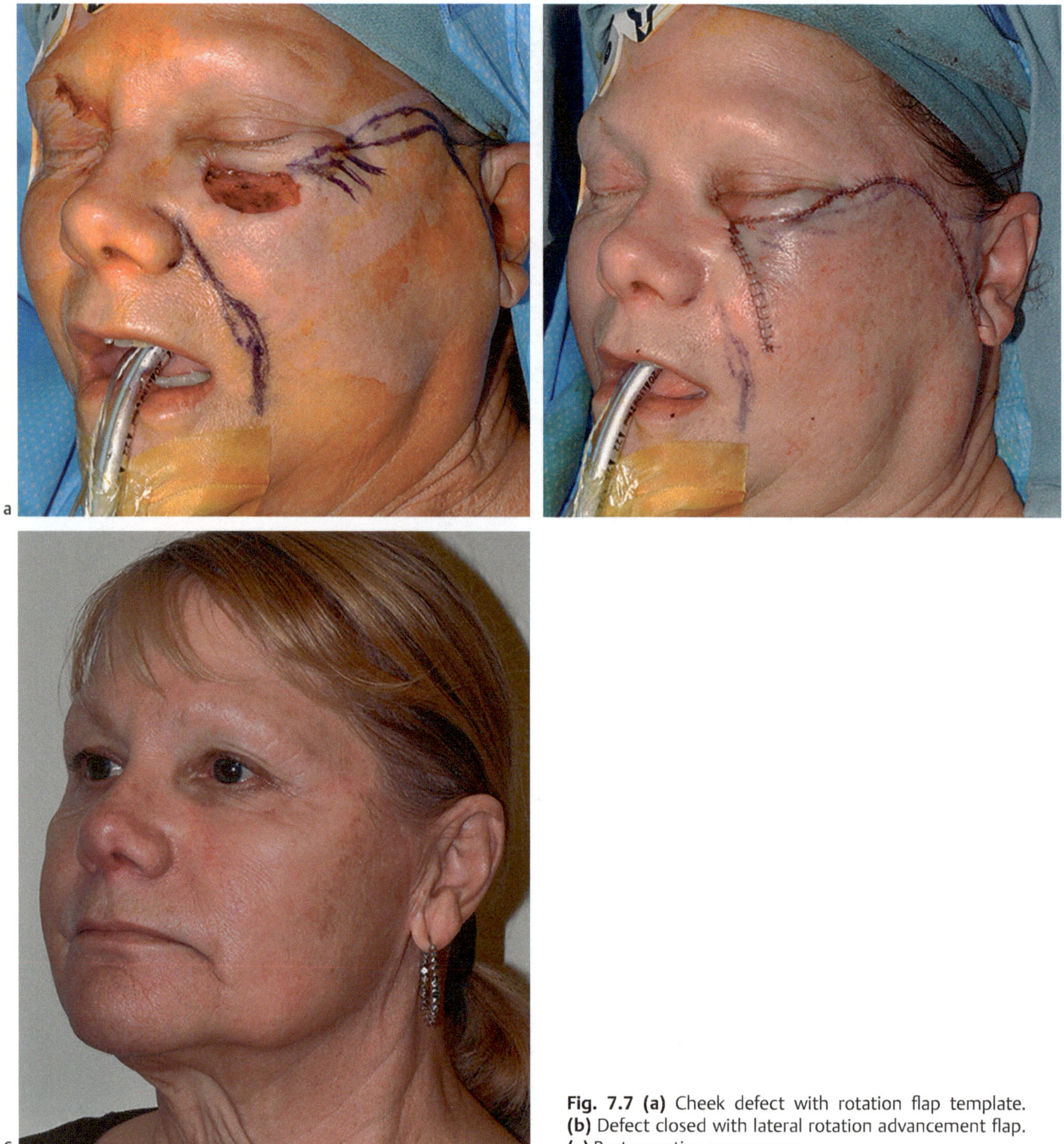

Fig. 7.7 (a) Cheek defect with rotation flap template. **(b)** Defect closed with lateral rotation advancement flap. **(c)** Postoperative appearance.

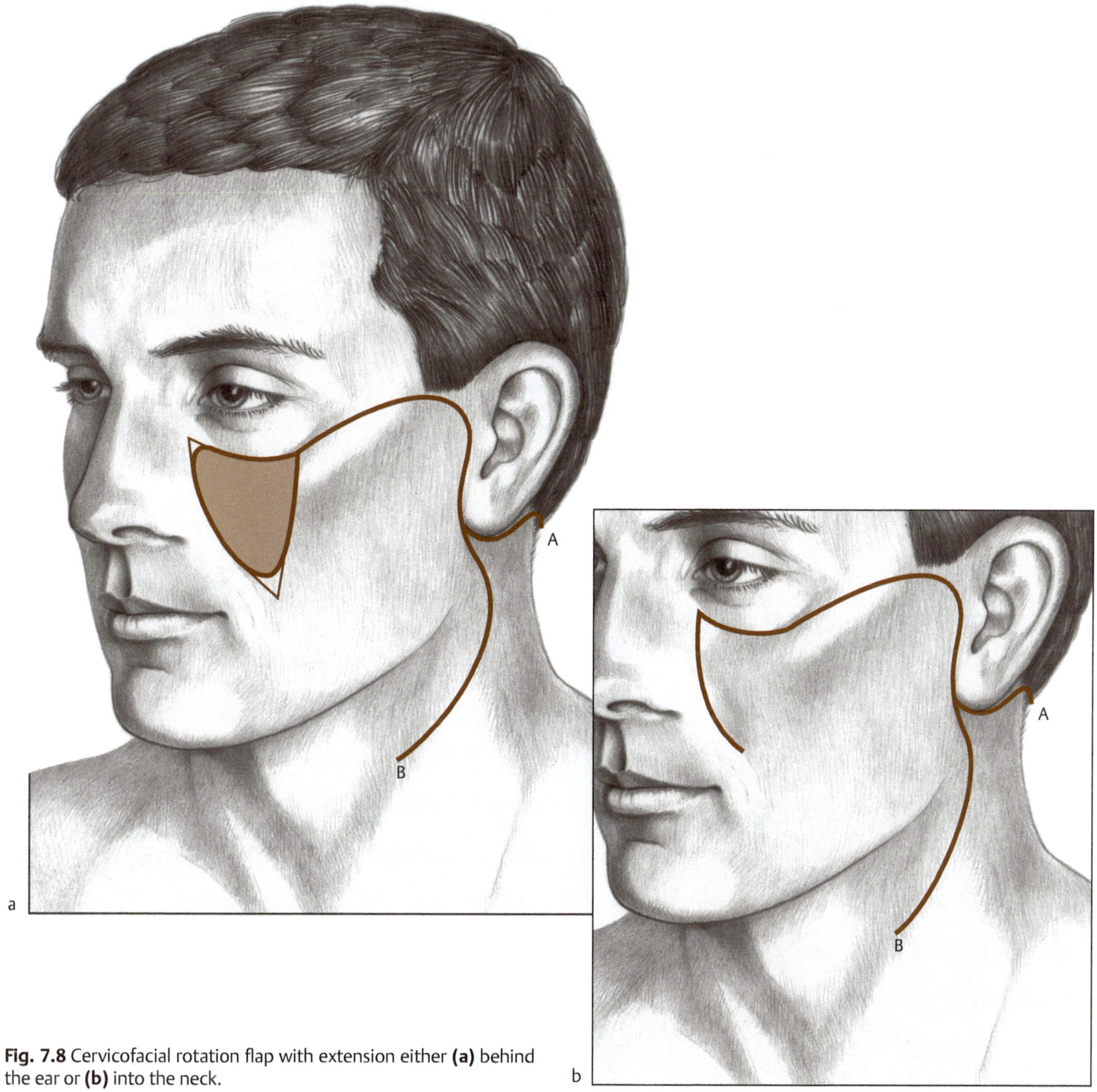

Fig. 7.8 Cervicofacial rotation flap with extension either **(a)** behind the ear or **(b)** into the neck.

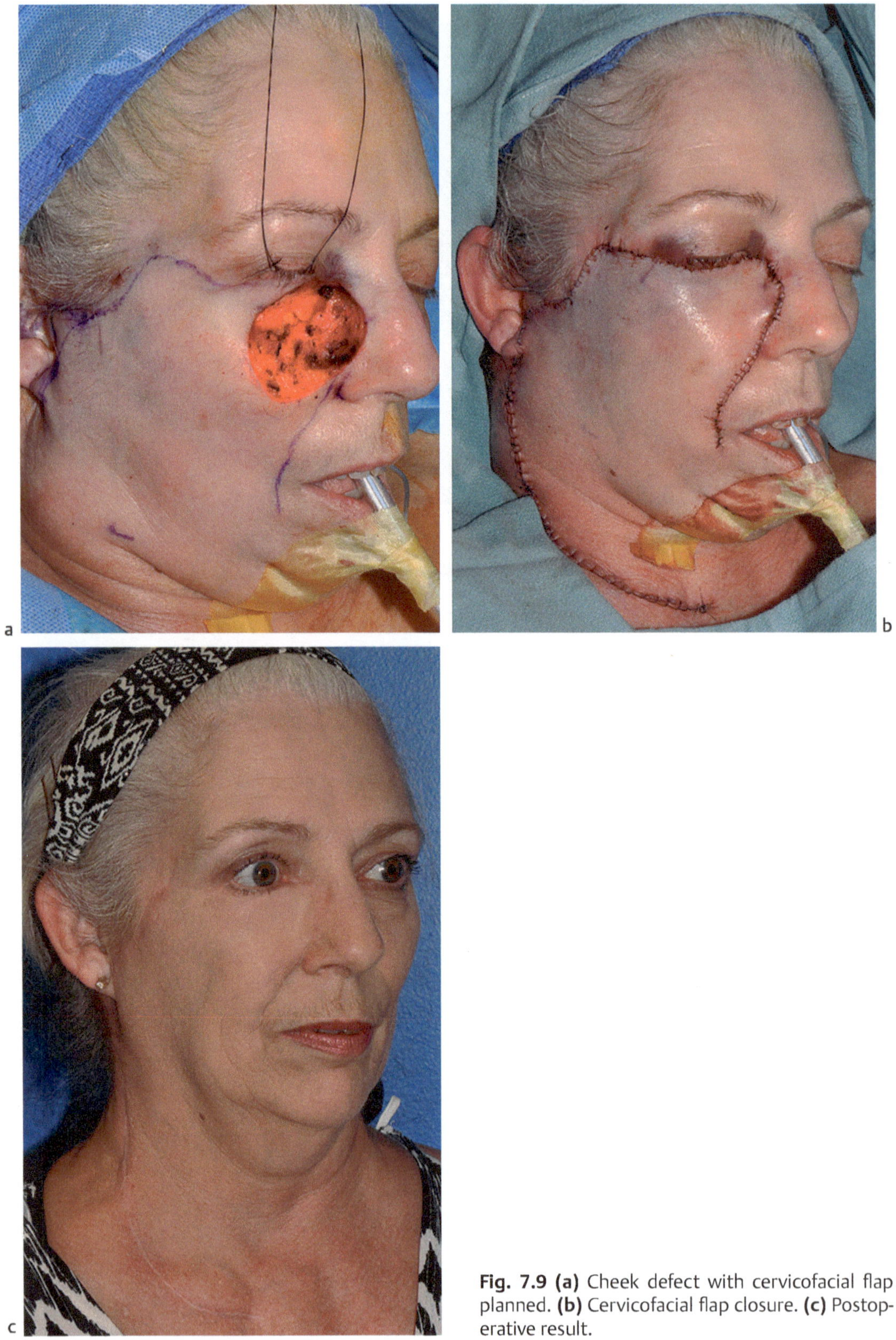

Fig. 7.9 (a) Cheek defect with cervicofacial flap planned. **(b)** Cervicofacial flap closure. **(c)** Postoperative result.

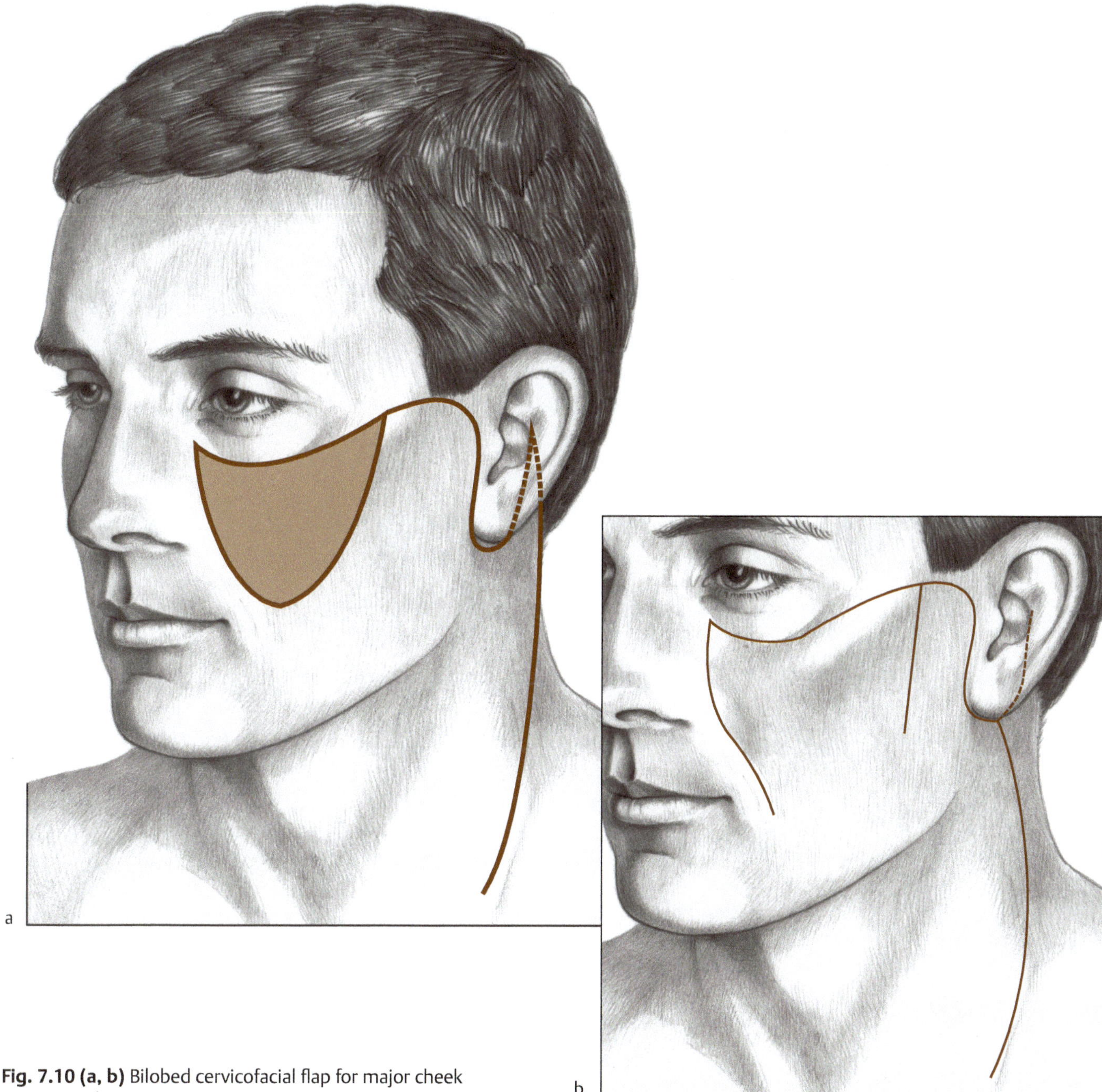

Fig. 7.10 (a, b) Bilobed cervicofacial flap for major cheek reconstruction.

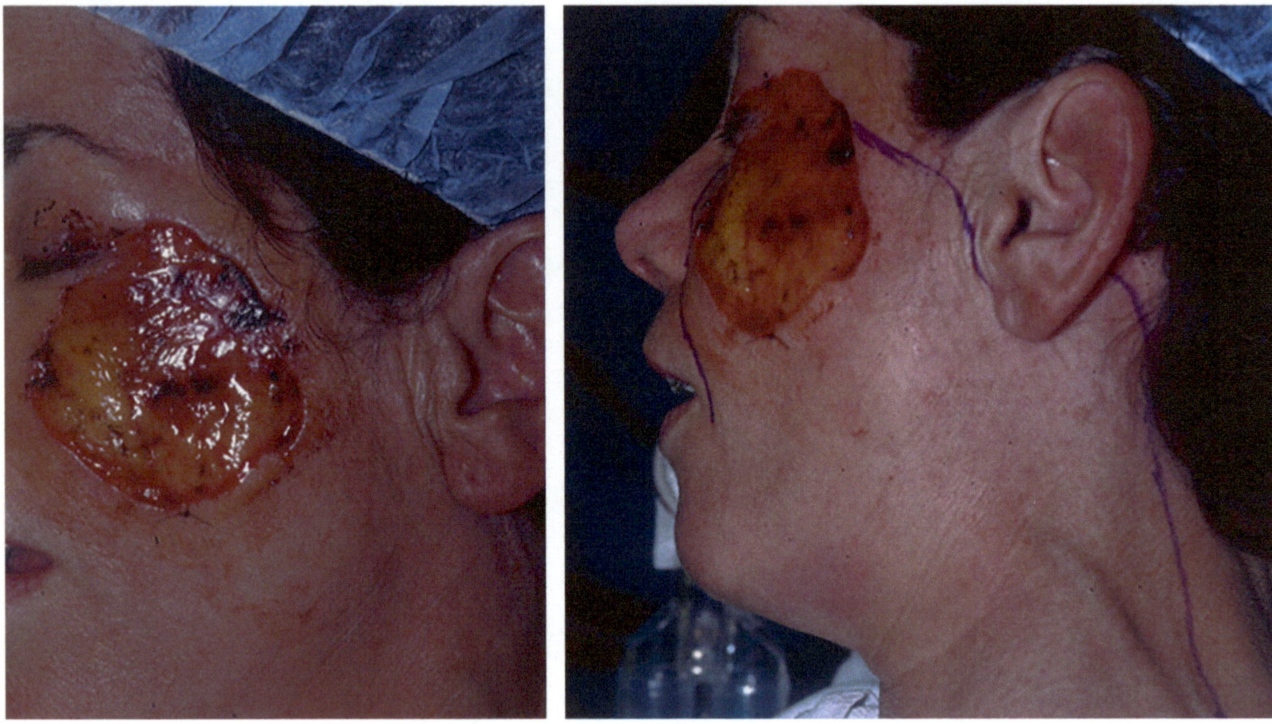

a b

Fig. 7.11 (a) Large medial cheek defect. **(b)** Bilobed cervicofacial flap planned.

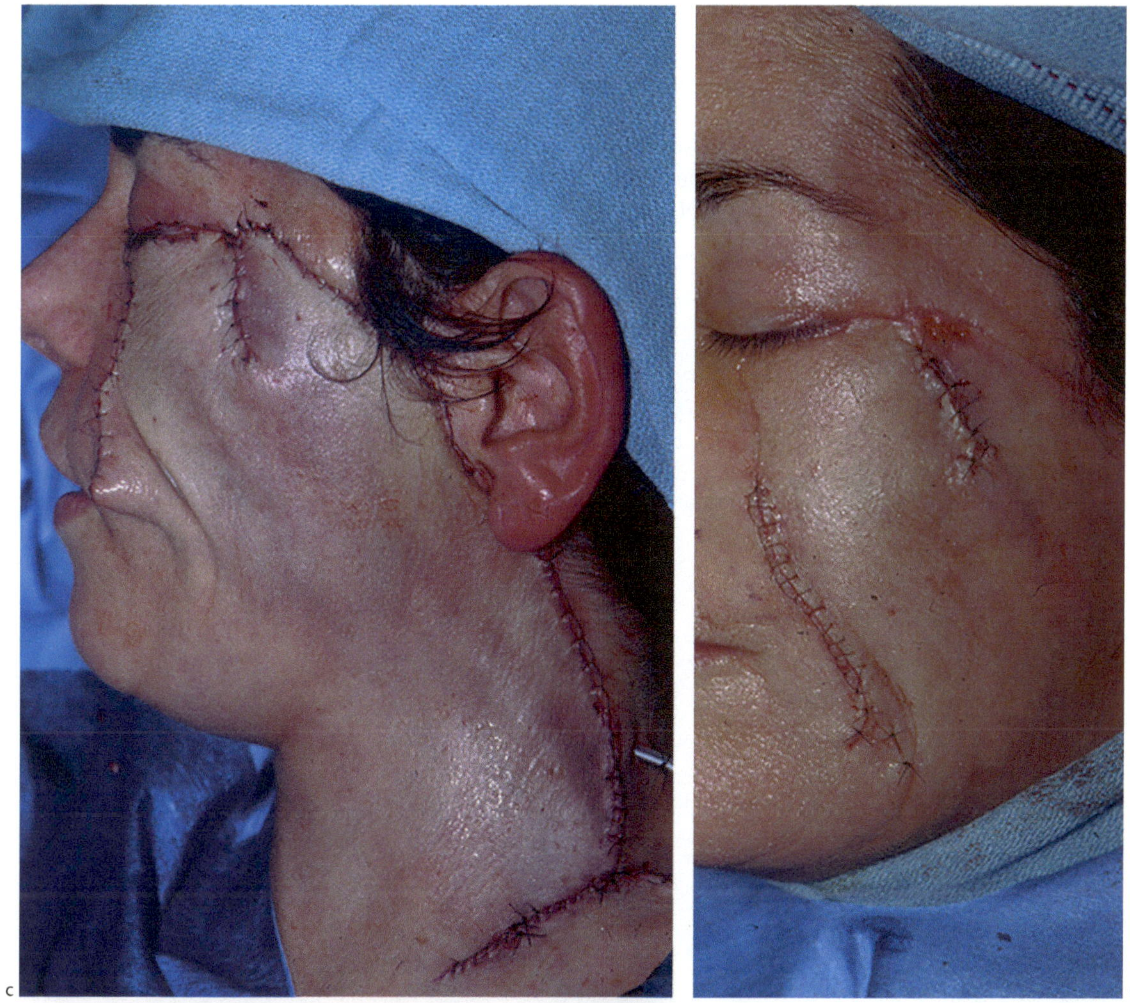

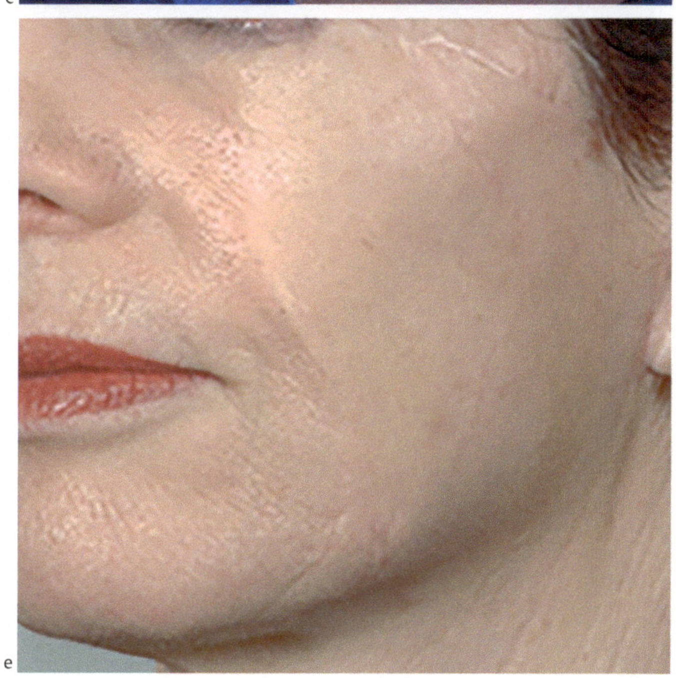

Fig. 7.11 (c) Flap at closure. **(d)** After secondary "dog-ear" excisions (not necessary in all cases). **(e)** Long-term postoperative result.

♦ Lateral Cheek Subunit

Most lateral cheek defects can be closed either primarily or with a cheek advancement flap similar to a rhytidectomy flap (**Fig. 7.12, Fig. 7.13,** and **Fig. 7.14**). Defects whose shape or positions are not well suited to an advancement flap are closed with some type of transposition flap. The classic rhombic flap is a good choice (**Fig. 7.15** and **Fig. 7.16**). Triangular defects or defects that are more horizontally oriented are appropriate for a cervical facial rotation flap. The entire lateral cheek subunit can be replaced with a cervicofacial rotation flap.

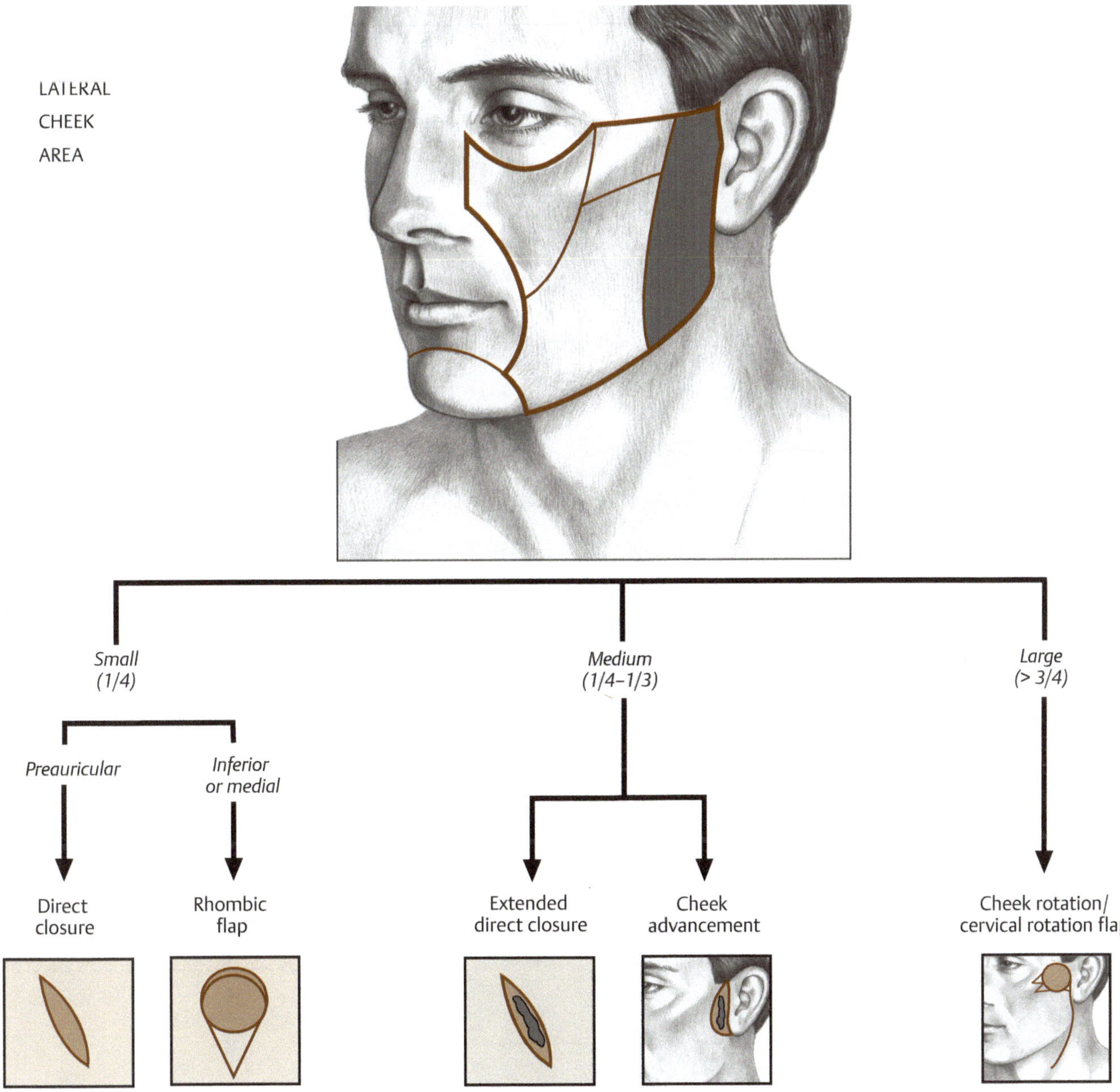

Fig. 7.12 Lateral cheek area.

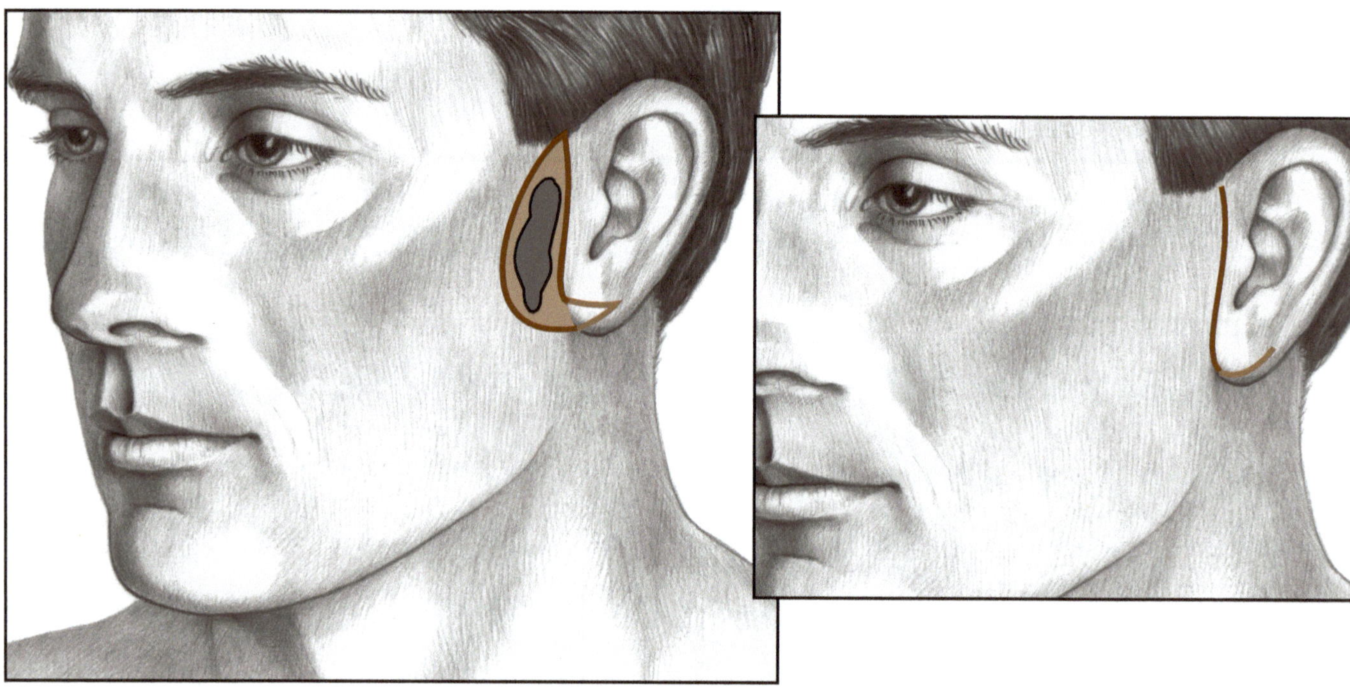

Fig. 7.13 Rhytidectomy-like flap for lateral cheek closure.

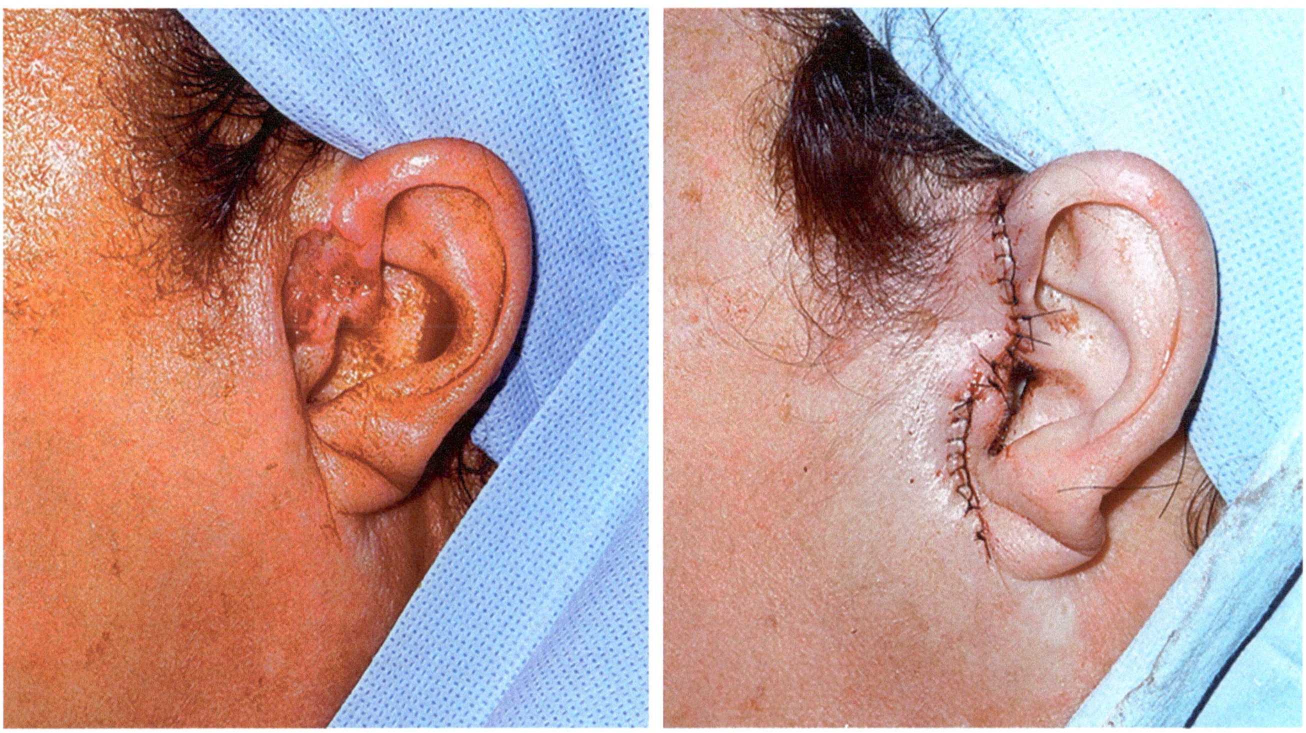

a b

Fig. 7.14 (a) Preauricular cheek defect. **(b)** After closure with direct cheek advancement, as in rhytidectomy.

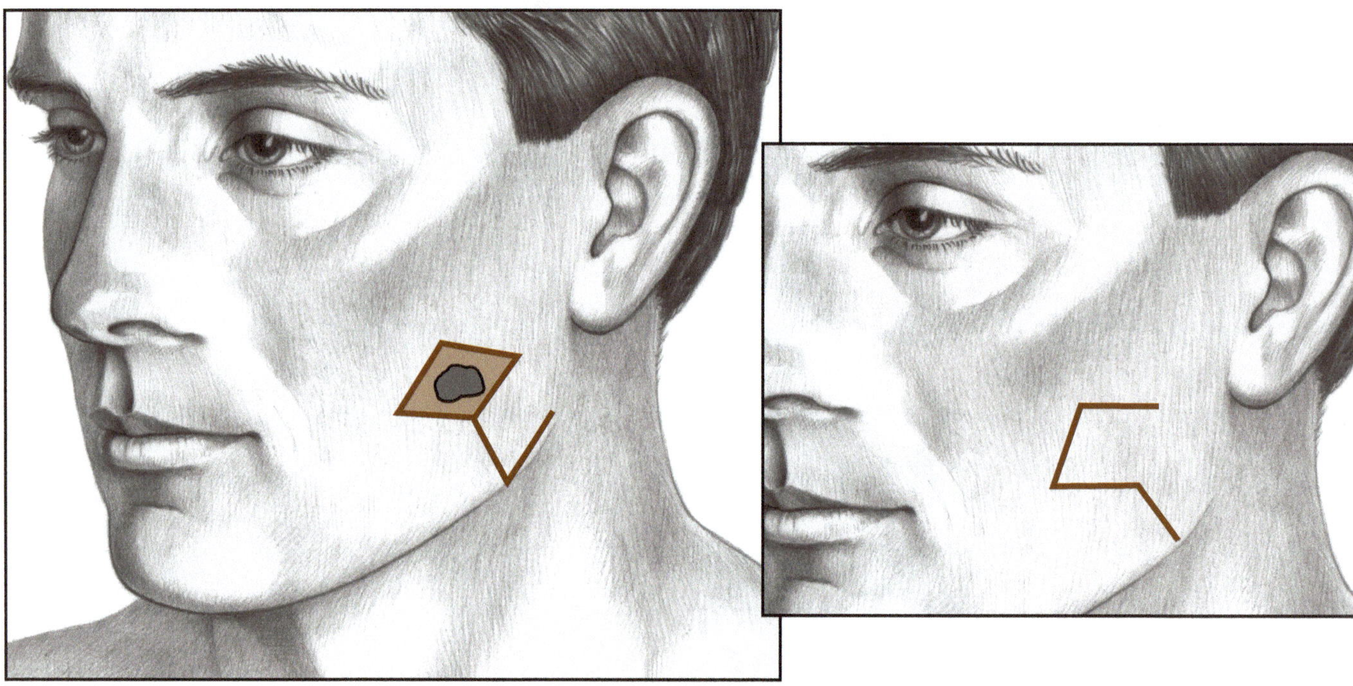

Fig. 7.15 Rhombic flap reconstruction of a lateral cheek defect.

a
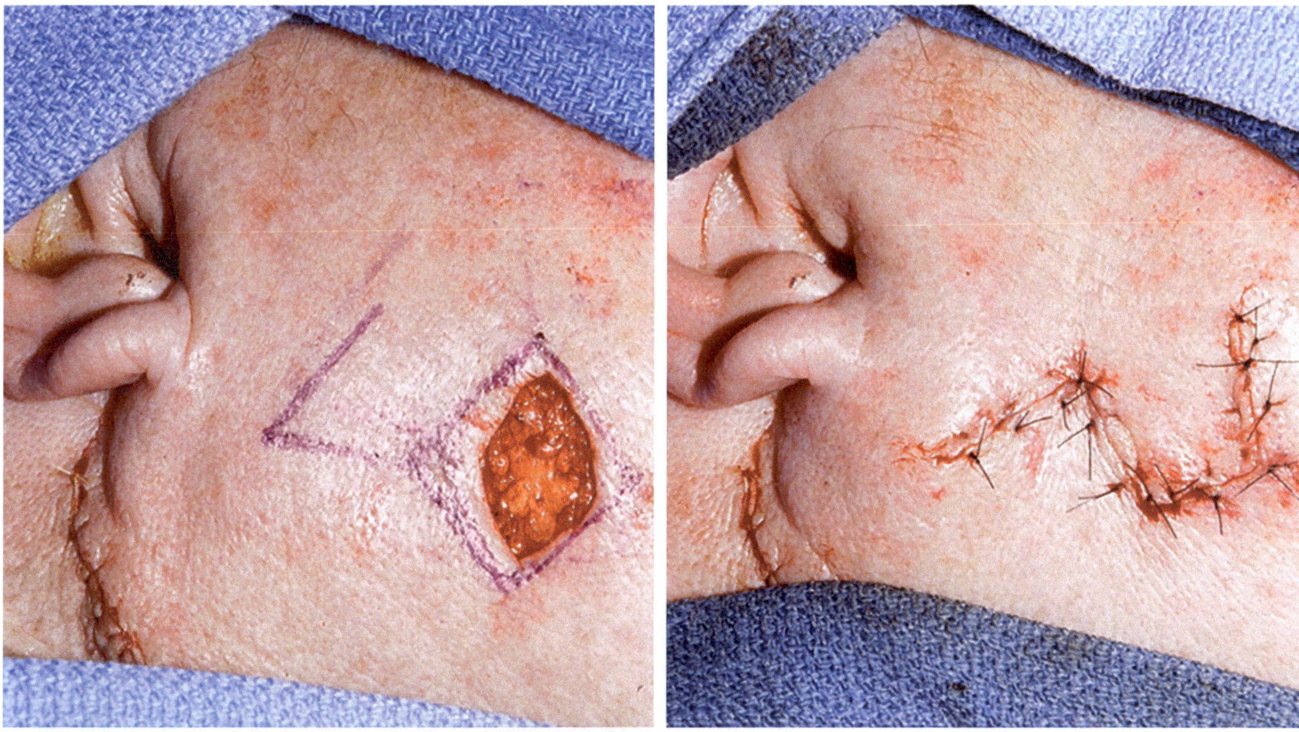
b

c
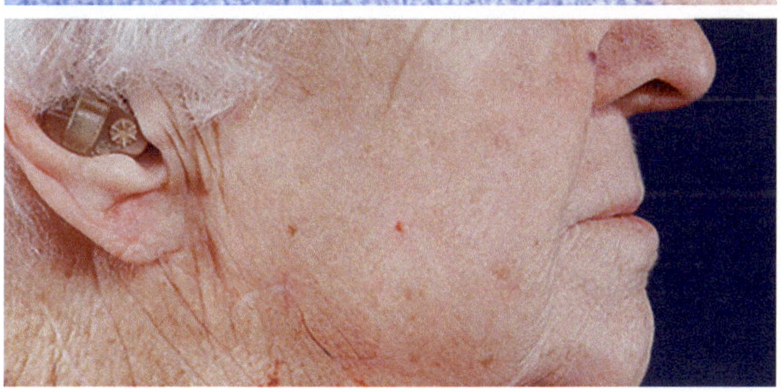

Fig. 7.16 (a) Rhombic flap planned for lateral cheek closure. **(b)** After closure. **(c)** Postoperative appearance.

Large lateral cheek defects are usually closed with a cervicofacial rotation flap (**Fig. 7.17**). The incisions can be carried either in a neck crease, as shown, or into the postauricular area (**Fig. 7.18**). An M-plasty can be used to avoid a standing cone formation without carrying the incision into the anterior cheek (**Fig. 7.19** and **Fig. 7.20**).

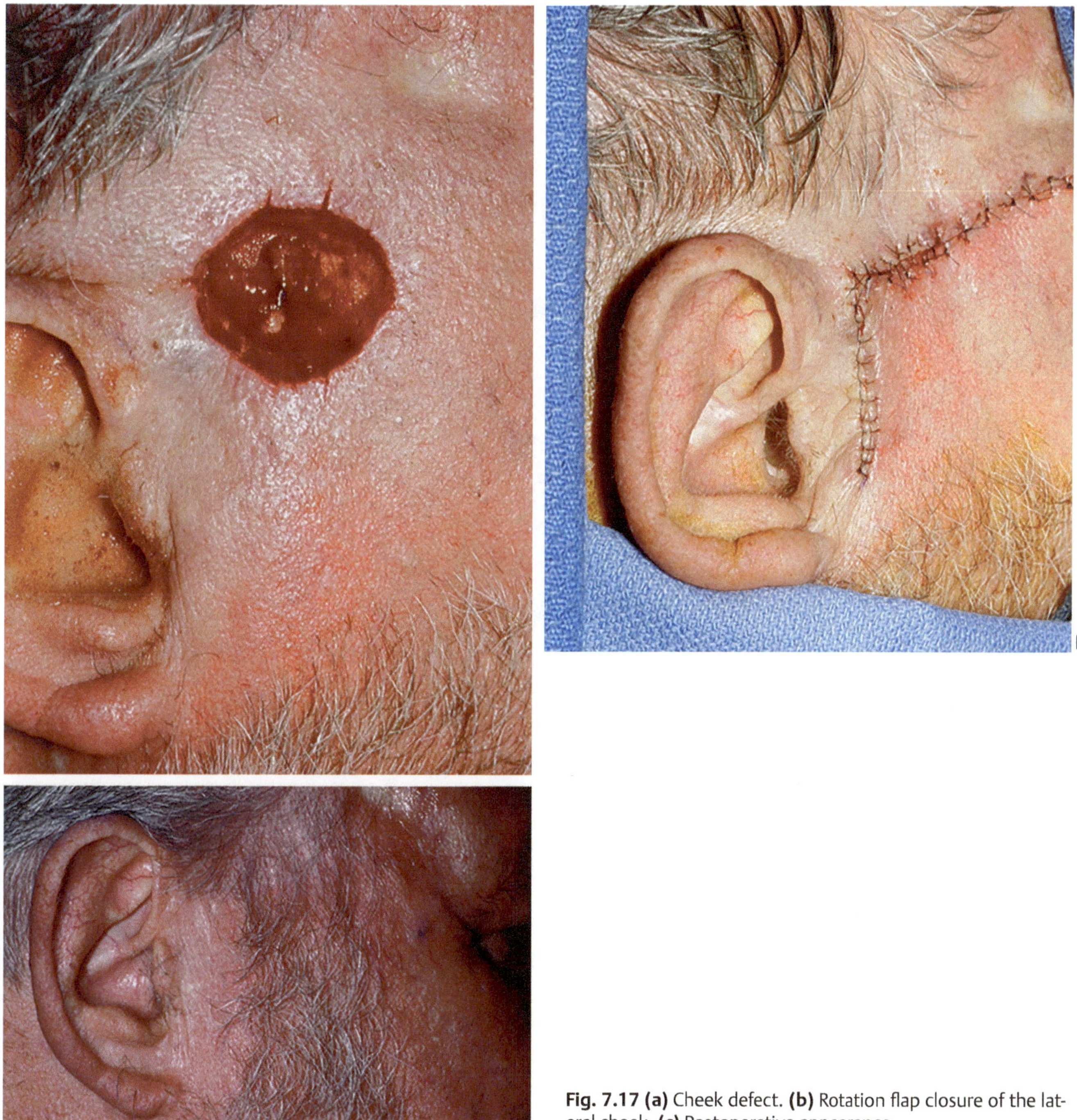

Fig. 7.17 (a) Cheek defect. **(b)** Rotation flap closure of the lateral cheek. **(c)** Postoperative appearance.

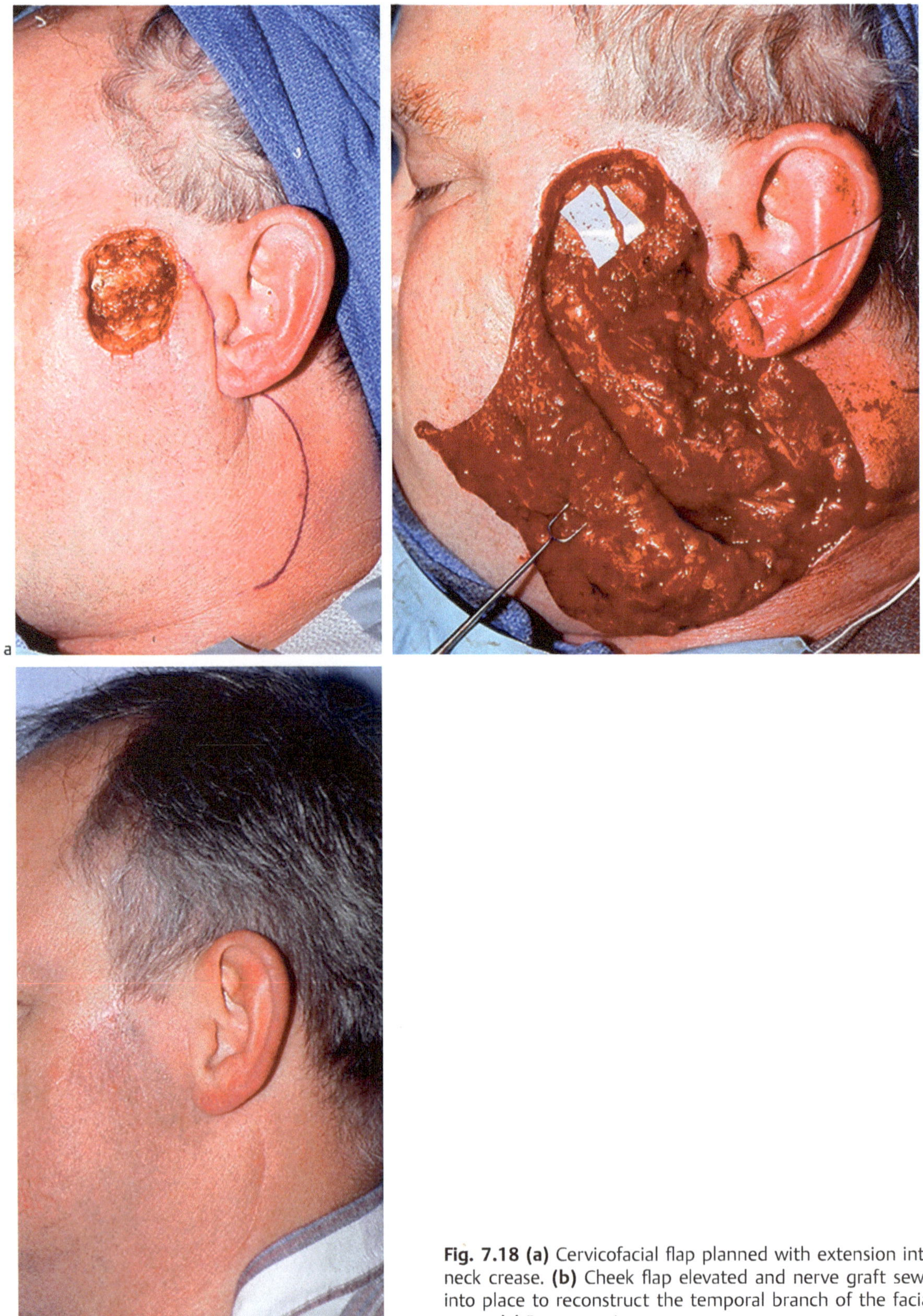

Fig. 7.18 (a) Cervicofacial flap planned with extension into neck crease. **(b)** Cheek flap elevated and nerve graft sewn into place to reconstruct the temporal branch of the facial nerve. **(c)** Postoperative appearance.

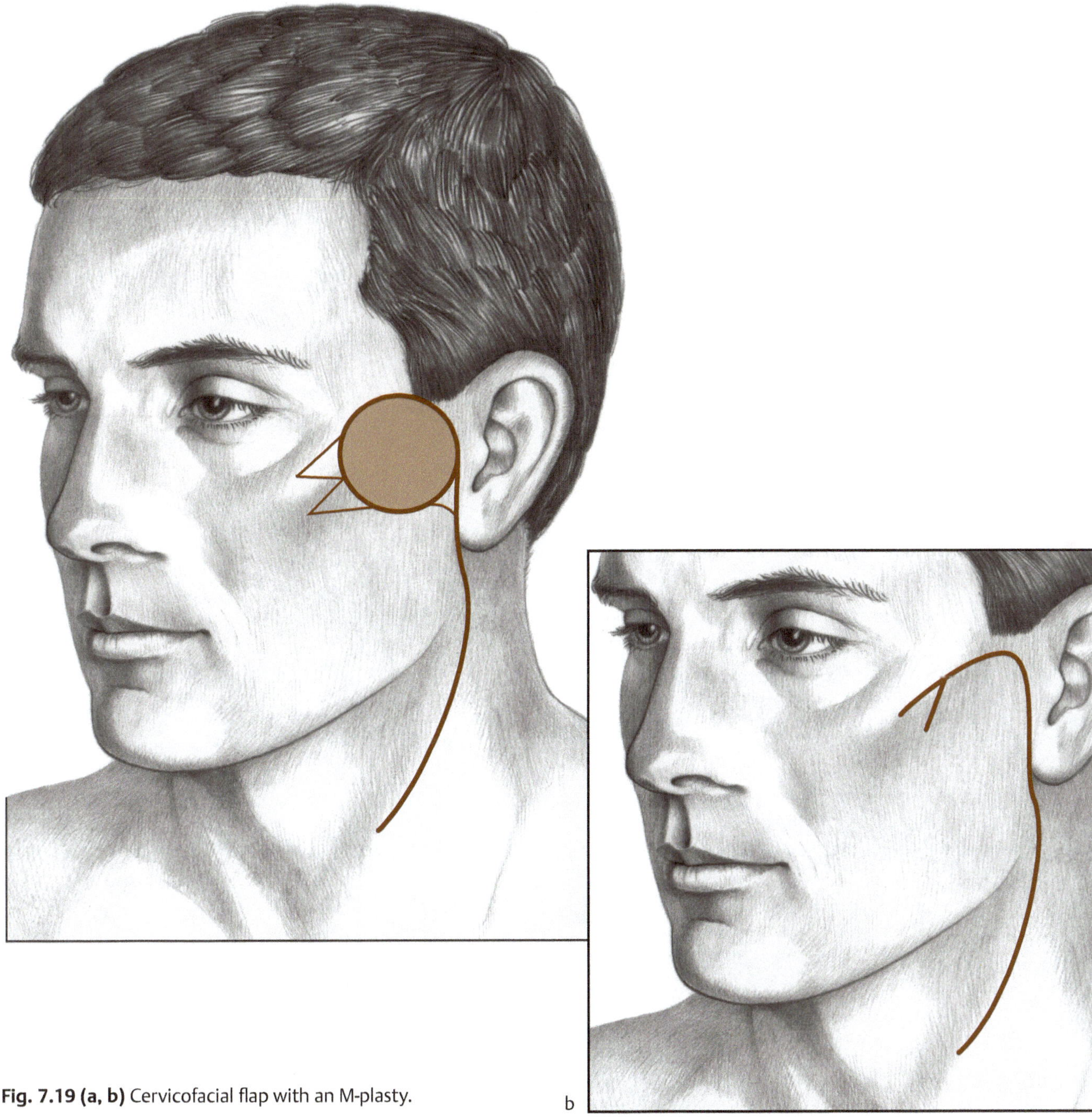

Fig. 7.19 (a, b) Cervicofacial flap with an M-plasty.

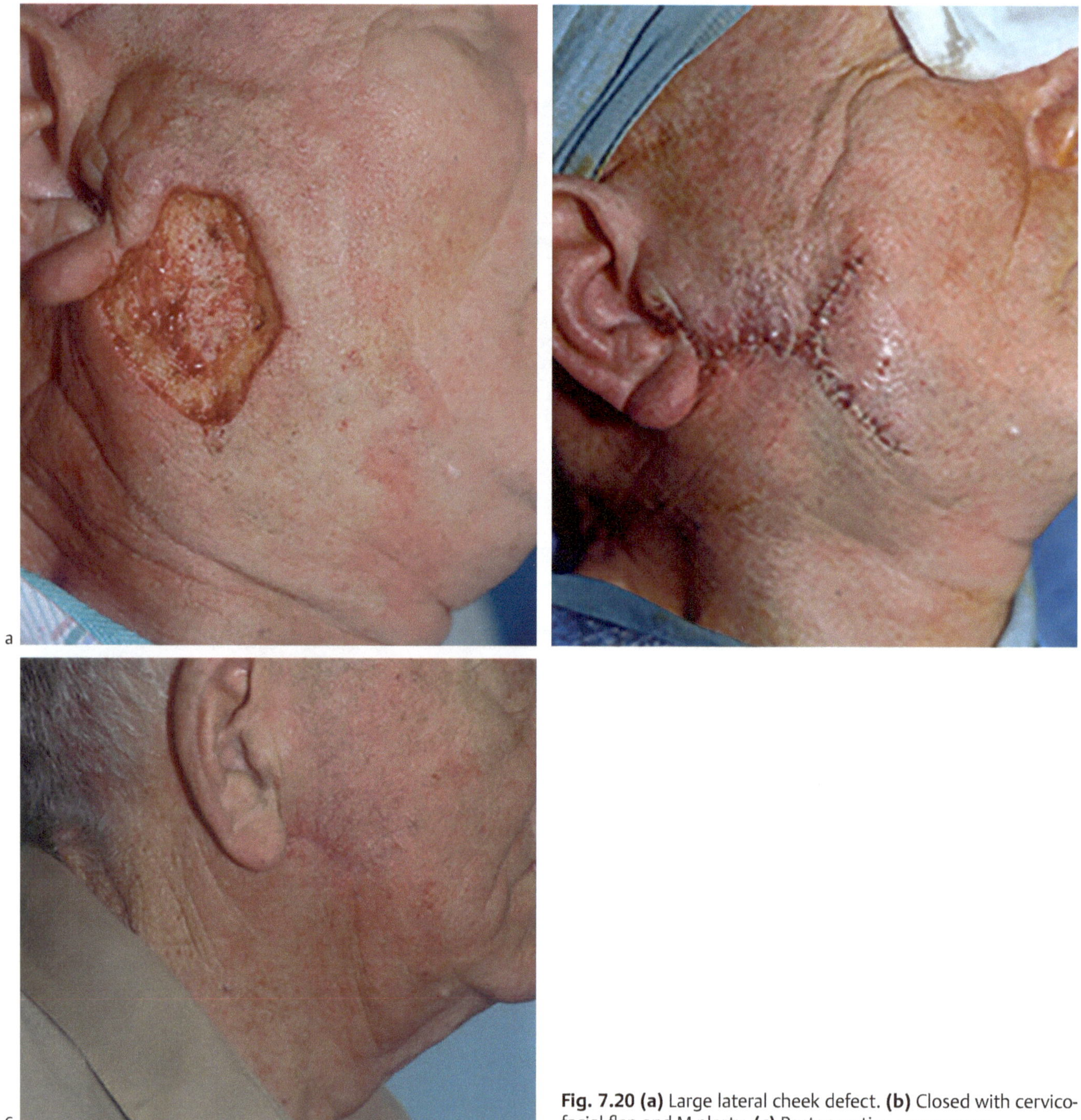

a b c

Fig. 7.20 (a) Large lateral cheek defect. **(b)** Closed with cervicofacial flap and M-plasty. **(c)** Postoperative appearance.

♦ Zygomatic Cheek Subunit

Defects of the zygomatic subunit can usually be repaired with primary closure, transposition flaps from the temporal forehead or lateral cheek, or cheek rotation or advancement flaps (**Fig. 7.21** and **Fig. 7.22**). Special care must be taken to elevate flaps in this region, as well as in the lateral subunit, in the plane just deep to the subdermal plexus to avoid damage to the frontal branch of the facial nerve, which is very superficial in this region. When the defect is close to the eyelid, suspension sutures of 3–0 or 4–0 long-lasting absorbable material should be placed at the lateral orbital rim to support the flap and prevent ectropion.

ZYGOMATIC

AREA

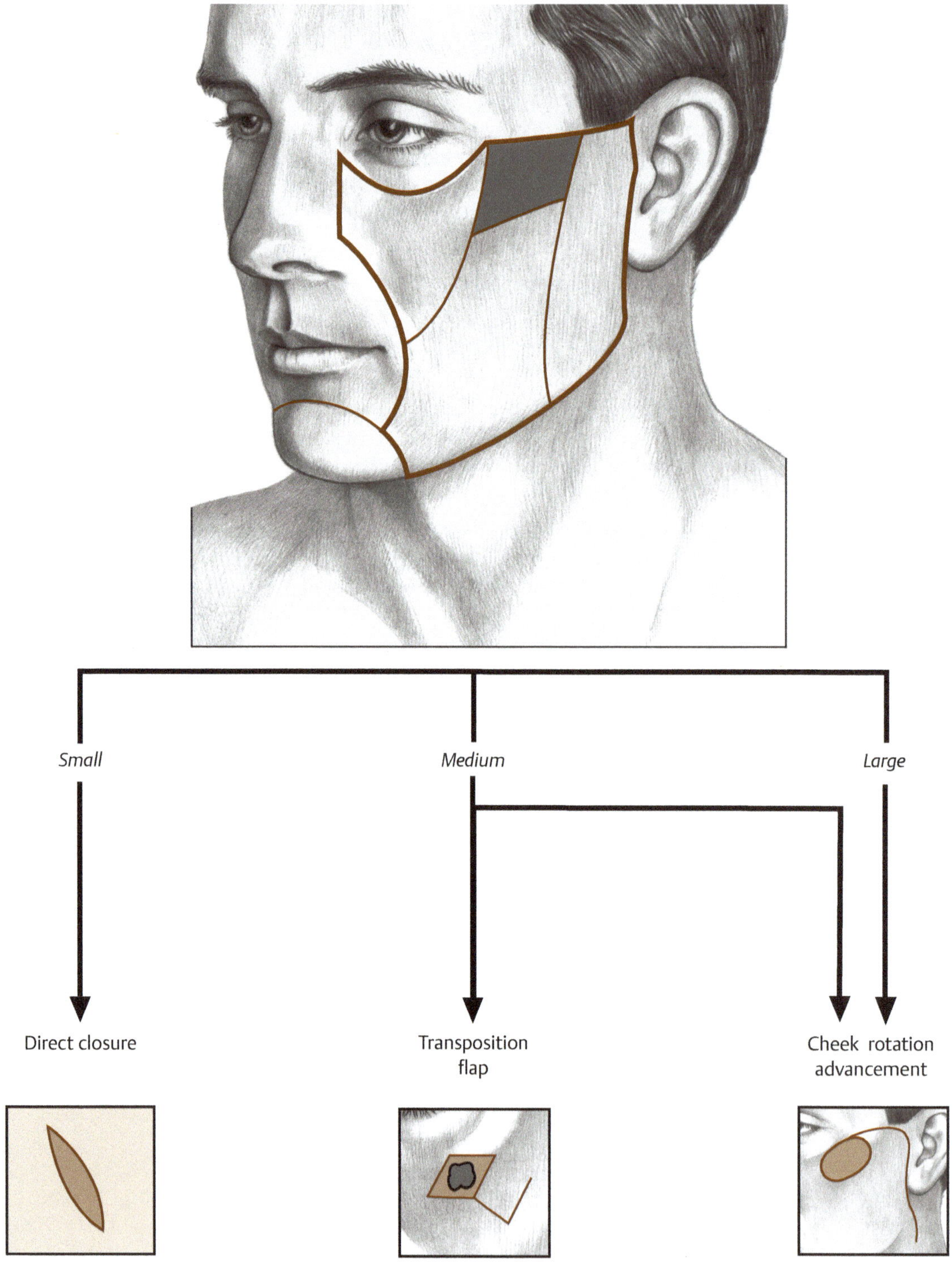

Fig. 7.21 Zygomatic area.

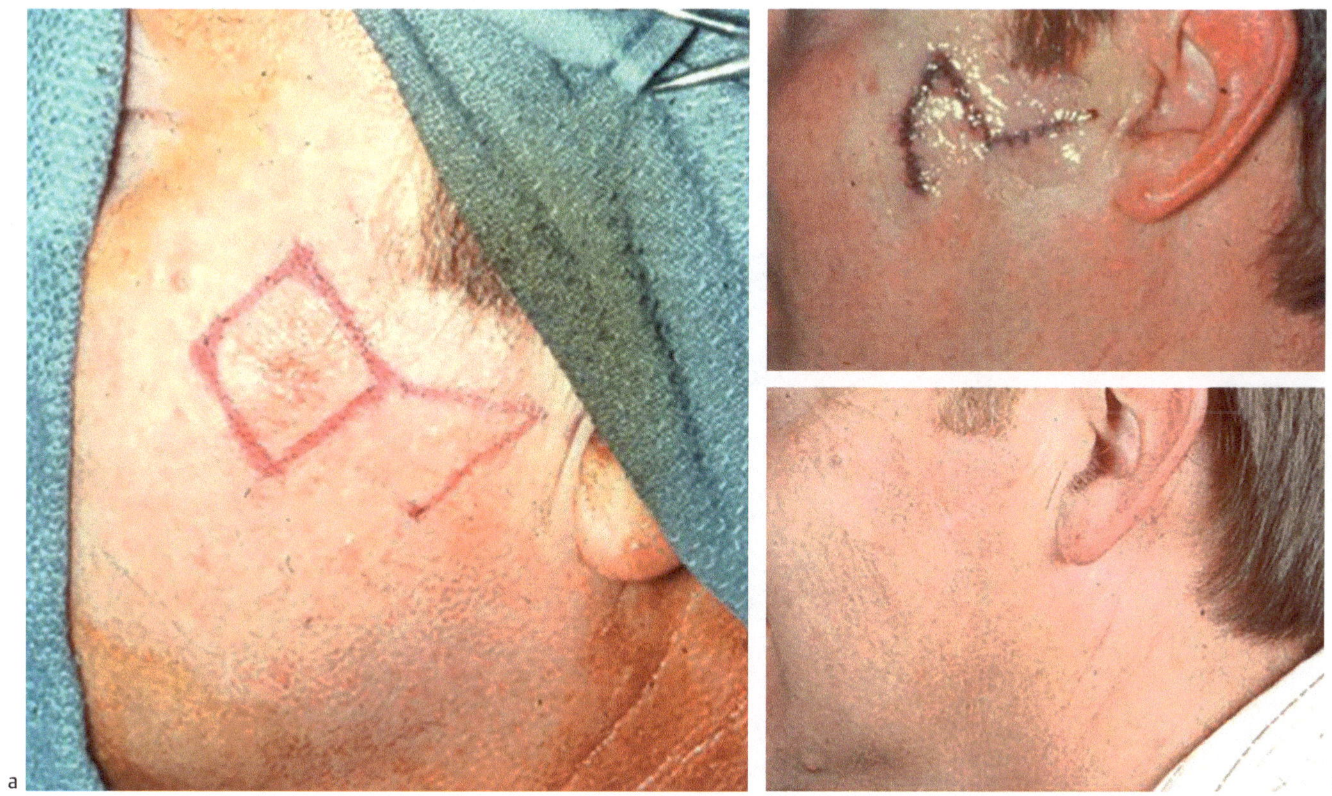

Fig. 7.22 **(a)** Rhombic flap planned for a zygomatic lesion. **(b)** After flap closure. **(c)** Postoperative result.

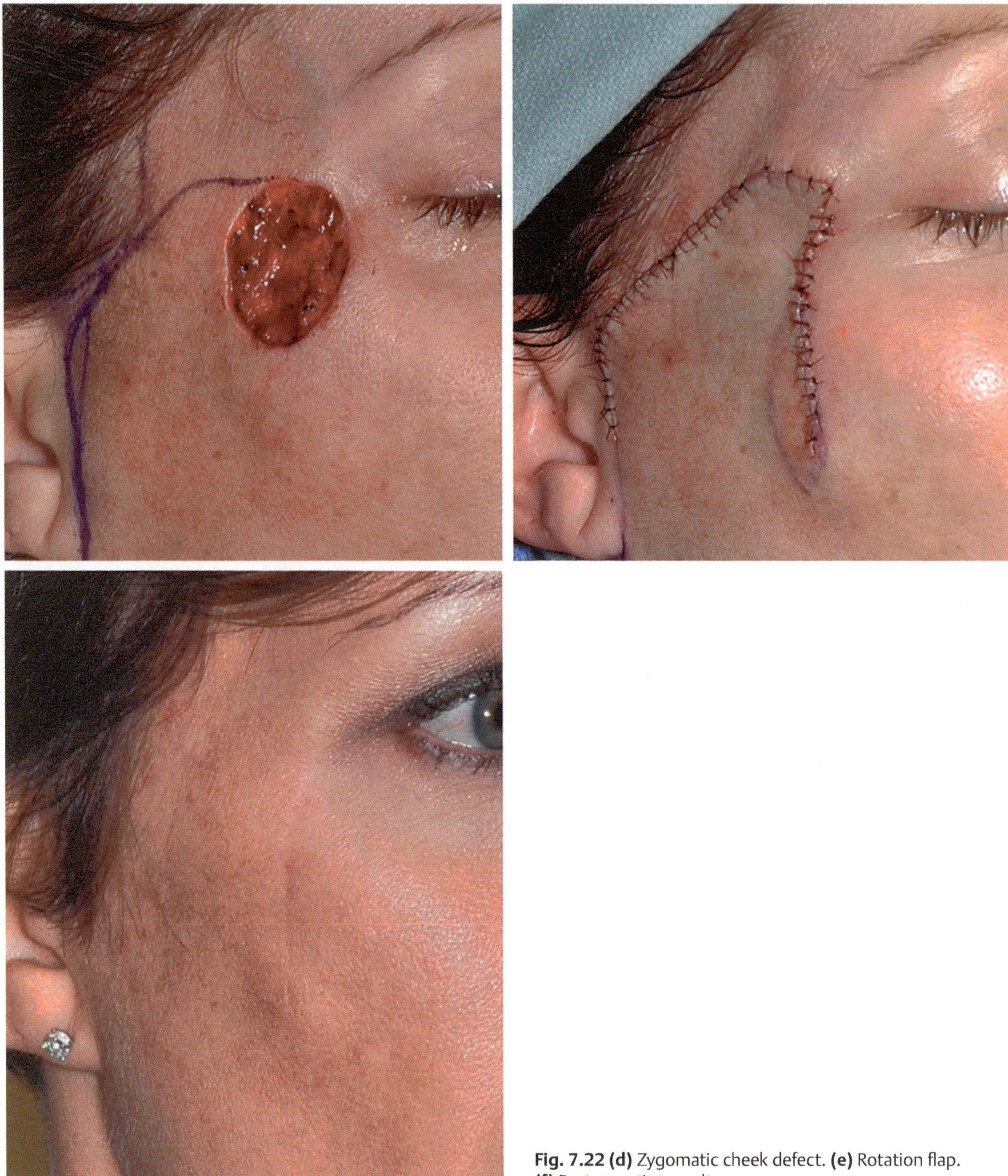

d

e

f

Fig. 7.22 (d) Zygomatic cheek defect. **(e)** Rotation flap. **(f)** Postoperative result.

♦ Buccal Cheek Subunit

Defects of the central cheek are closed primarily in the relaxed skin tension lines when possible (**Fig. 7.23**). Small-to-medium central cheek defects are closed with the rhombic, note, or bilobed flap (**Fig. 7.24** and **Fig. 7.25**). Each of these flaps is elevated in the plane just deep to the subdermal plexus. The largest defects are usually closed with a cervicofacial rotation flap. Full-thickness defects of the buccal region of the cheek are usually closed with regional flaps or free flaps and are beyond the scope of this book.

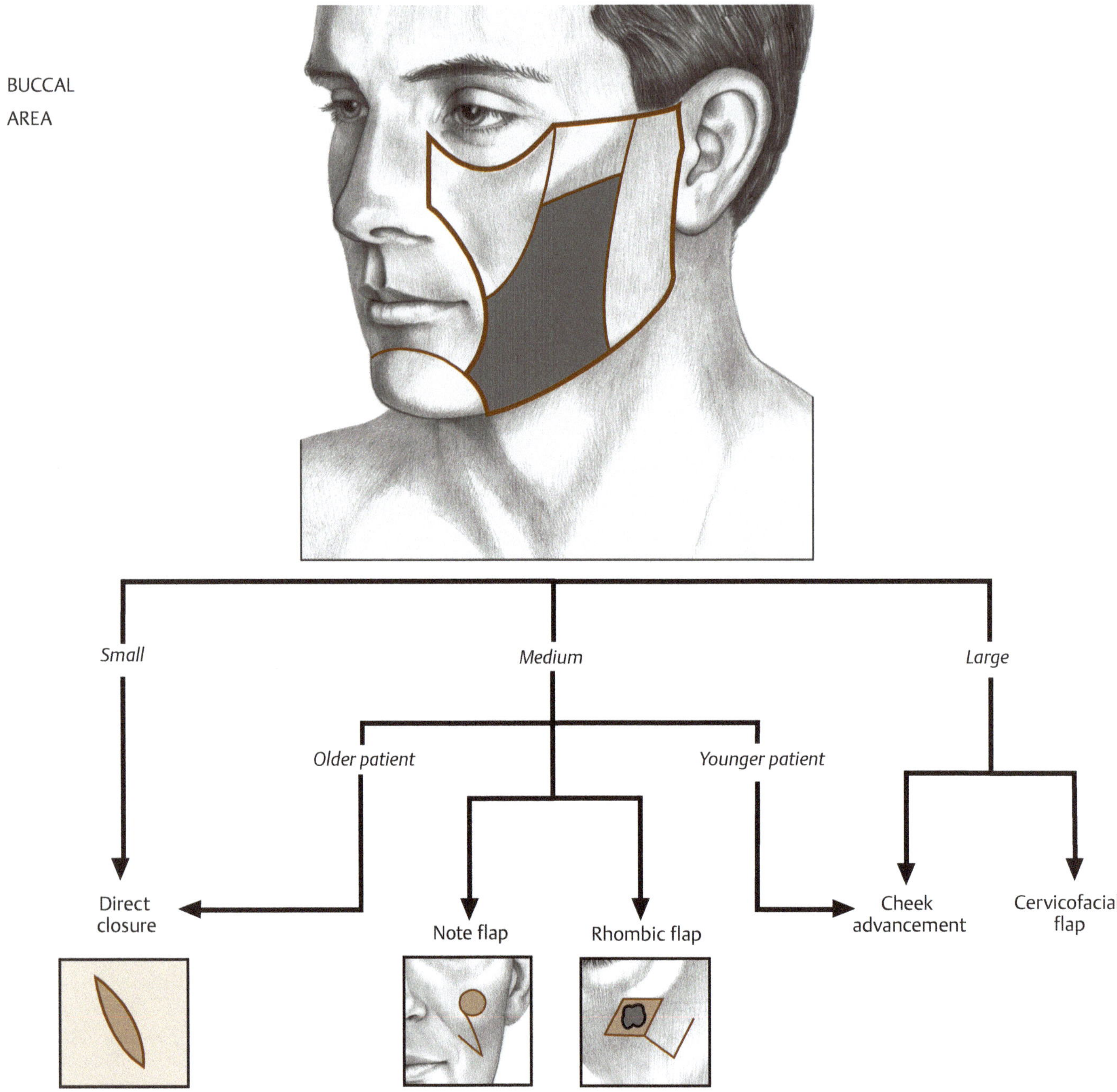

Fig. 7.23 Buccal area.

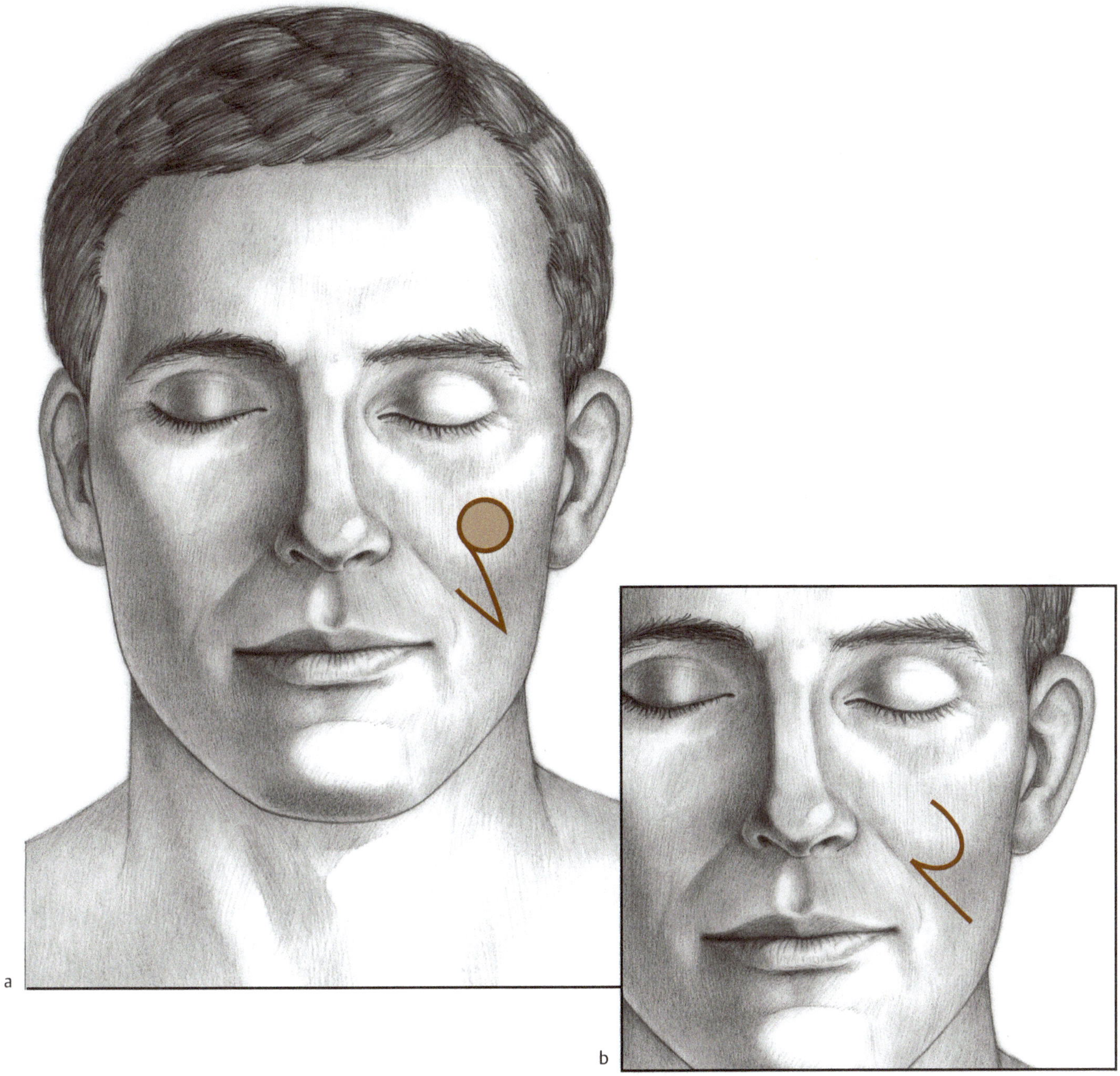

Fig. 7.24 (a, b) Note flap of the cheek.

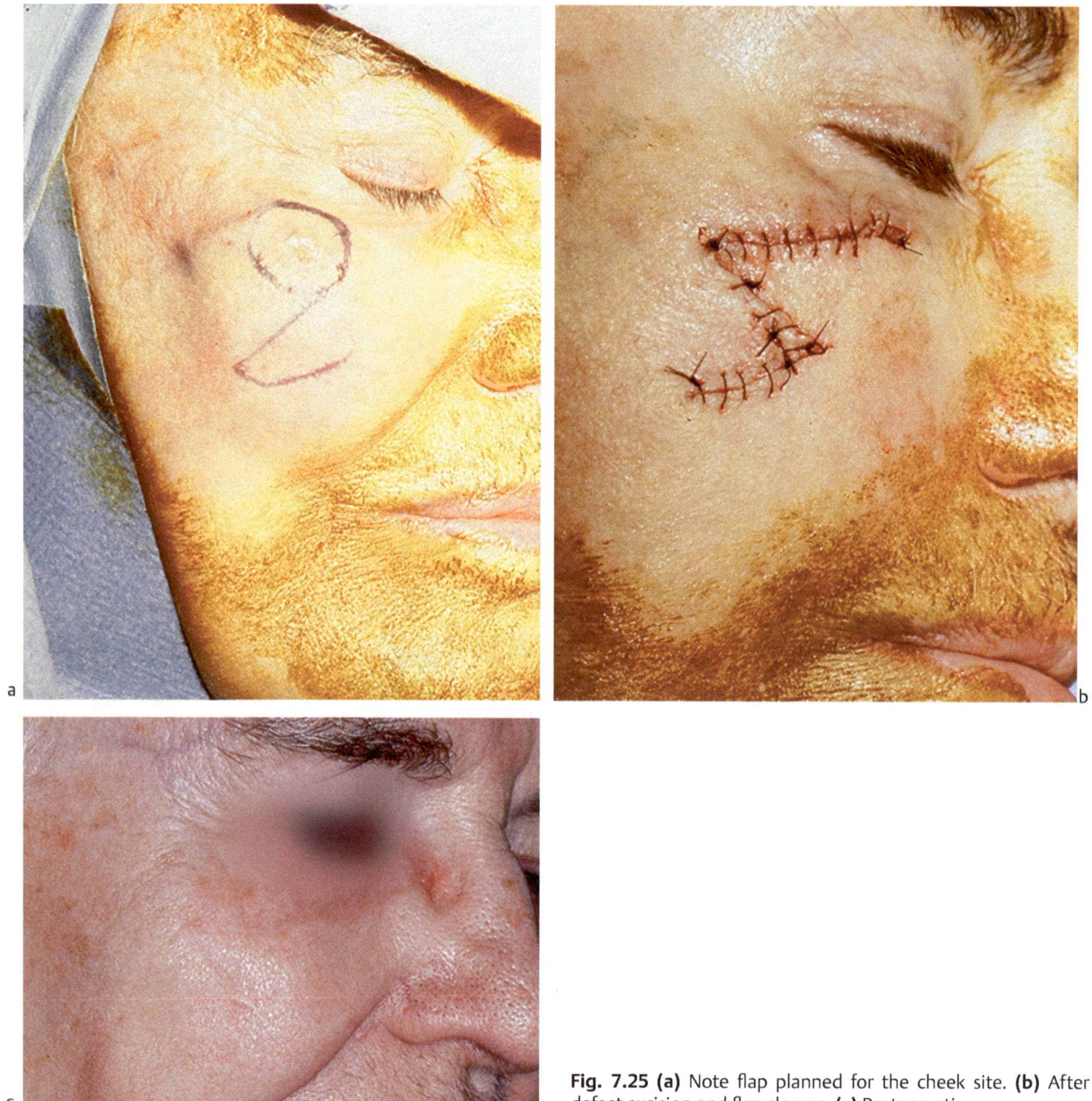

Fig. 7.25 (a) Note flap planned for the cheek site. **(b)** After defect excision and flap closure. **(c)** Postoperative appearance.

♦ Cheek/Lower Eyelid and Cheek/Nose Defects

The combined cheek/lower eyelid and cheek/nose defects are common enough that they deserve mention. Defects of both the cheek and lower eyelid are best reconstructed with a combination of a cheek rotation advancement flap for anterior lamella reconstruction and either a tarsal-conjunctival flap or a nasal-septal mucochondrial composite graft for posterior lamella reconstruction (**Fig. 7.26**). The nasal-septal composite graft is commonly too thick to optimally reconstruct the posterior lamella, but it should be kept in mind as an alternative in cases where a tarsal-conjunctival flap is not available or practical. When a composite graft is used, the cartilage should be shaved to thin it. The cheek rotation advancement flap should be appropriately thinned in the region of the lower eyelid for better tissue match. Also, the use of periosteal-dermal suspension sutures in the medial and lateral canthal regions is extremely important to prevent ectropion.

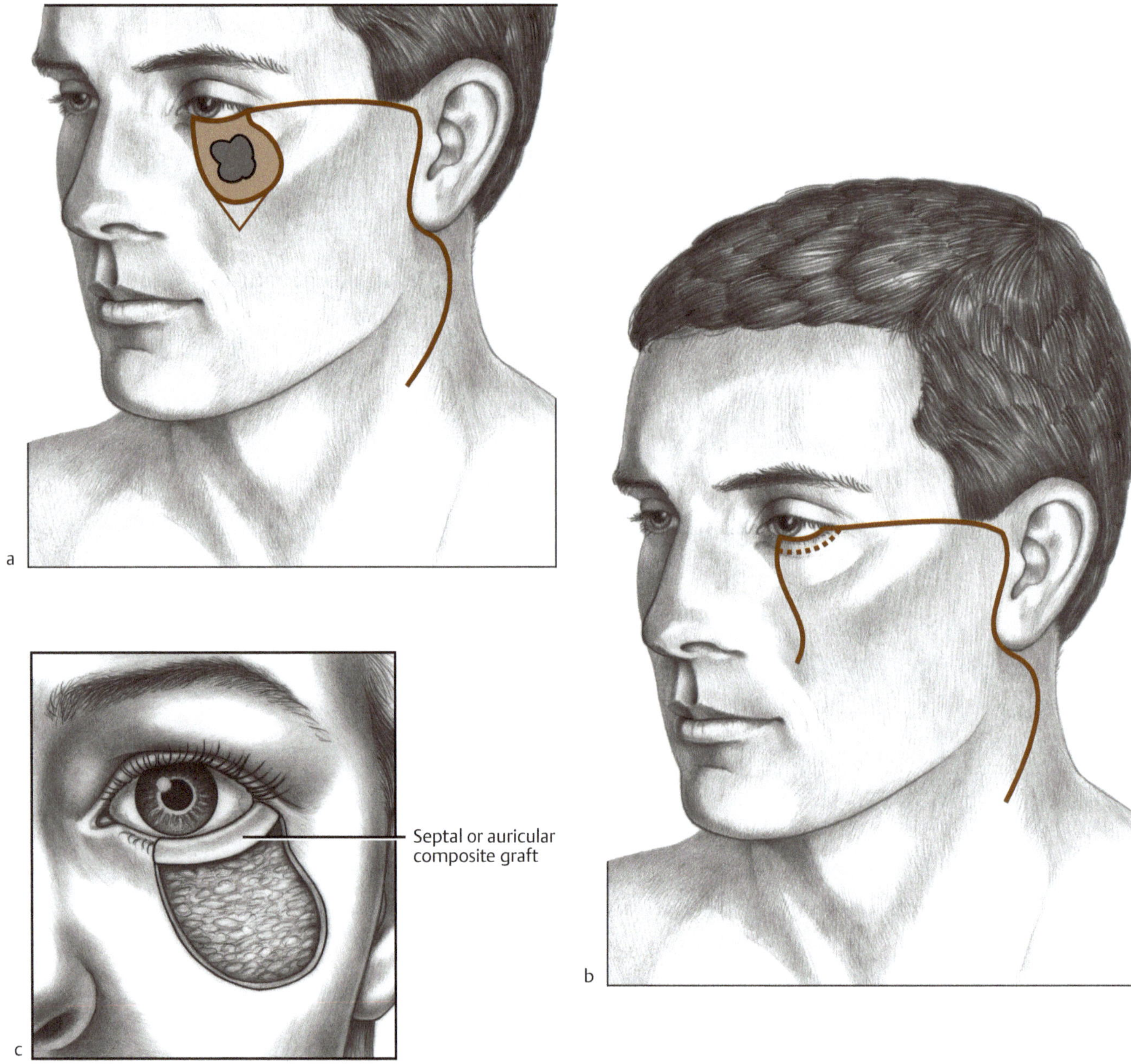

Fig. 7.26 (a-c) Cervicofacial rotation flap for combined cheek and lower eyelid reconstruction.

The cheek/nose combination defect should usually be reconstructed with separate techniques to avoid blunting of the nasofacial groove. Often, the less involved subunit may be treated with simple local tissue advancement and dermal-periosteal sutures to prevent blunting of the groove. This is followed by a second flap for the more involved subunit. Large defects of the region are best reconstructed with a forehead flap for the nasal defect and a cheek rotation advancement flap for the cheek defect (**Fig. 7.27** and **Fig. 7.28**). If the cheek defect is too large, a bilobed cervicofacial flap is an option (**Fig. 7.29**). Again, both of these flaps should be fixed to the nasofacial groove with dermal-periosteal sutures. These patients should be warned of the possible need for later revision of this junction.

Finally, some patients with combined cheek and eyelid or cheek and nose defects also have had partial maxillectomies. We have found that the underlying maxilla can be reliably reconstructed with split calvarial bone grafts and maxillofacial plates at the time of flap reconstruction. When these bone grafts are used to reconstruct the maxilla, they do not need intrasinus lining, as the mucosa of the sinus tends to regenerate over the grafts. Yet intranasal lining should be reconstructed, as this area does not tend to regenerate mucosa as quickly, and the exposed grafts are prone to resorption.

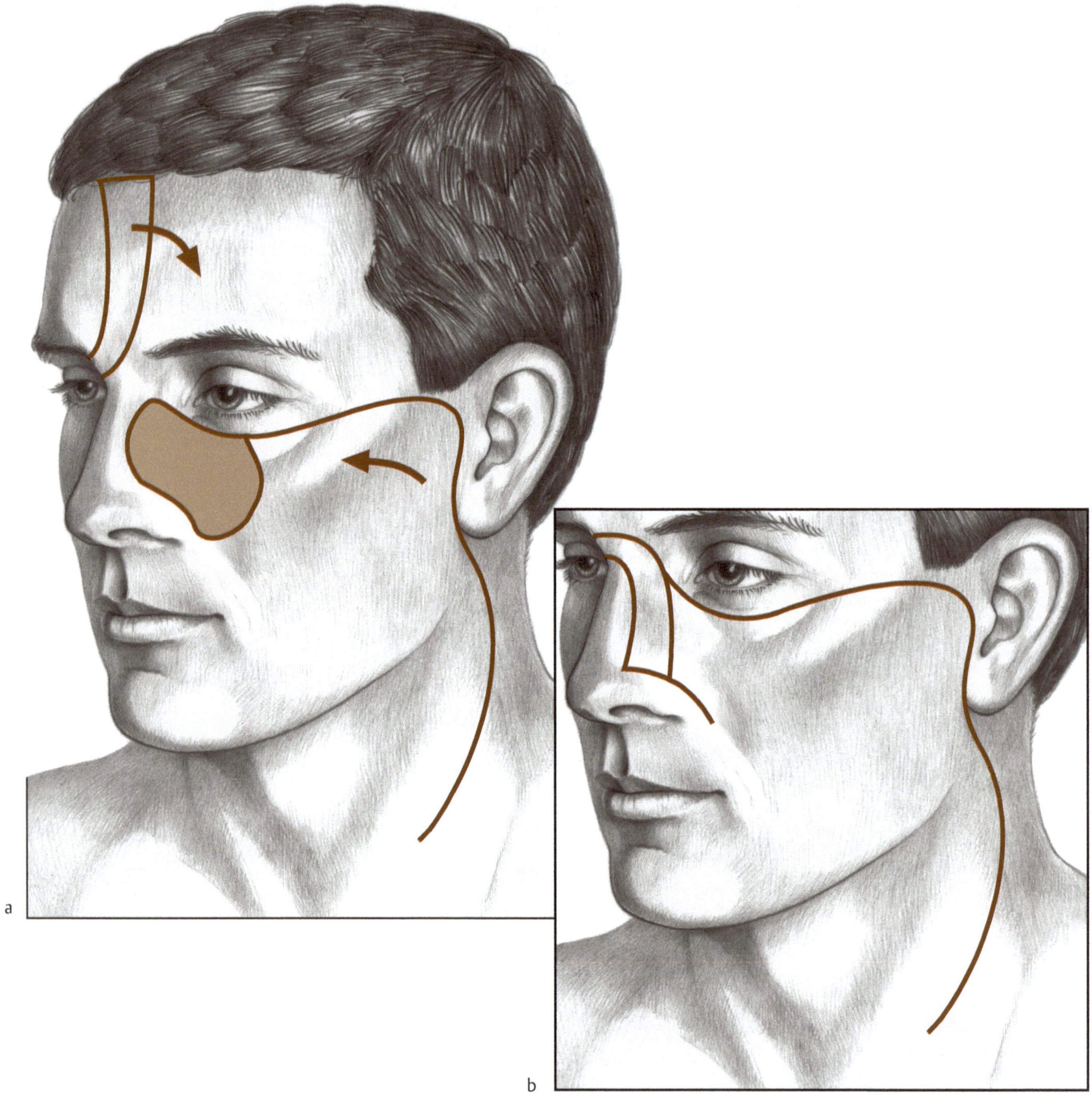

Fig. 7.27 (a, b) Forehead flap and cheek flap for a combined nasal-and-cheek defect.

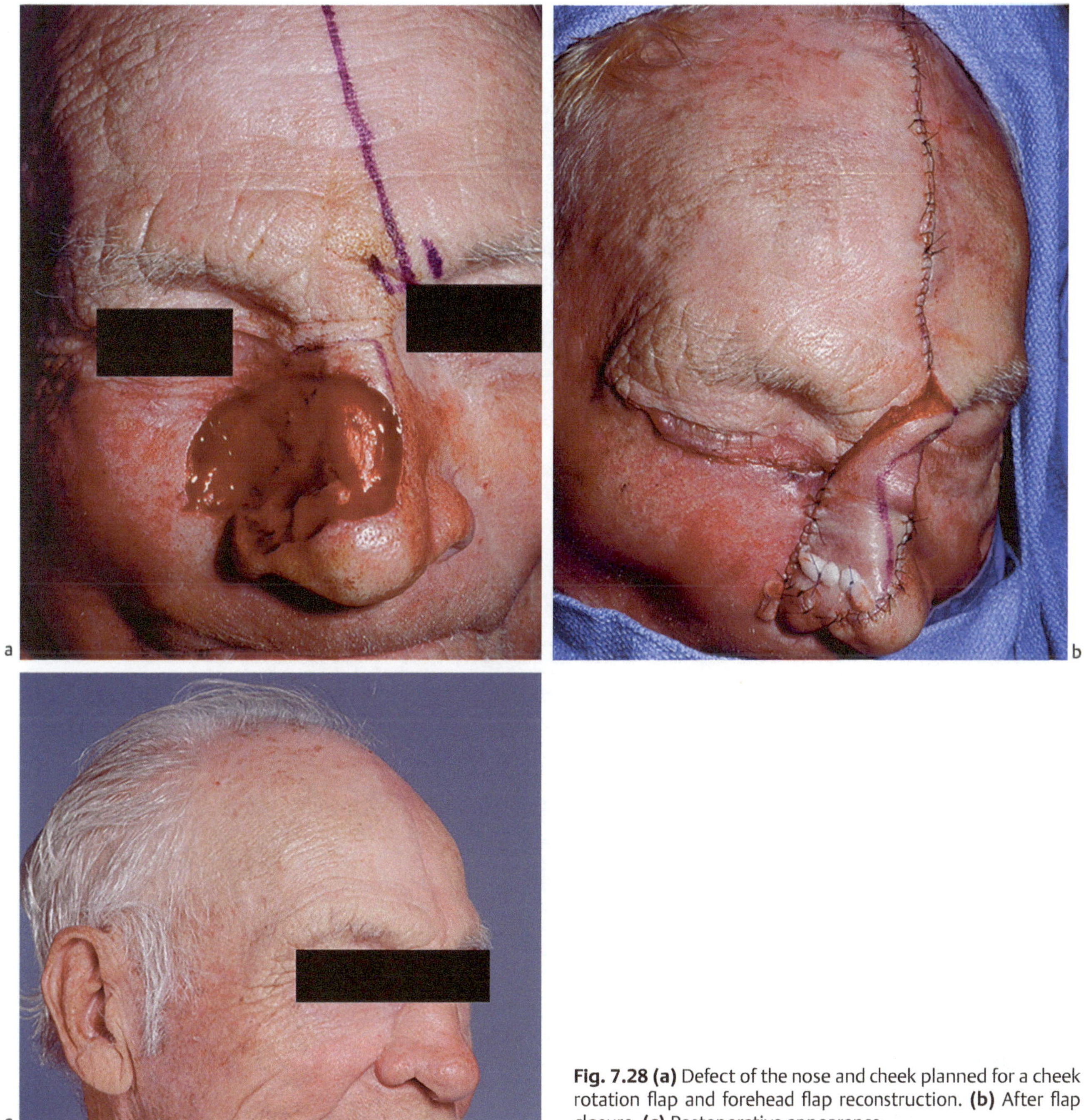

Fig. 7.28 **(a)** Defect of the nose and cheek planned for a cheek rotation flap and forehead flap reconstruction. **(b)** After flap closure. **(c)** Postoperative appearance.

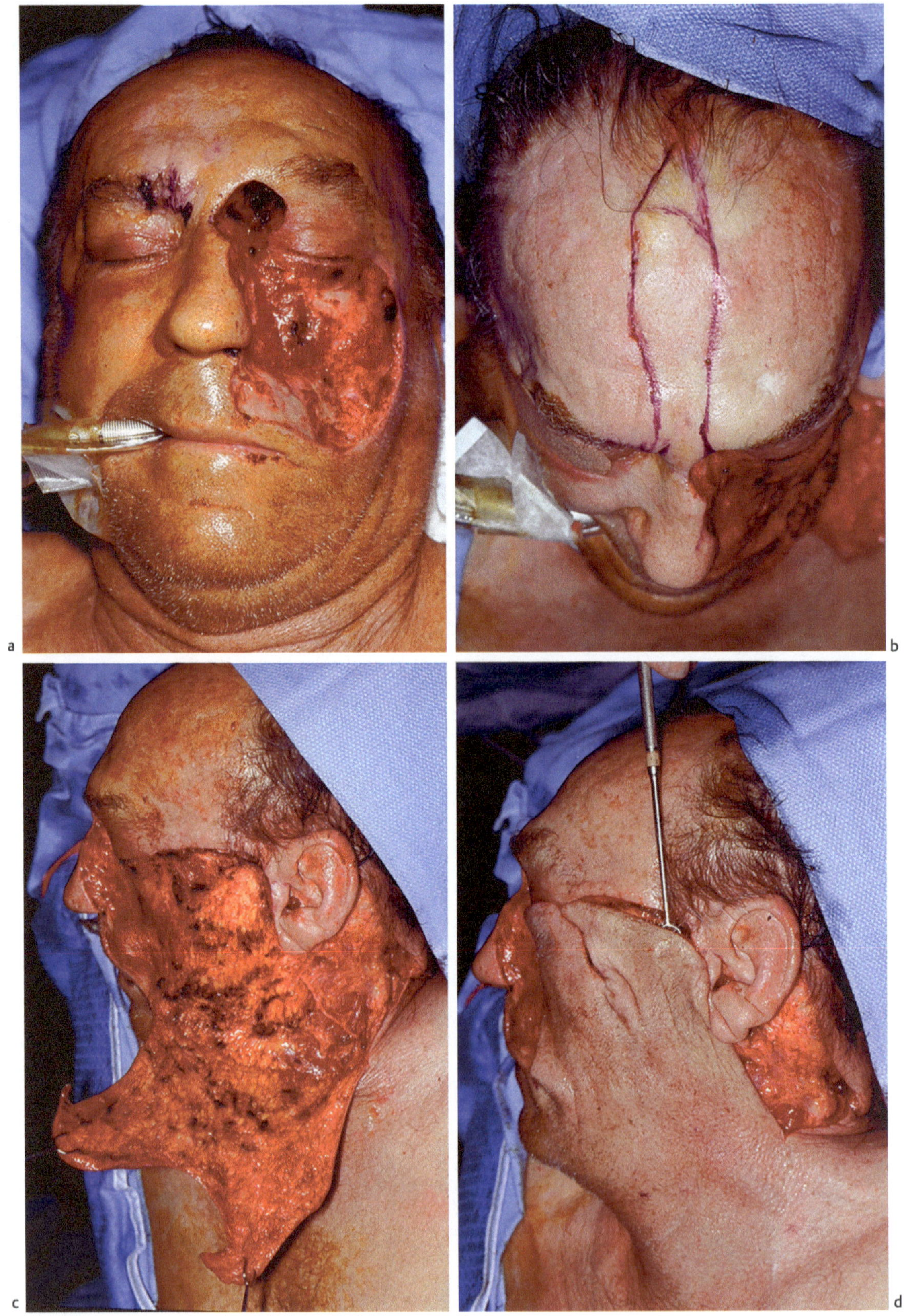

Fig. 7.29 (a) Large cutaneous defect of the cheek, eyelid, and nose. **(b)** Large paramedian forehead flap for nasal reconstruction. The donor site of the forehead will be closed primarily in the midline because of the patient's high hairline. **(c)** Large bilobed cervicofacial flap elevated. **(d)** Bilobed flap transposed into place.

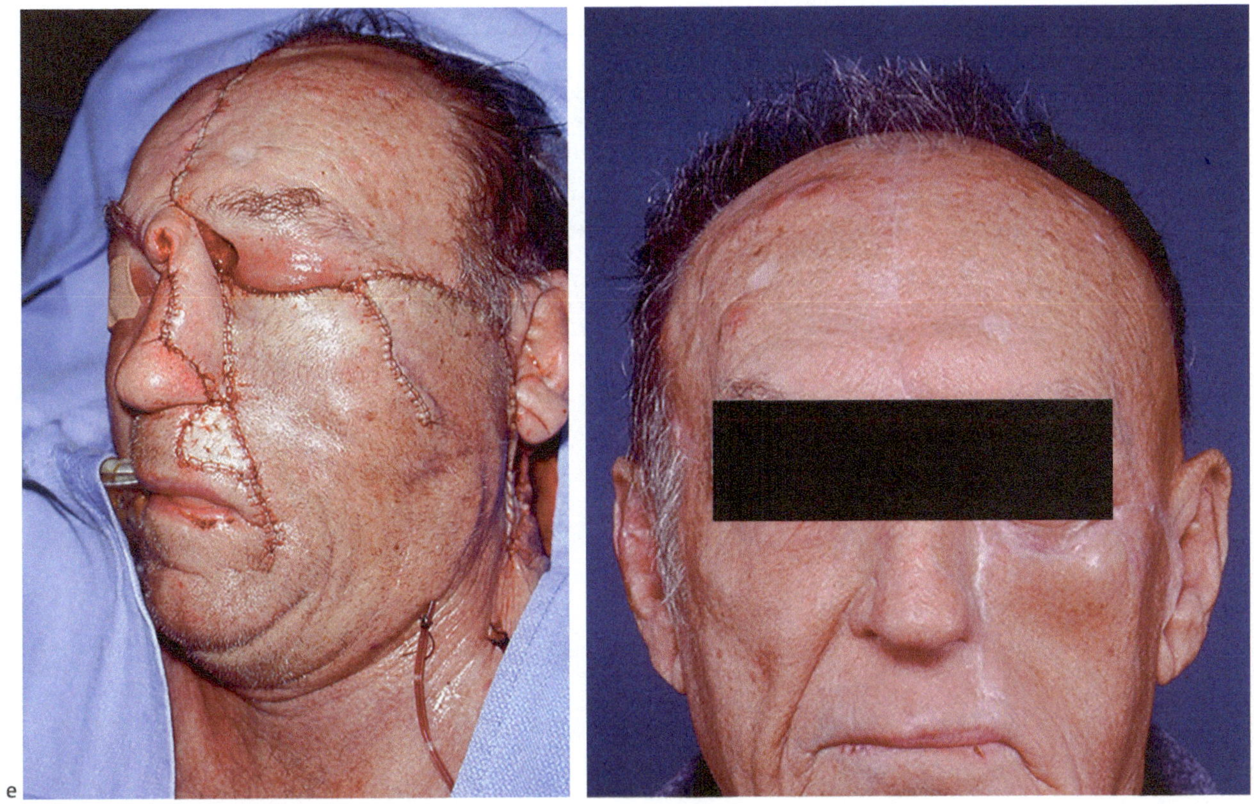

Fig. 7.29 (e) Flap is closed in place. The upper lip was reconstructed with a full-thickness skin graft. (f) Postoperative appearance.

Suggested Reading

Becker FF. Rhomboid flap in facial reconstruction: new concept of tension lines. Arch Otolaryngol 1979;105(10):569–573

Borges AF. The rhombic flap. Plast Reconstr Surg 1981;67(4):458–466

Cook TA, Davis RE. Cheek reconstruction. Oper Tech Otolaryngol—Head Neck Surg 1993;4:31–36

Cook TA, Israel JM, Wang TD, Murakami CS, Brownrigg PJ. Cervical rotation flaps for midface resurfacing. Arch Otolaryngol Head Neck Surg 1991;117(1):77–82

Davison SP, Sherris DA, Meland NB. An algorithm for maxillectomy defect reconstruction. Laryngoscope 1998;108(2):215–219

Juri J, Juri C. Cheek reconstruction with advancement-rotation flaps. Clin Plast Surg 1981;8(2):223–226

Larrabee WF Jr, Trachy R, Sutton D, Cox K. Rhomboid flap dynamics. Arch Otolaryngol 1981;107(12):755–757

Weisberger EC, Hanke W. Reconstruction of full-thickness defects of the cheek. Arch Otolaryngol 1983;109(3):190–194

8 Ears

Summary

This chapter focuses on the specific considerations with respect to ear reconstruction. Ear reconstruction is classically complex, given the cartilage framework and intimate relationship of the skin with the perichondrium. This chapter provides a reconstruction algorithm based on the defect location from more basic primary closure of earlobe defects, to complete reconstruction using cartilage grafting and staged flaps. Specific attention is also provided with respect to the intimate relationship of perichondrium and reconstruction choice.

Keywords: helical advancement, tubed pedicle flap, helical rim, concha, bolster, star wedge excision, postauricular flap, cartilage harvest

The ear is composed of a framework of unique elastic cartilage that is extremely flexible. Laterally, this framework is covered by an inelastic, thin skin with scant, underlying subcutaneous tissue. The skin on the lateral ear is adherent to the perichondrium and thus reveals the contours of the underlying ear cartilage in great detail. On the medial surface, the skin has a greater amount of subcutaneous tissue and is much less adherent to the underlying perichondrium. Because of the extremely complex contour of the auricle, subunit division and reconstruction are not practical. Rather, the ear is more effectively divided by areas of concavity or convexity in considering reconstruction (**Fig. 8.1**).

Cartilage present in the concavities of the ear is less critical to the appearance of the ear and can be used as grafting material for other areas of the face. Cartilage grafts from the conchal bowl can be used for nose and eyelid reconstruction. Composite grafts from the superior helix are of value for nasal reconstruction. Cutaneous-perichondrial grafts from the conchal bowl are useful for nasal reconstruction; these grafts of skin and perichondrium can be used to repair partial-thickness defects of the ala and will contract minimally.

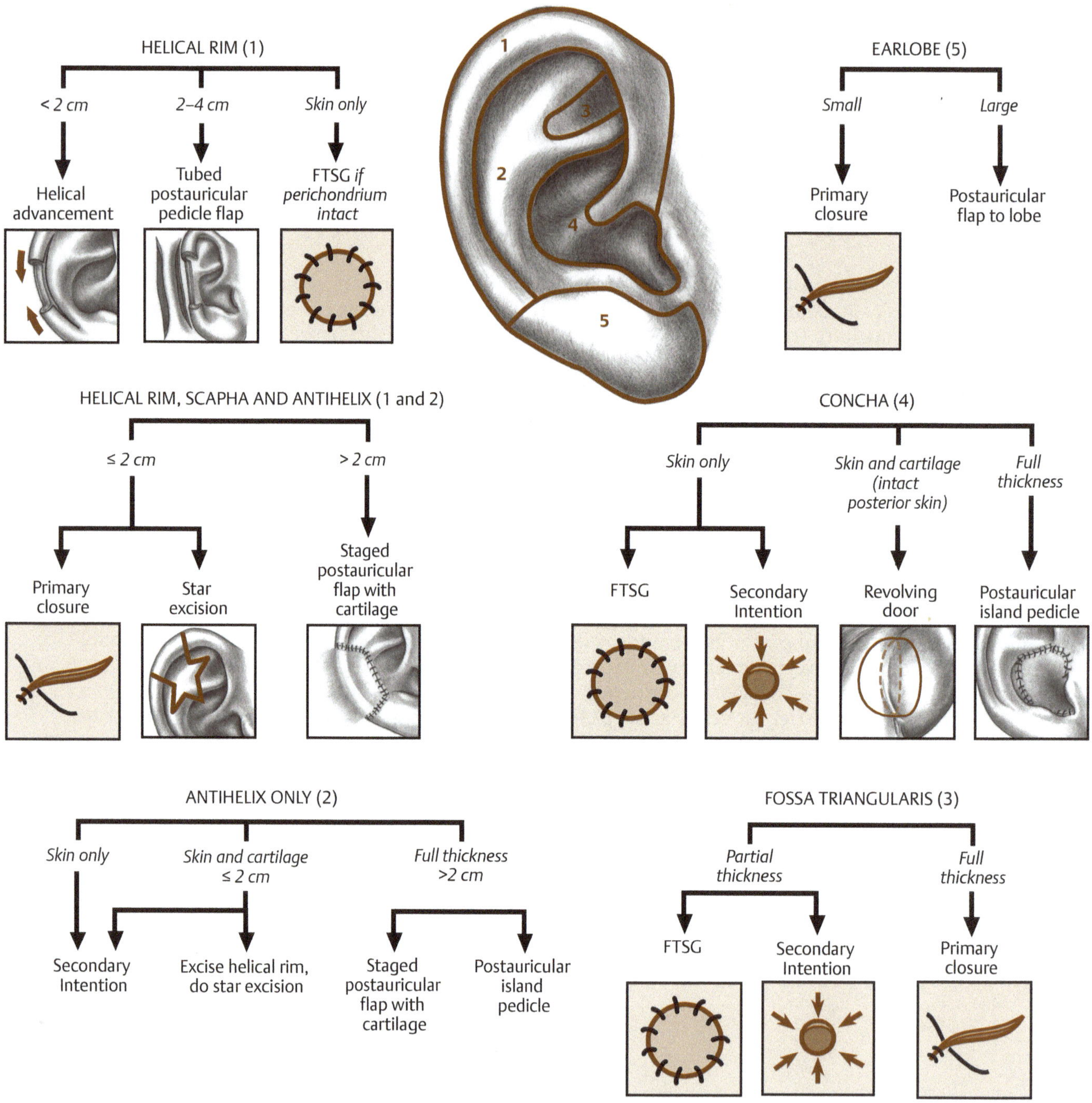

Fig. 8.1 Division of the ear. FTSG, full-thickness skin graft.

The location, depth, and size of the ear defect are all factors that must be considered in choosing appropriate reconstructive options. Defects that involve skin only and are located in a concave region of the ear can often be allowed to heal by secondary intention with acceptable cosmetic results. Skin defects overlying convexities tend to heal less well by secondary intention, though some patients will accept the results to avoid surgery. Small defects over a convexity of the ear can be repaired with a full-thickness skin graft (FTSG) or by mobilization of adjacent skin from a concave region, which can, in turn, be allowed to heal by secondary intention (**Fig. 8.2**).

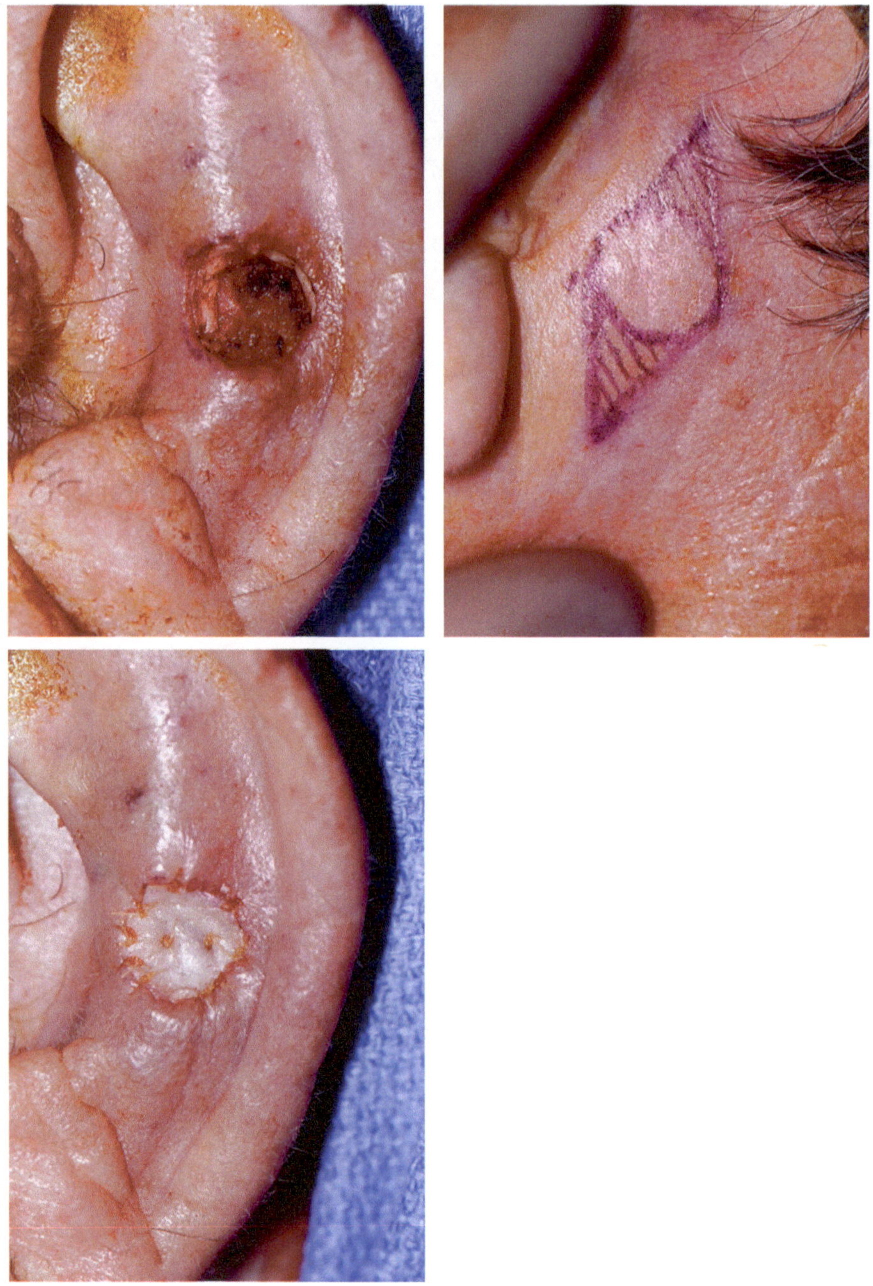

Fig. 8.2 (a) Defect of a convex portion of the ear. **(b)** Postauricular skin is a good donor site for full-thickness skin grafts (FTSGs). **(c)** FTSG sewn into place.

Defects of the concha that include loss of anterior skin and cartilage can be treated with either an FTSG or a "revolving door" postauricular flap (**Fig. 8.3** and **Fig. 8.4**). The "revolving door" flap recruits the postauricular skin as an island pedicle flap to reconstruct the anterior concha. Approximately one-third of the skin is taken from the back of the auricle and two-thirds from the skin posterior to the sulcus. The donor site is closed primarily.

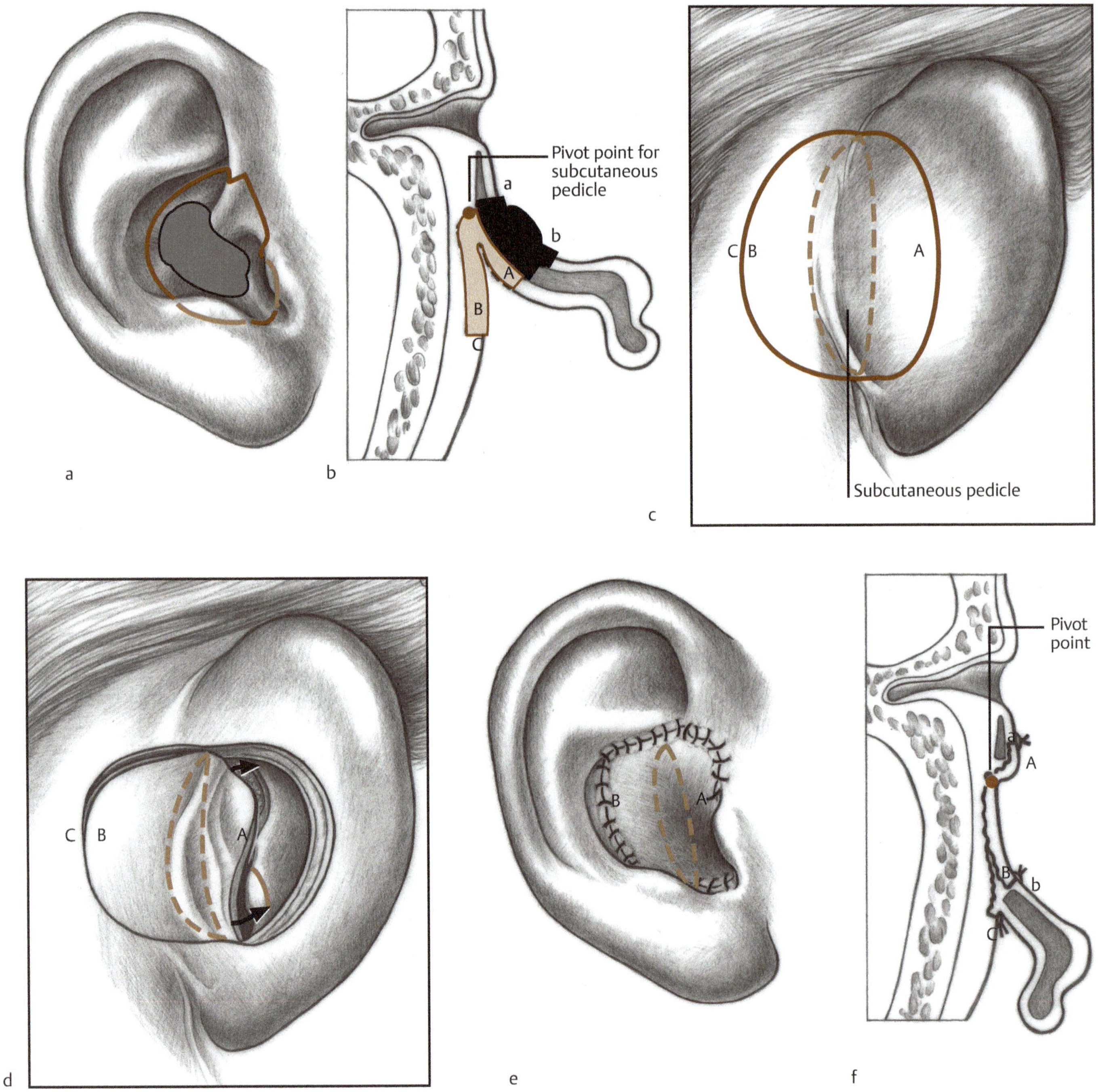

Fig. 8.3 (a–f) Postauricular revolving door flap.

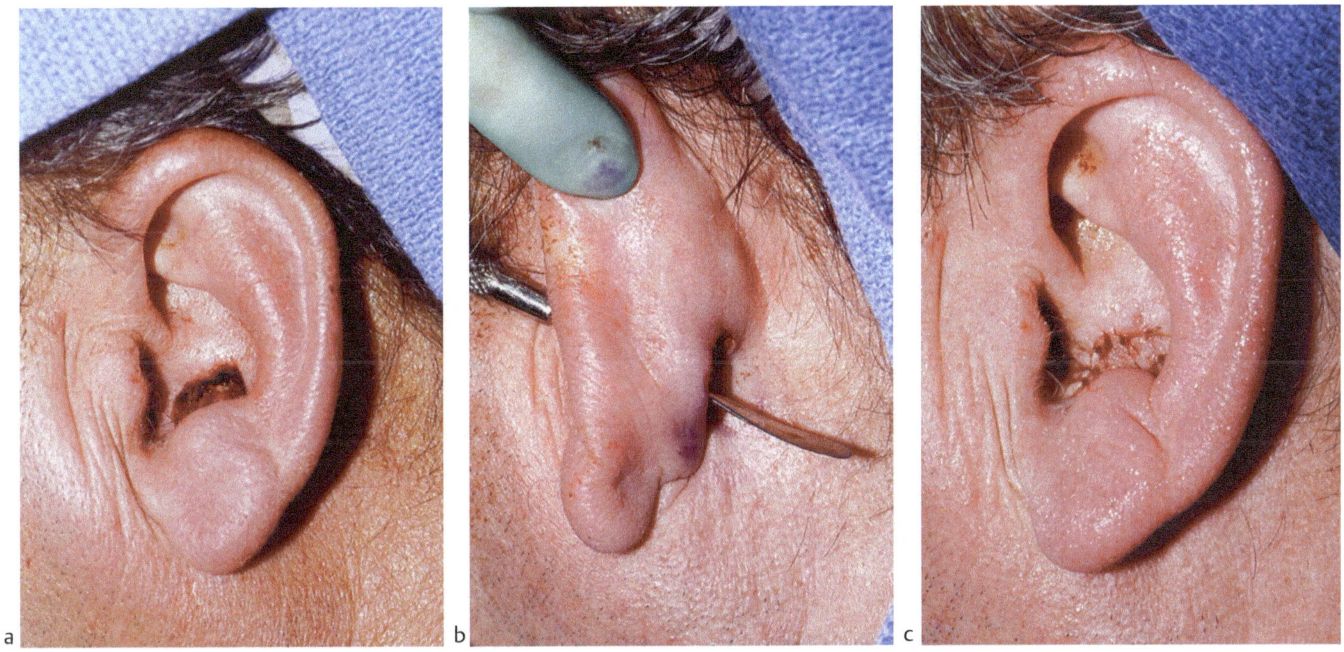

Fig. 8.4 (a) Conchal bowl defect involving anterior skin and cartilage. **(b)** A through-and-through defect is produced after an incision is made in the postauricular skin, and the flap is pulled forward into the defect. **(c)** The flap is sewn in place, and the postauricular skin is closed onto itself.

Through-and-through defects of the concha are repaired with a staged postauricular island flap. In the first stage, an island pedicle flap based on the postauricular skin is created, and its margins sutured to the skin of the anterior defect. At a second stage, 3 or more weeks later, the base of the flap with abundant subcutaneous tissue is severed, and the resulting defect is repaired with a combination of primary closure and an FTSG.

Skin-only defects involving the helix or ear margin may be repaired with local skin flaps from the adjacent postauricular surface. Such defects of the lobule or anterior helix can be repaired with a one-stage flap, whereas defects on the midportion may require a staged procedure, with severance of the flap base at 3 weeks.

A tear of the earlobe is common and is usually secondary to an earring pulled through the base of a pierced ear. A simple closure may result in notching at the earlobe margin; therefore, a small Z-plasty is incorporated in the repair (**Fig. 8.5**). Each limb of the Z-plasty only needs to be the width of a no. 15 blade. The patient should not pierce the ear for 3 to 6 months postoperatively, or the defect may recur. Clip-on earrings can be worn in the interim.

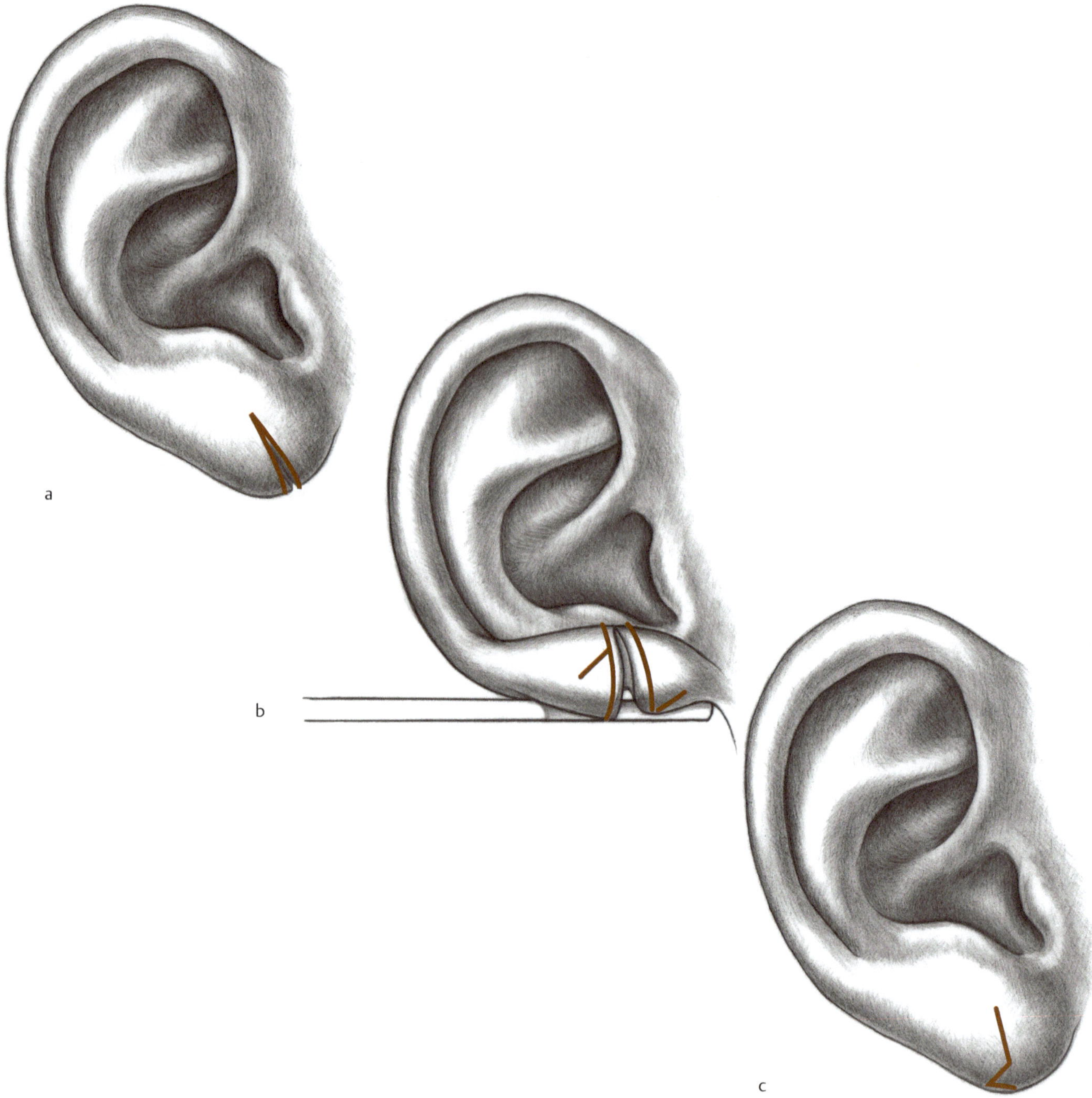

Fig. 8.5 (a–c) Z-plasty repair of the torn earlobe defect.

More extensive earlobe defects can be reconstructed with a flap of postauricular skin (**Fig. 8.6**). Subcutaneous tissue to the depth of the mastoid periosteum is elevated with the flap to better reconstruct the thick natural lobule. The deep layer of the flap is tailored prior to closure. Septal cartilage may be placed between the flaps to prevent contracture of the reconstructed earlobe.

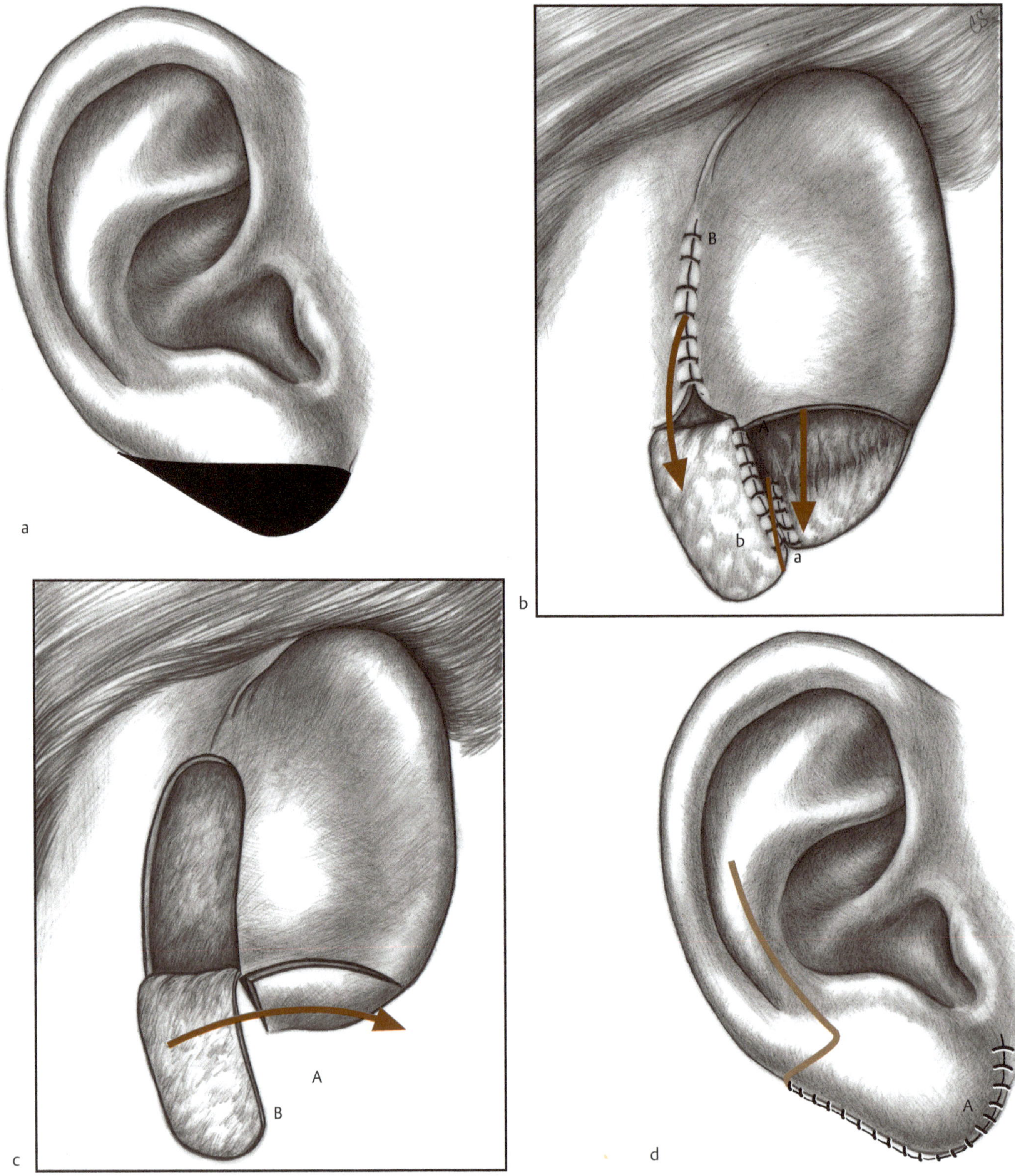

Fig. 8.6 (a–d) Earlobe reconstruction.

Defects involving both skin and cartilage of the helical rim that are < 2 cm are repaired using helical rim and advancement flaps (**Fig. 8.7** and **Fig. 8.8**). These flaps are elevated along the helix and may consist of one long flap or two shorter flaps, depending on the direction(s) from which tissue can be advanced. The flaps are cut through anterior skin and cartilage only. The postauricular skin is undermined widely to allow tissue advancement. The flaps are then advanced with a vascular supply from both the helical base and postauricular skin. The cartilage is reapproximated with 5–0 or 6–0 absorbable sutures with the knots tied medially. After closure of the two helical flaps, redundant postauricular skin is excised. Burow triangles of cartilage may need to be excised opposite the flaps to lower closing tension. The skin is closed with 6–0 monofilament permanent sutures.

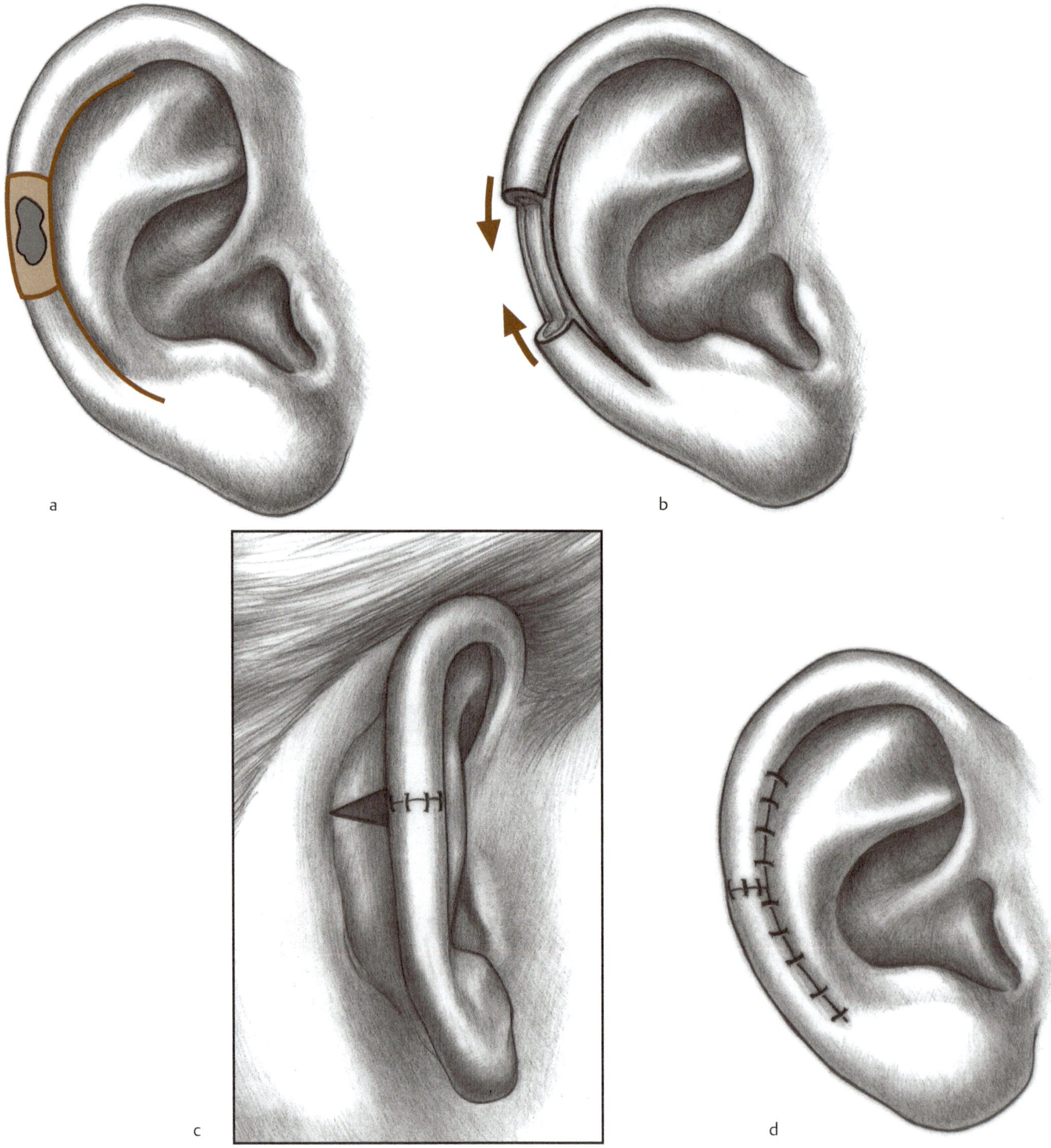

Fig. 8.7 (a–d) Bilateral helical advancement flaps.

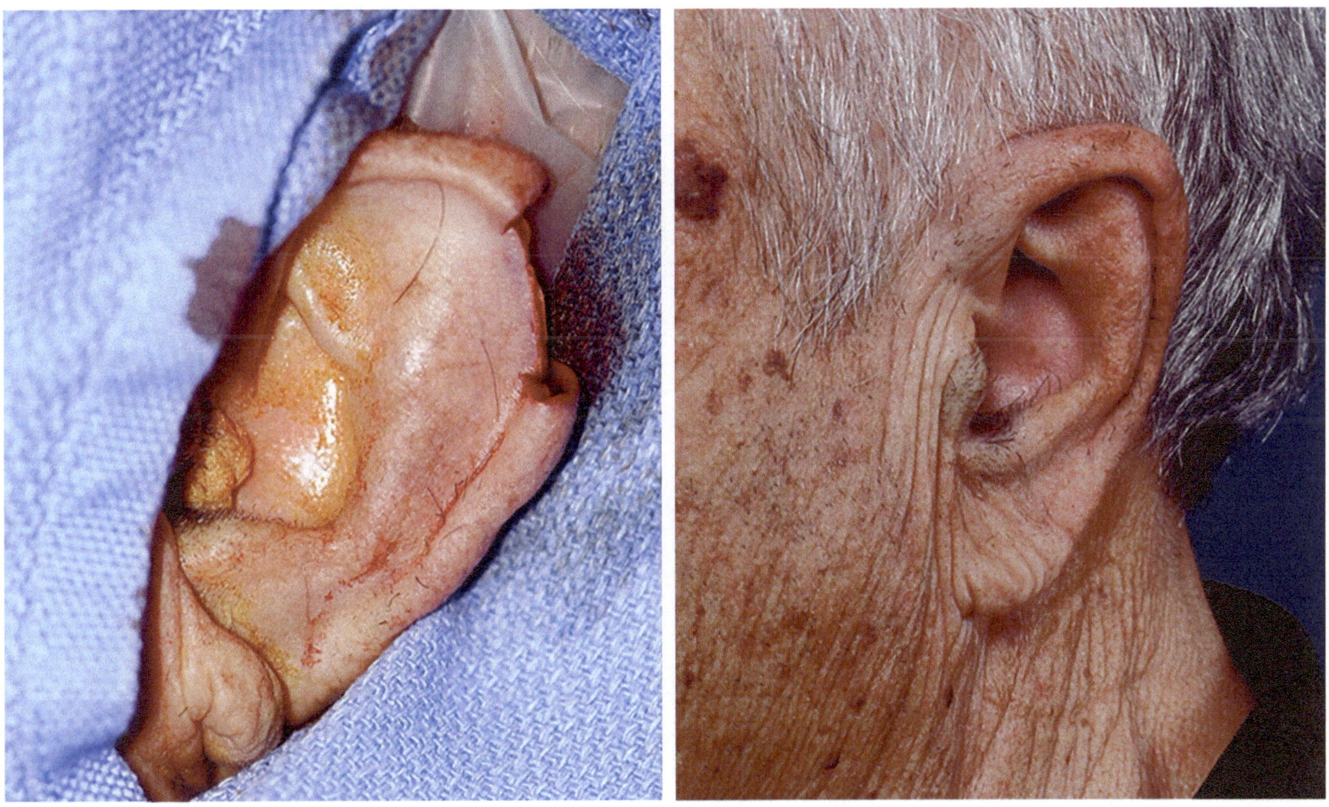

a b

Fig. 8.8 (a) Full-thickness defect of the helical rim. **(b)** Postoperative appearance.

Extensive defects of the helix involving both skin and cartilage are repaired with a tubed-bipedicled postauricular flap (**Fig. 8.9** and **Fig. 8.10**). At the first stage, a bipedicled flap of postauricular skin is created and tubed on itself over a cartilage graft from the ipsilateral or contralateral concha. It is usually necessary to recruit essentially the entire width of skin from the auricular sulcus to the hairline. Three weeks after primary surgery, the superior end of the flap is cut and transferred to the defect site. As much of the flap as possible is sutured to the donor site, leaving it pedicled inferiorly. The inferior pedicle both facilitates venous drainage and provides improved arterial blood supply. Three or more weeks later, the base of the pedicle is severed and inset. The donor area can be skin grafted if it cannot be closed primarily.

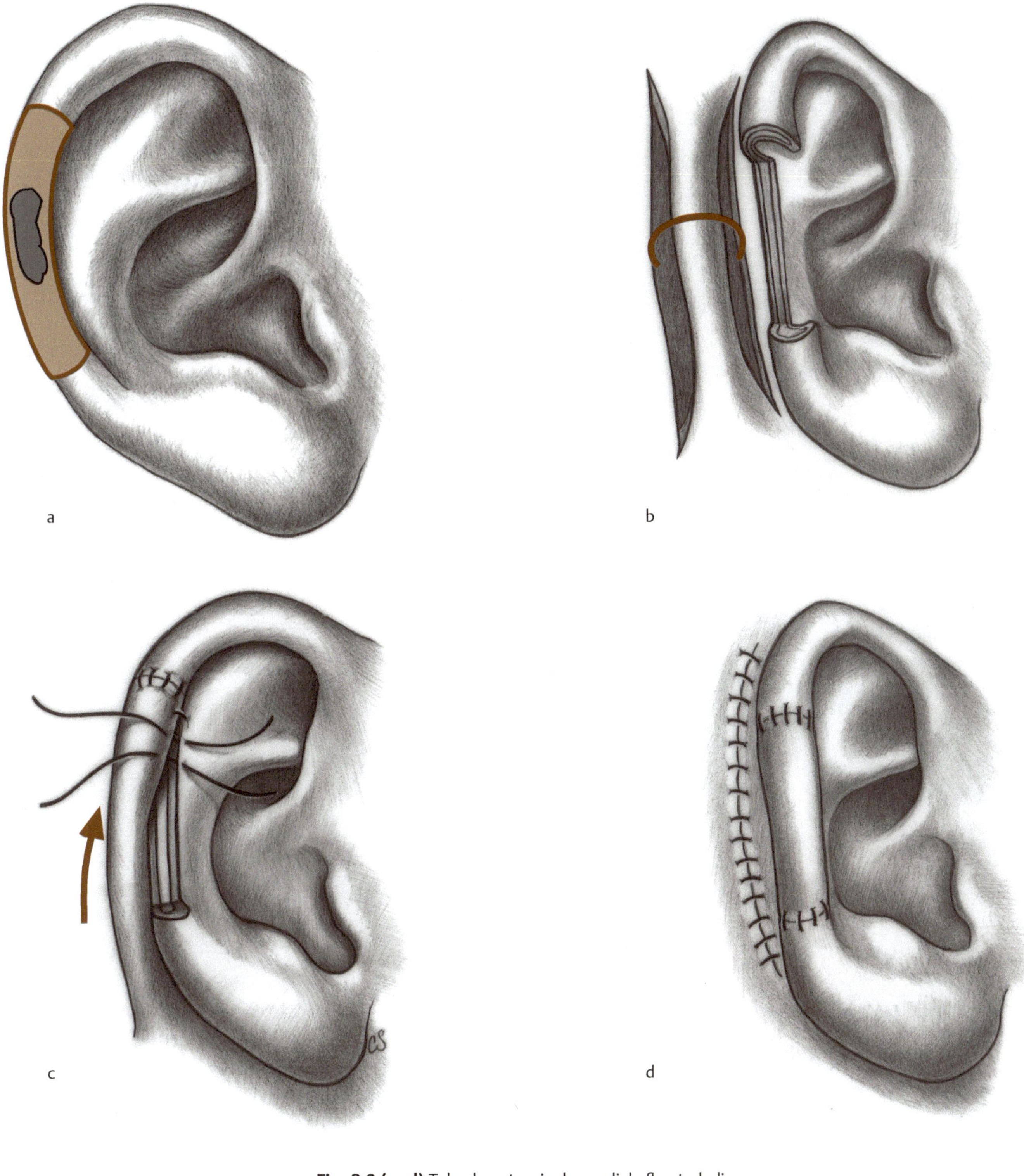

a b c d

Fig. 8.9 (a–d) Tubed postauricular pedicle flap to helix.

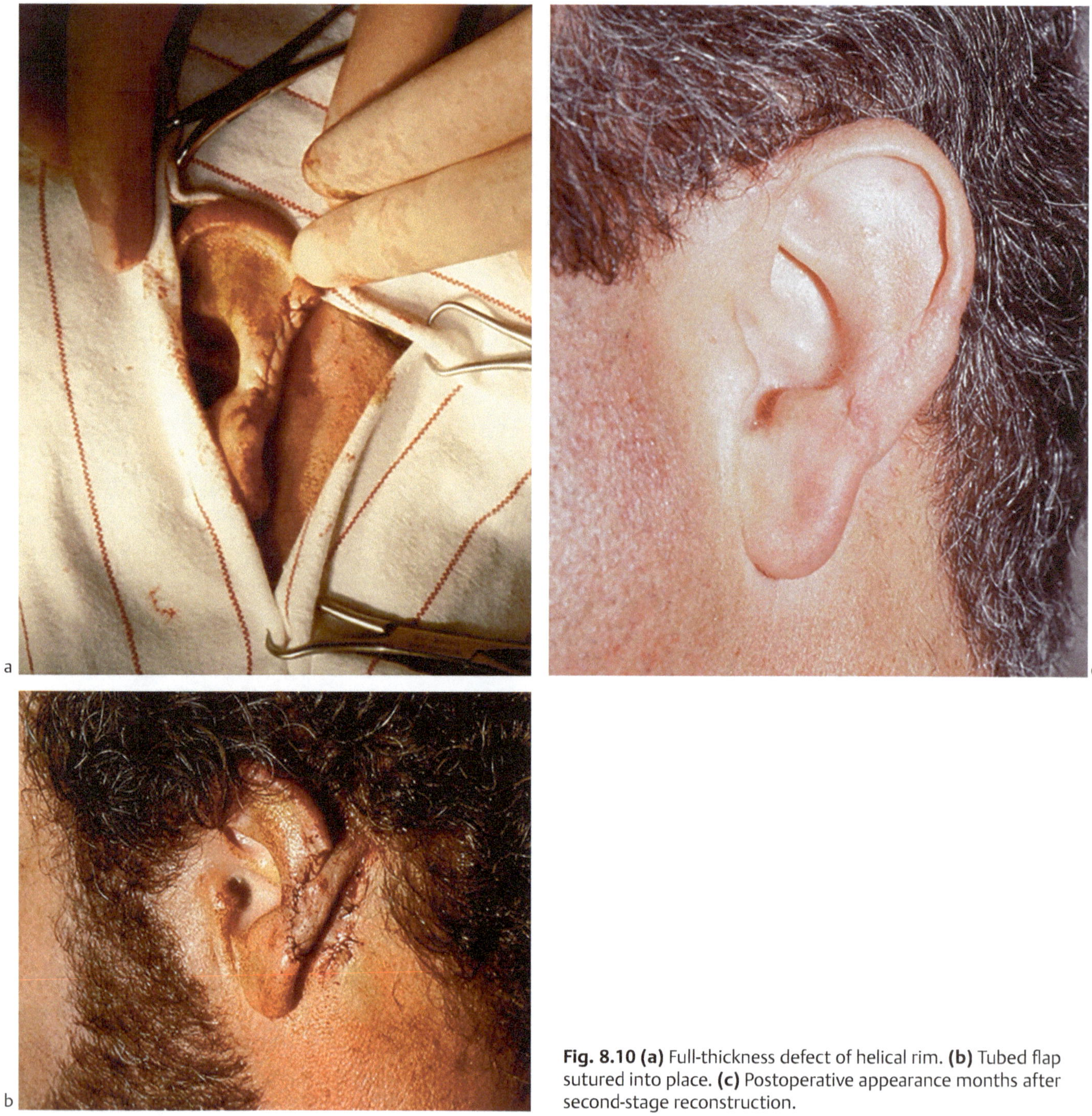

Fig. 8.10 (a) Full-thickness defect of helical rim. **(b)** Tubed flap sutured into place. **(c)** Postoperative appearance months after second-stage reconstruction.

Full-thickness defects involving both the helix and adjacent tissue of the antihelix, and no larger than 25% of the ear, can be repaired primarily. A star-shaped excision is necessary to prevent excessive wound-closing tension and buckling of the cartilage (**Fig. 8.11** and **Fig. 8.12**). After completion of the resection, the wound is closed by first approximating the auricular cartilage with 5–0 long-lasting absorbable sutures employed in a through-and-through manner that incorporates the perichondrium. Knots are tied on the medial surface of the ear to lessen the chance of extrusion. Skin closure is with 5–0 or 6–0 nylon, with sutures removed at 5 to 7 days. This usually results in the creation of an ear with excellent contour but noticeably smaller than the contralateral ear.

In larger helical rim defects, a wedge can be excised to make the ear slightly small and to allow for helical advancement flap closure (**Fig. 8.13**). This approach represents a combination of the wedge excision technique and the helical rim advancement flap.

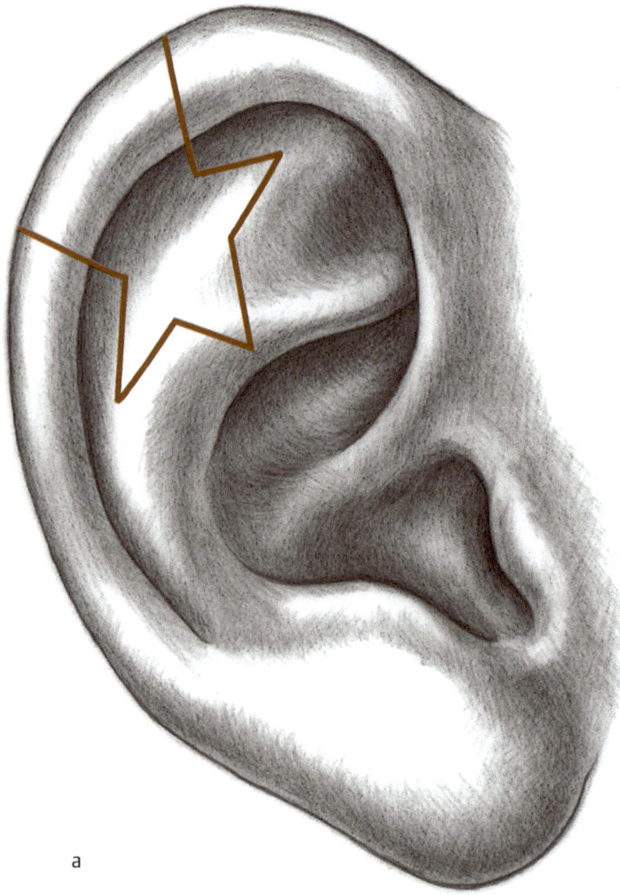

a

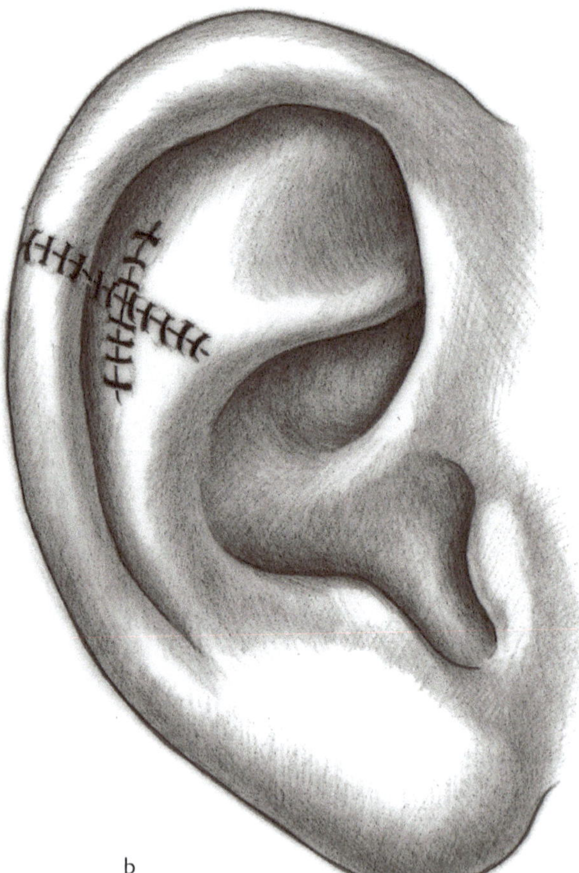

b

Fig. 8.11 (a, b) Star-shaped wedge excision.

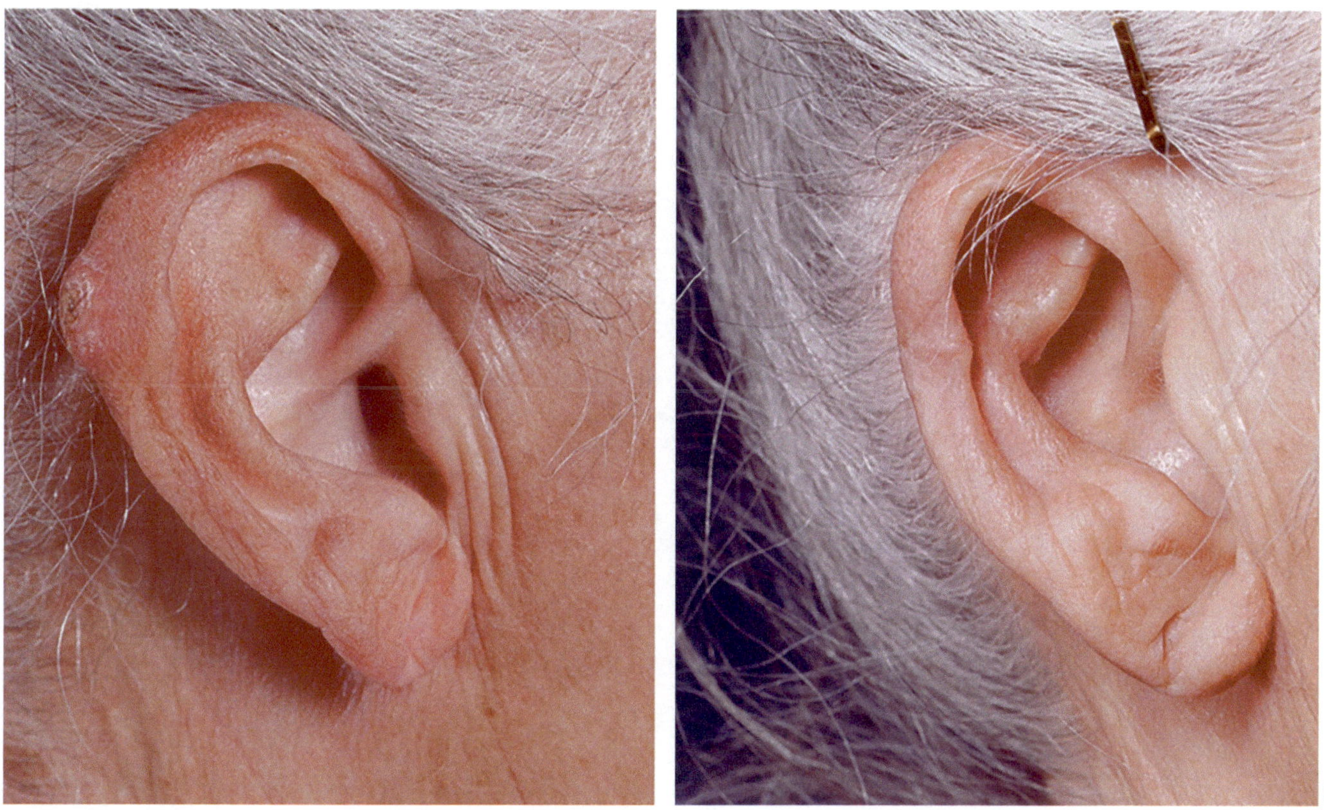

Fig. 8.12 (a) Lesion of the helical rim. **(b)** After star-shaped excision with primary repair.

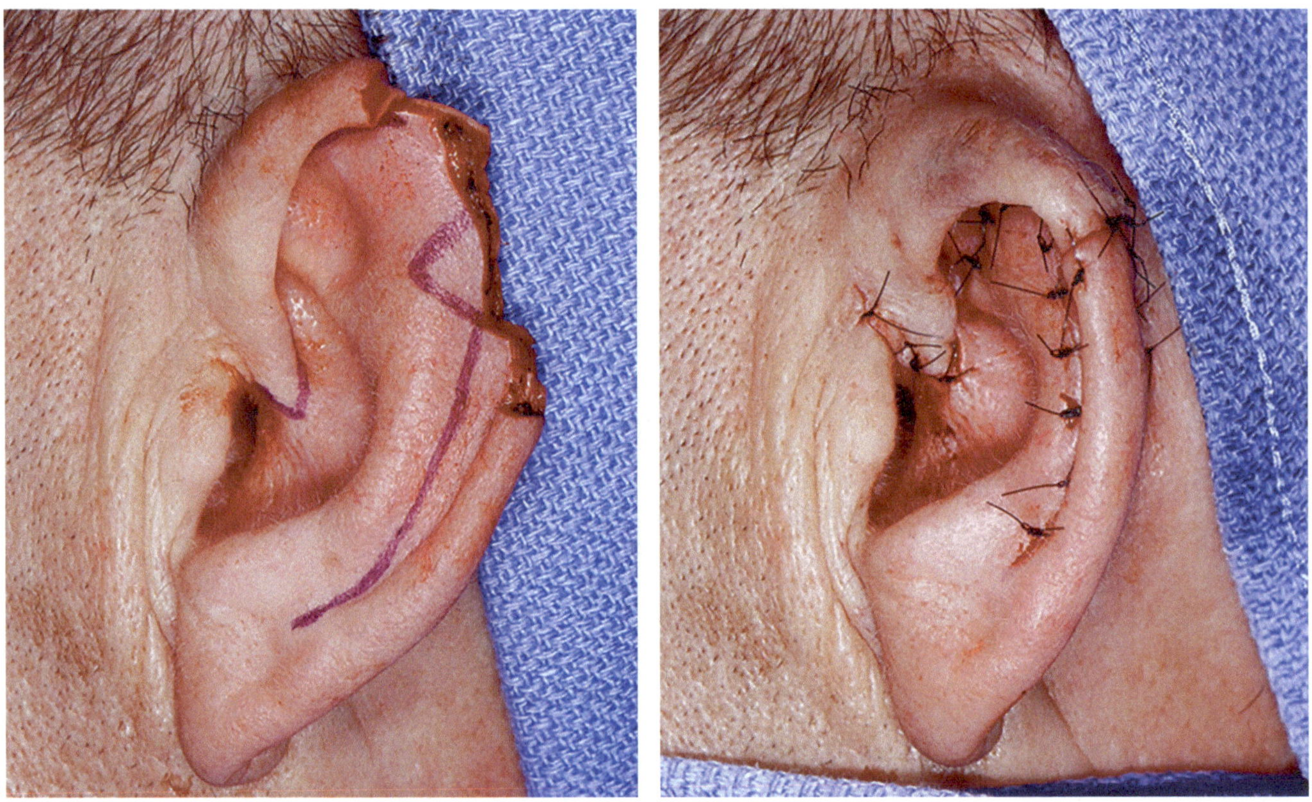

Fig. 8.13 (a) Defect planned for combined wedge excision and helical advancement flaps. **(b)** After closure, the auricle appears somewhat smaller, but the contour is excellent.

More extensive defects involving the middle third of the helix, antihelix, and portions of the concha are usually repaired with staged postauricular flaps (**Fig. 8.14**). At the first stage, a cartilage graft from a rib is designed and sutured to the remaining auricular cartilage defect. The postauricular flap is then advanced over this graft and sutured to the anterior skin of the defect. The postauricular sulcus is preserved when possible. After 3 weeks, the flap base is severed, and the remainder of the flap is used to create the posterior helix (see dotted lines in **Fig. 8.14a**). The dotted lines represent the point of secondary incision. The skin is then flipped onto the back of the ear at the second stage. The remaining defect is closed with a skin graft. Bolsters or a triangular fixation suture may be required to help create the sulcus between the helix and the antihelix.

Extensive auricular reconstructions are performed with rib cartilage grafts, the temporoparietal fascia flap, and, occasionally, tissue expansion. These reconstructions are beyond the scope of this book, and readers are referred to the work of Brent.

Suggested Reading

Antia NH, Buch VI. Chondrocutaneous advancement flap for the marginal defect of the ear. Plast Reconstr Surg 1967;39(5):472–477

Brent B. Reconstruction of traumatic ear deformities. Clin Plast Surg 1978;5(3):437–445

Brent B, Byrd HS. Secondary ear reconstruction with cartilage grafts covered by axial, random, and free flaps of temporoparietal fascia. Plast Reconstr Surg 1983;72(2):141–152

Bumsted RM. Methods of therapy and reconstruction of malignant auricular neoplasms. Facial Plast Surg 1987;5(1):19–27

Bumsted RM, Ceilley RI. Auricular malignant neoplasms. Identification of high-risk lesions and selection of method of reconstruction. Arch Otolaryngol 1982;108(4):225–231

Chen C, Chen ZJ. Reconstruction of the concha of the ear using a postauricular island flap. Plast Reconstr Surg 1990;86(3):569–572

Converse JM. Traumatic deformities of the auricle. In: Surgical Treatment of Facial Injuries. Baltimore: Williams & Wilkins; 1974:11289–11334

Field LM. The single-pedicle retroauricular advancement flap. J Dermatol Surg Oncol 1988;14(7):722–727

Krespi YP, Ries WR, Shugar JMA, Sisson GA. Auricular reconstruction with postauricular myocutaneous flap. Otolaryngol Head Neck Surg 1983;91(2):193–196

Mellette JR Jr. Ear reconstruction with local flaps. J Dermatol Surg Oncol 1991;17(2):176–182

Millard DR Jr. Reconstruction of one-third plus of the auricular circumference. Plast Reconstr Surg 1992;90(3):475–478

Sanniec K, Harirah M, Thornton J. Ear Reconstruction after Mohs Cancer Excision: Lessons Learned from 327 Consecutive Cases. Plast Reconstr Surg 2019;144(3):719-729

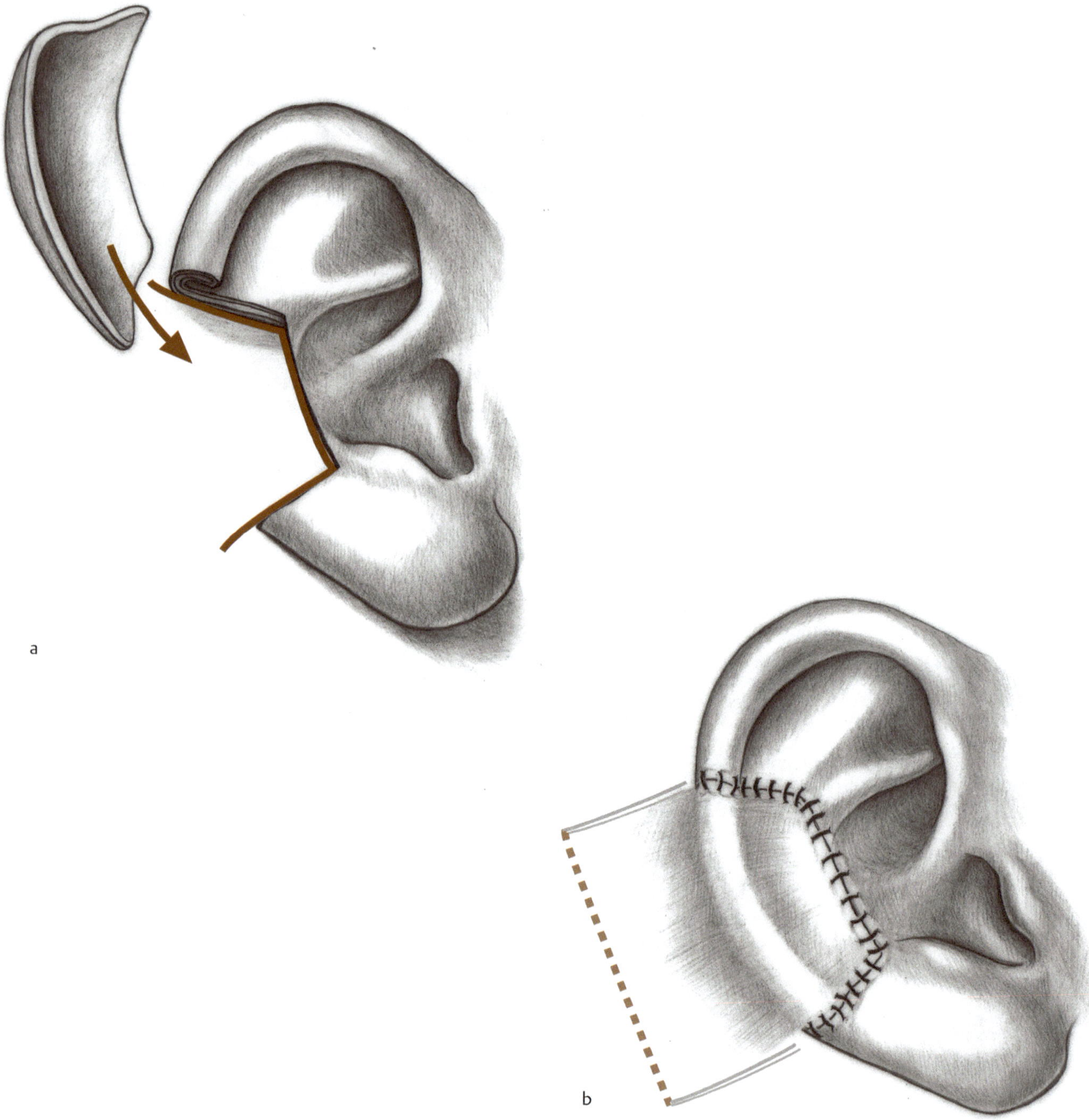

a

b

Fig. 8.14 (a, b) Postauricular flap with cartilage graft.

9 Lips and Chin

Summary

This chapter focuses on reconstruction of lip and chin defects with the goal of provide oral competence for speech and oral feeding. Lip reconstruction algorithm is directed by size with smaller defects predominantly closed with primary closure and larger defects requiring closure with well-designed flaps. The oral commissure is of added challenge and such reconstruction principles are discussed in this chapter.

Keywords: estlander flap, Abbe flap, bilateral advancement flap, karapandzic flap, Bernard–Burow flap, Gilles fan flap, oral commissure, vermilion border

The lower third of the face is dominated by the lips, which serve as the focal point for both spoken and expressive communications. Reconstruction is influenced by both functional and aesthetic considerations. The goals of perioral reconstruction are oral competency, adequate oral access, mobility, and normal anatomical proportions. When all reconstructive goals cannot be met, oral competency and access take priority.

The lip is composed of three layers: mucosa, orbicularis oris muscle, and skin. With age, there is a decrease in the skin thickness and perioral elasticity. The resulting lip redundancy is accentuated by loss of dentition and premaxillary bone. In many cases, these changes provide excess tissue for reconstruction.

The orbicularis oris muscle comprises the bulk of the lips and lacks bony attachments. Blood supply to the lips is from the superior and inferior labial branches of the facial artery. The main arterial branches are between the intraoral mucosa and the orbicularis oris muscle.

The lips and the surrounding perioral region form the oral (labial) facial aesthetic unit (**Fig. 9.1**). The upper lip region is divided into two lateral subunits and one medial subunit, each of which should be reconstructed as a totality when possible. The lower lip region is comprised of one skin subunit. The mucosal lips are each a separate subunit. The chin is a separate aesthetic unit, separated from the lower lip by the mental crease, bordered laterally by an extension of the crease and inferiorly by the inferior border of the mandible. Because of the close proximity of the chin and the relative rarity of cutaneous defects of the chin, this unit will be discussed in this chapter.

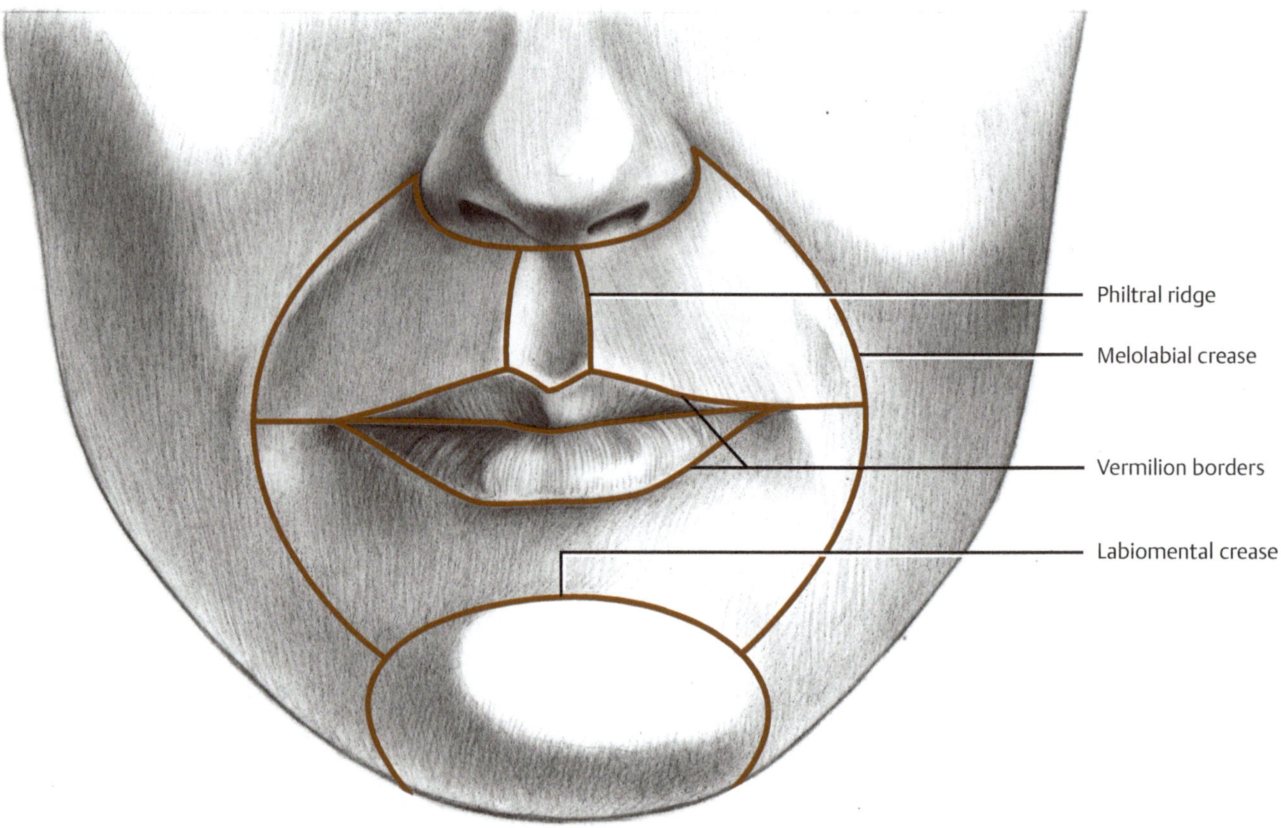

Fig. 9.1 Aesthetic subunits of the lip.

♦ Lower Lip and Chin

Partial Thickness

Because the majority of lower lip carcinomas involve the vermilion, their excision usually involves a full-thickness resection. In addition to the treatment of tumors (especially squamous cell carcinoma), leukoplakia or actinic damage of the lower lip mucosa is common and should be treated with a vermilionectomy (**Fig. 9.2**). The mucosa is excised from the mucocutaneous junction posteriorly as far as the lesion extends and to the depth of the orbicularis oris musculature. The mucosa on the buccal surface of the lip is then sharply and bluntly undermined and advanced to the previous mucocutaneous junction. Minimizing the amount of mucosa sharply elevated maximizes the preservation of cutaneous sensory innervation to the mucosa and future lip sensation. This procedure can be done on the upper or lower lips or to re-create the mucosa of the lip in total lip reconstruction. If there is not enough local mucosa for advancement, a pedicled flap can be elevated from the ventral surface of the anterior tongue. This flap is left pedicled on the dorsal anterior tongue for 10 to 14 days prior to division and inset. Using the undersurface of the tongue avoids placing the irregular surface of the dorsal tongue onto the lips.

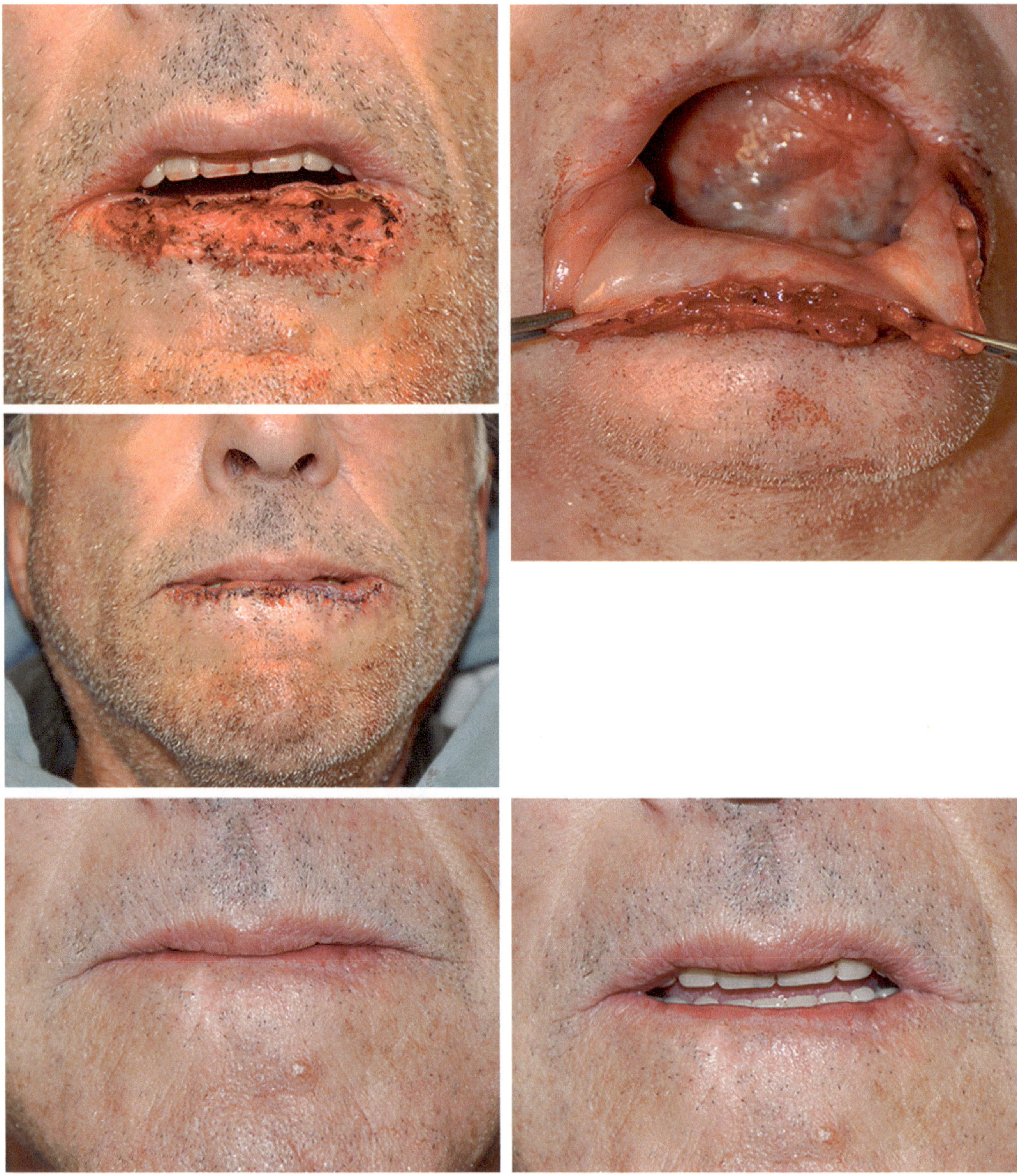

Fig. 9.2 (a) Lower lip lesion. **(b)** Lower lip vermilion mucosal advancement. **(c)** Appearance after closure. **(d)** Postoperative appearance mouth closed. **(e)** Postoperative appearance mouth open.

Skin-only defects of the lower lip are less common and can usually be closed primarily or with local skin flaps (**Fig. 9.3**). Lesions adjacent to the labiomental crease or the vermilion are closed using the A-to-T flap (**Fig. 9.4**). The releasing incisions are placed in the labiomental crease or the vermilion border, respectively, depending on the location of the lesion. The primary defect is then closed parallel to relaxed skin tension lines (RSTLs).

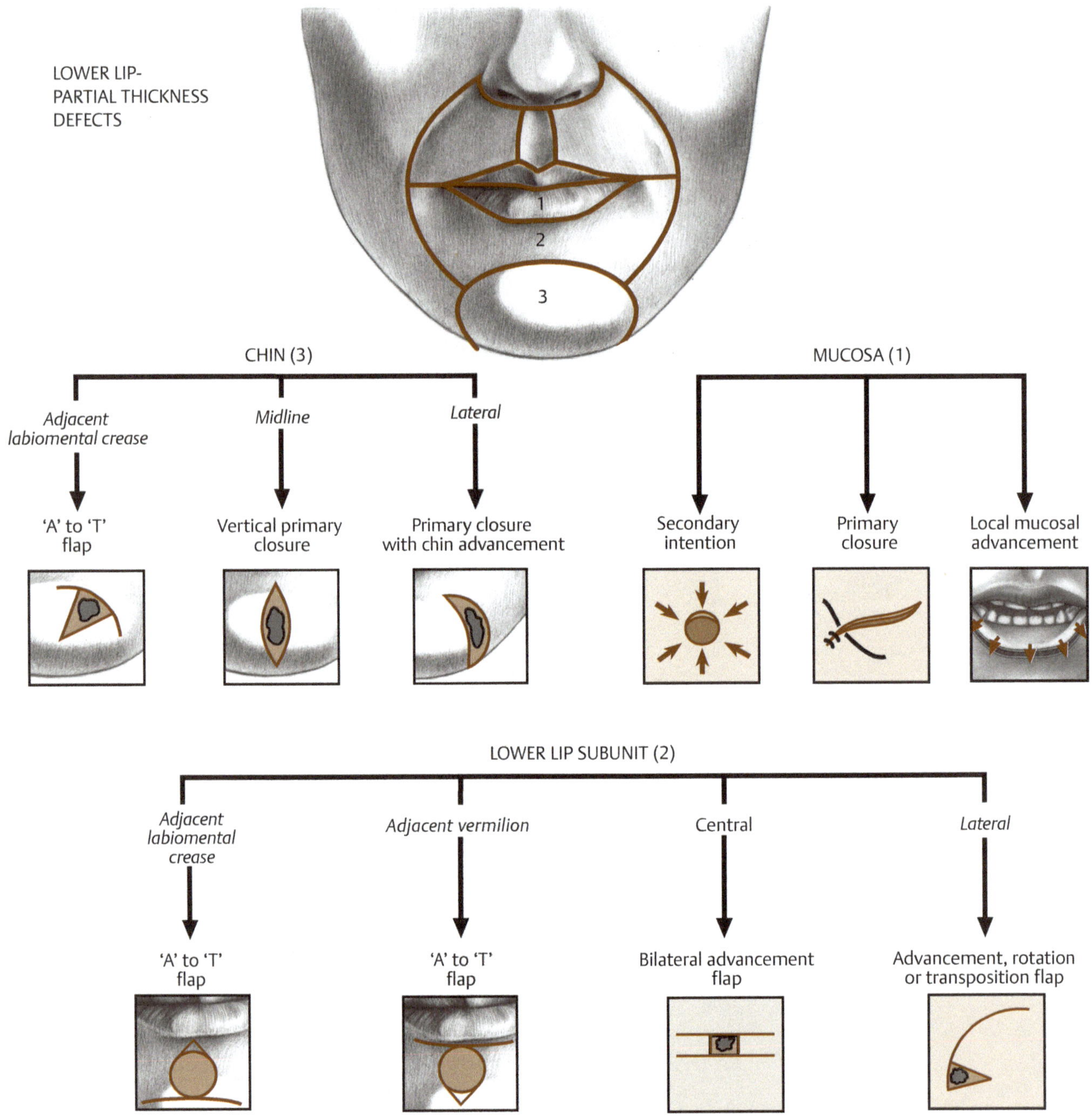

Fig. 9.3 Lower lip: partial-thickness defects.

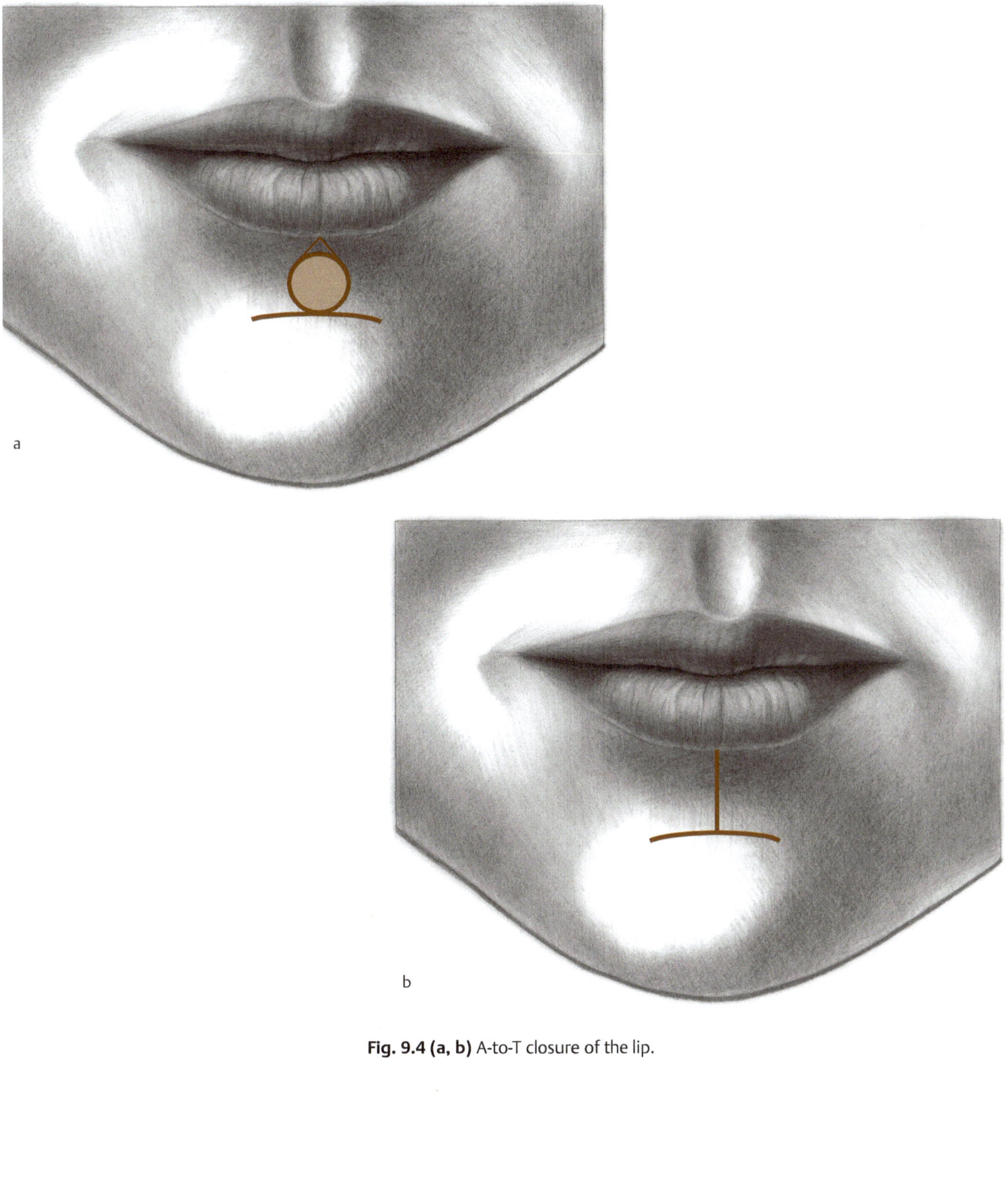

Fig. 9.4 (a, b) A-to-T closure of the lip.

Central superficial lesions of the lower lip are closed with unilateral or bilateral advancement flaps, incised in the labiomental crease and at the vermilion border, and extended onto the cheek skin as needed. Burow triangle excisions may be necessary along either of these incisions for proper wound closure. Lateral lower lip defects not corresponding to the described defects can be closed with either advancement or rotation flaps.

Defects of the chin adjacent to the labiomental crease can be closed with an A-to-T flap of appropriate depth (**Fig. 9.5** and **Fig. 9.6**). Defects of the chin in the midline can be closed with a primary vertical or horizontal closure (**Fig. 9.7**). Soft tissue can be debulked in the midline to make the chin symmetric. If the mandible is asymmetric or overly protuberant, the bone can be reduced to facilitate closure. If the defect is located off to one side, the chin can be advanced to the deficient side and contoured appropriately with subcutaneous dissection (**Fig. 9.8**). Fat "flip-flop" flaps can be used to maintain symmetry. If significant subcutaneous tissue is lost, chin augmentation with an implant may be necessary at a later time.

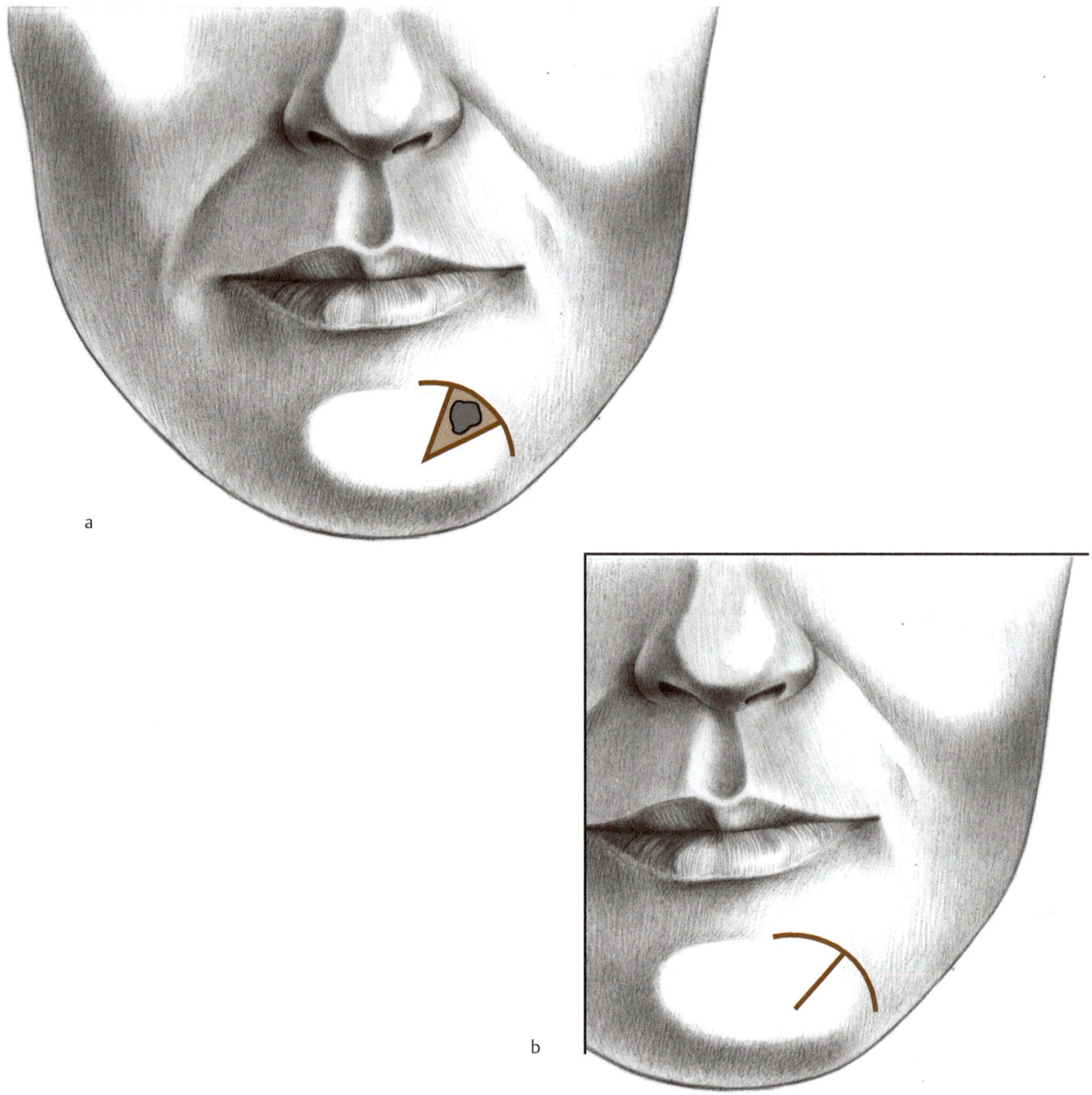

Fig. 9.5 (a, b) A-to-T closure of the chin.

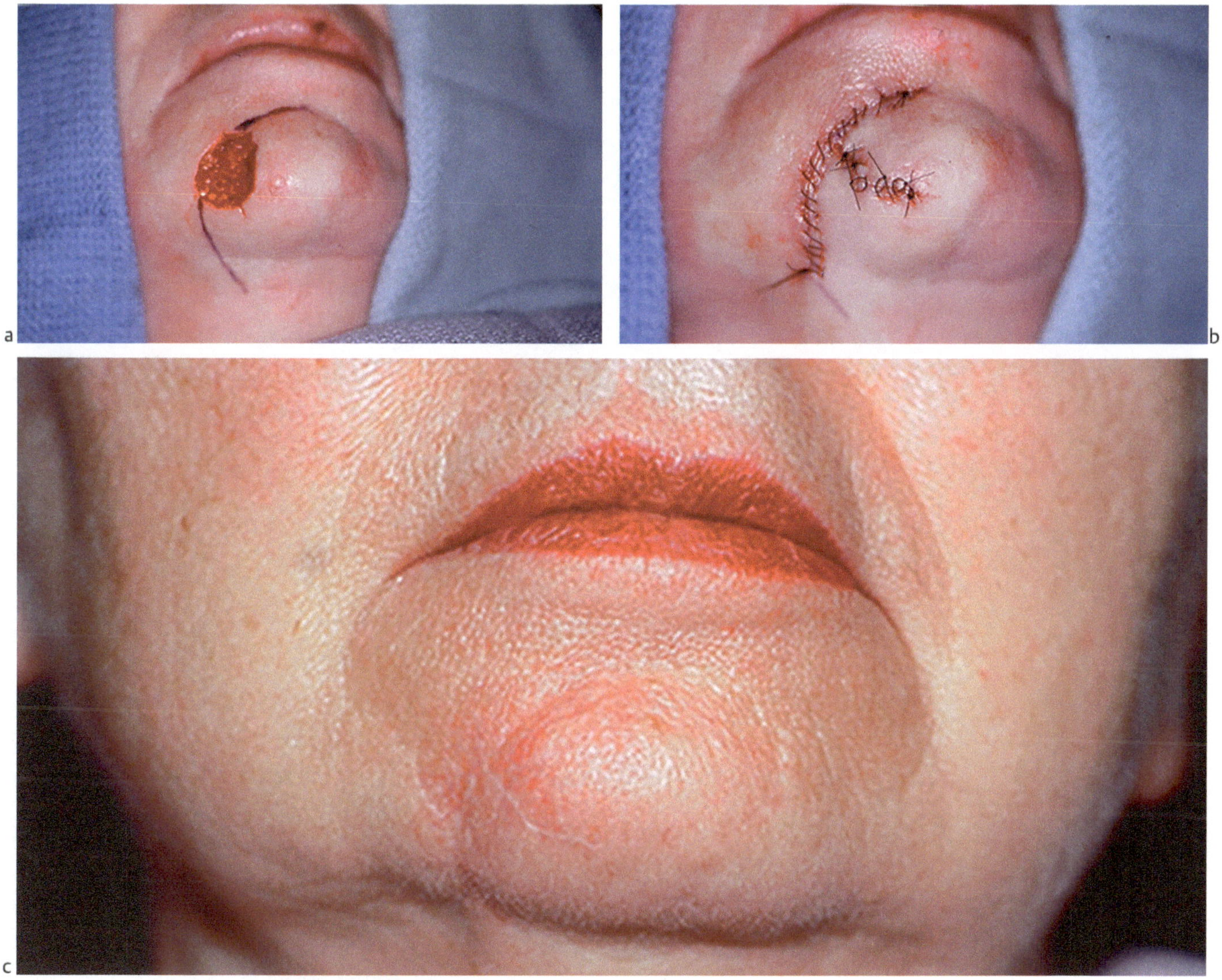

Fig. 9.6 **(a)** A-to-T flap planned for the chin. **(b)** After closure. **(c)** Late postoperative appearance.

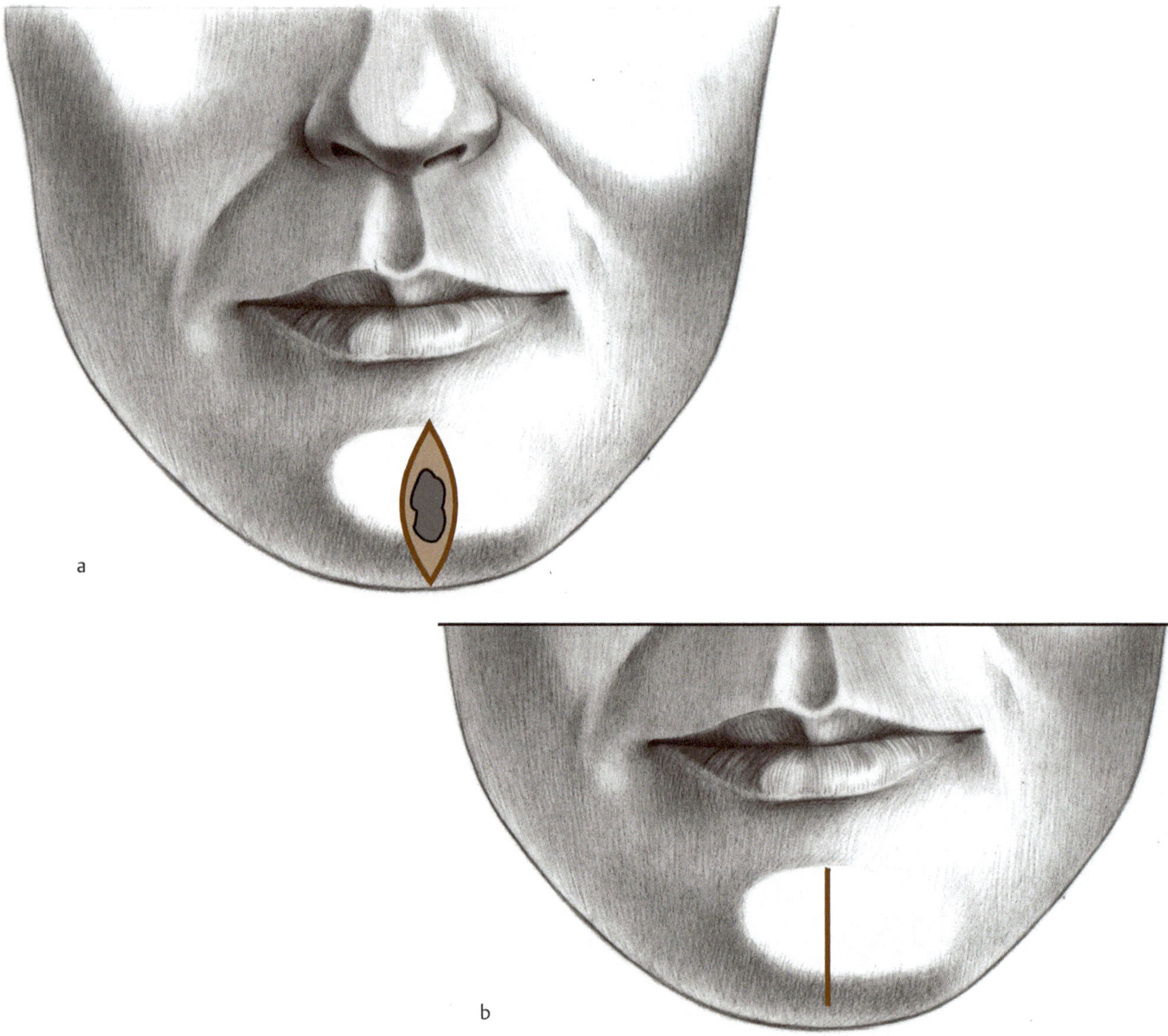

Fig. 9.7 (a, b) Primary midline chin closure.

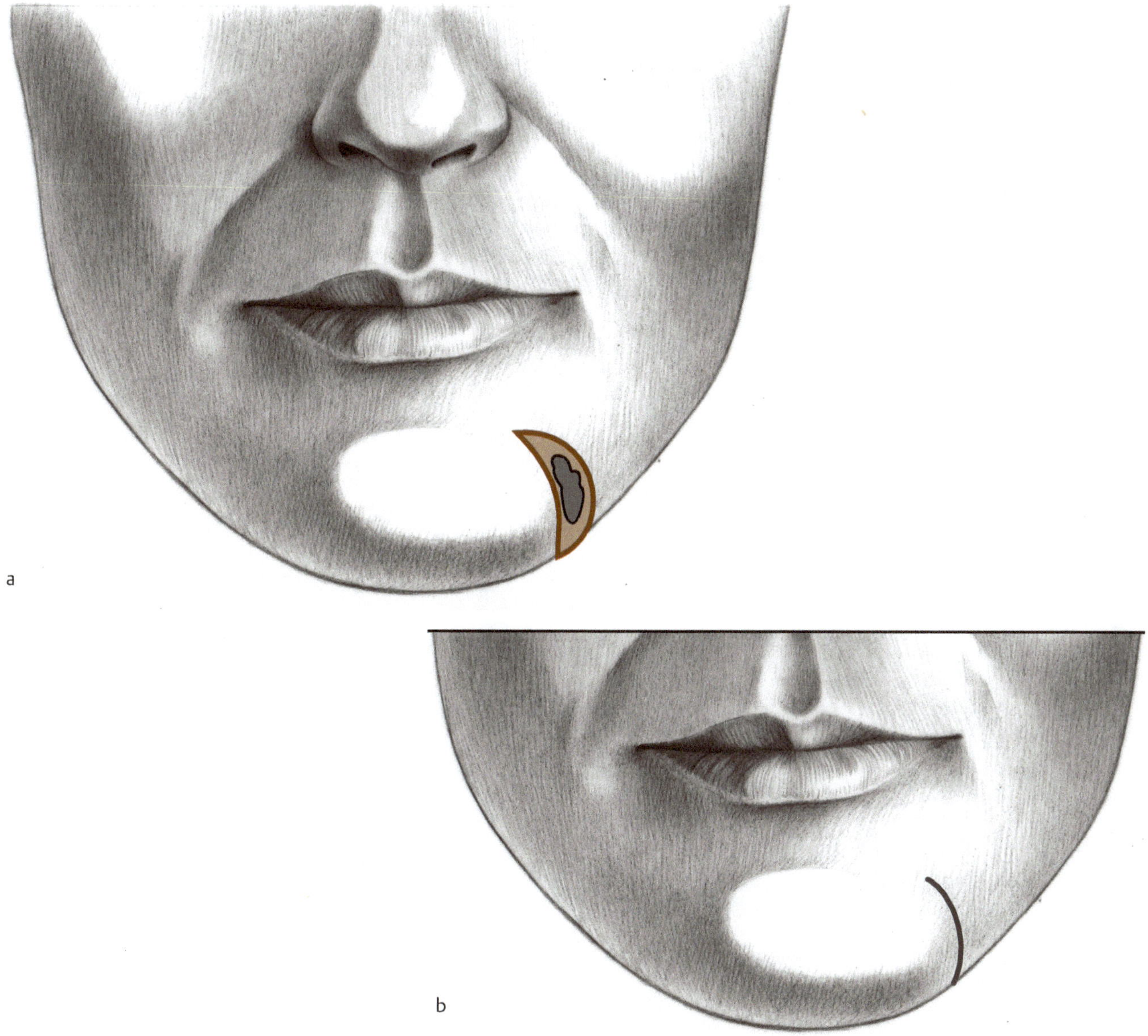

Fig. 9.8 (a, b) Lateral closure of the chin.

Full Thickness

Because of the great elasticity of the lower lip, full-thickness lesions involving one-fourth to one-third of the lower lip can be excised and repaired primarily (**Fig. 9.9**). For the smallest lesions, a standard V excision is often used. The V excision should not cross the labiomental crease and should be planned so as to parallel RSTLs (**Fig. 9.10**). The mucocutaneous junction should be tattooed or scratched prior to all full-thickness lip excisions, to facilitate exact alignment of this important surface landmark at the end of the procedure. The wound is closed in three layers of mucosa, muscle, and skin. The anterior vermilion border should be approximated with the first cutaneous suture. The muscle layer is approximated with 3–0 and 4–0 absorbable sutures. The skin is closed with 5–0 or 6–0 nonabsorbable sutures, and the mucosa is loosely closed with absorbable sutures.

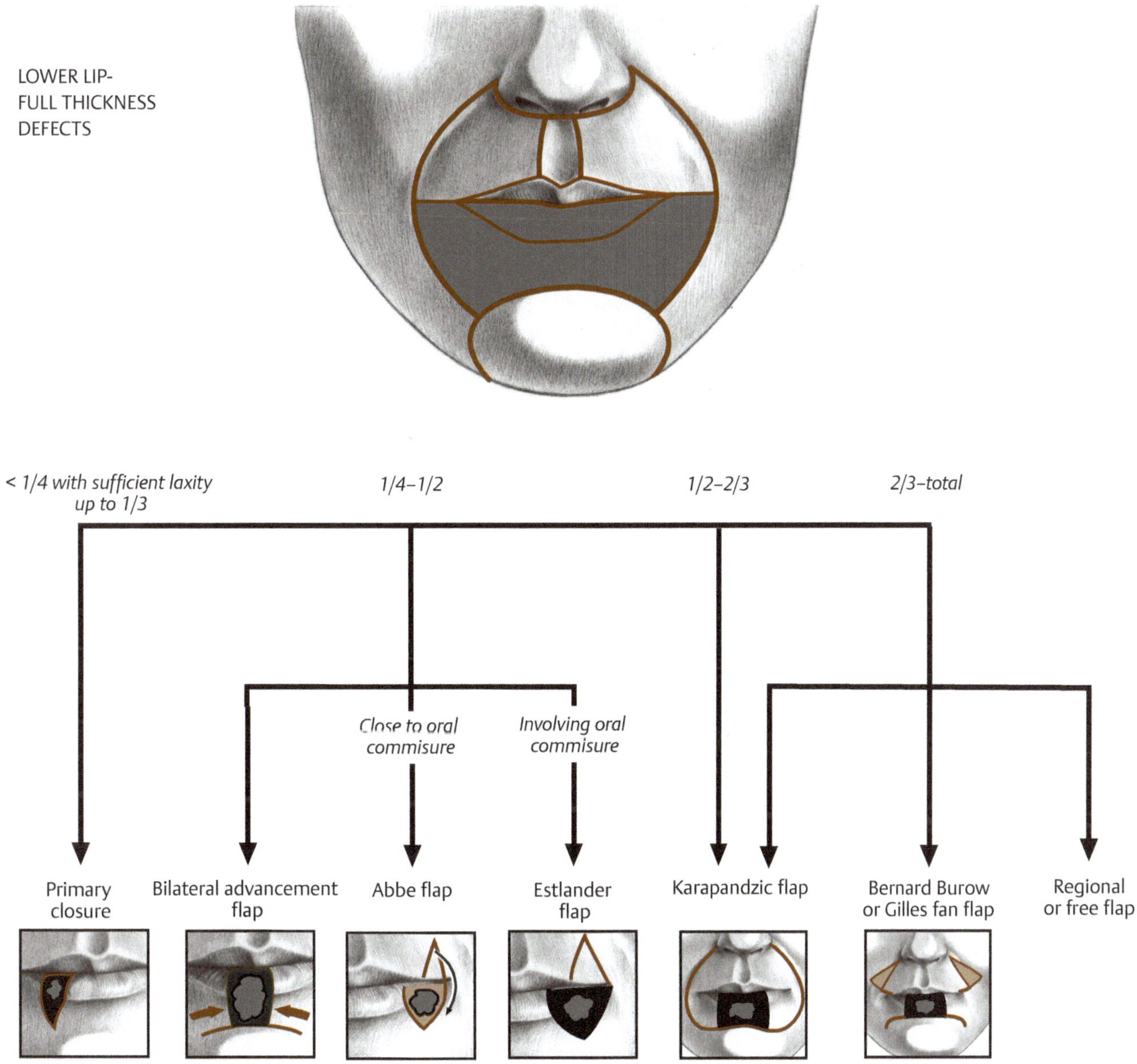

Fig. 9.9 Lower lip: full-thickness defects.

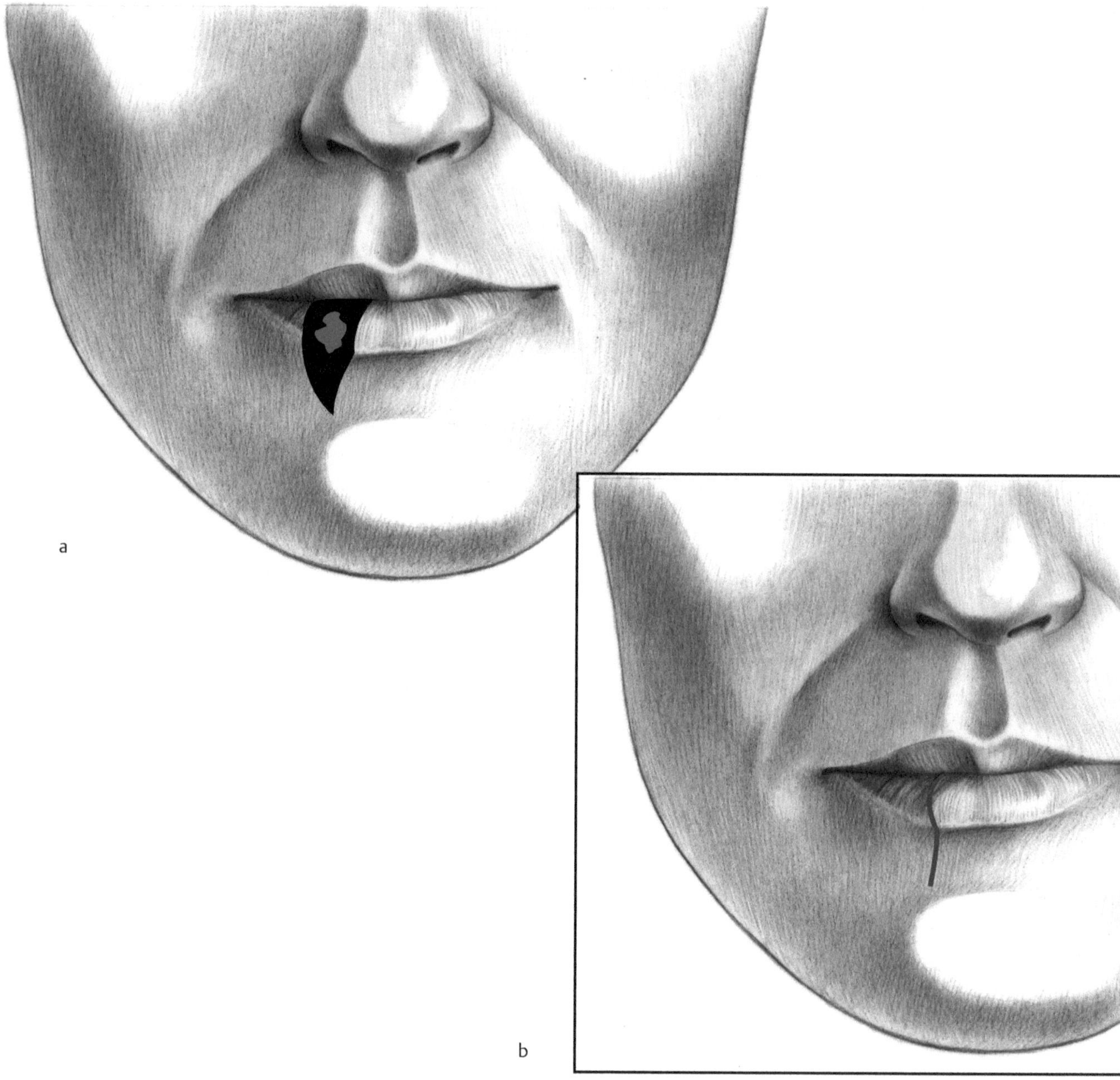

a

b

Fig. 9.10 (a, b) Wedge excision of the lower lip.

For more centrally located tumors occupying up to one-half the lower lip, a rectangular excision with full-thickness bilateral advancement flaps incised in the labiomental sulcus will facilitate closure (**Fig. 9.11** and **Fig. 9.12**). Burow triangle excisions at the labiomental sulcus may be necessary for proper wound alignment (**Fig. 9.13**). The wound is closed in three layers.

It is helpful to visualize lower lip reconstruction as a spectrum from wedge excision to bilateral advancement flaps to Abbe flaps and/or the Bernard–Burow repair. One can begin with a wedge excision and if there is excessive tension or distortion create bilateral advancement flaps. If there is a need to do a simultaneous excision of the vermilion, mucosa can be advanced from the oral surface of the advancement flaps. Although for defects of intermediate size one would normally use an Abbe flap, occasionally a unilateral Bernard–Burow is indicated. This would be the case, for instance, in someone for whom a staged repair was logistically impossible.

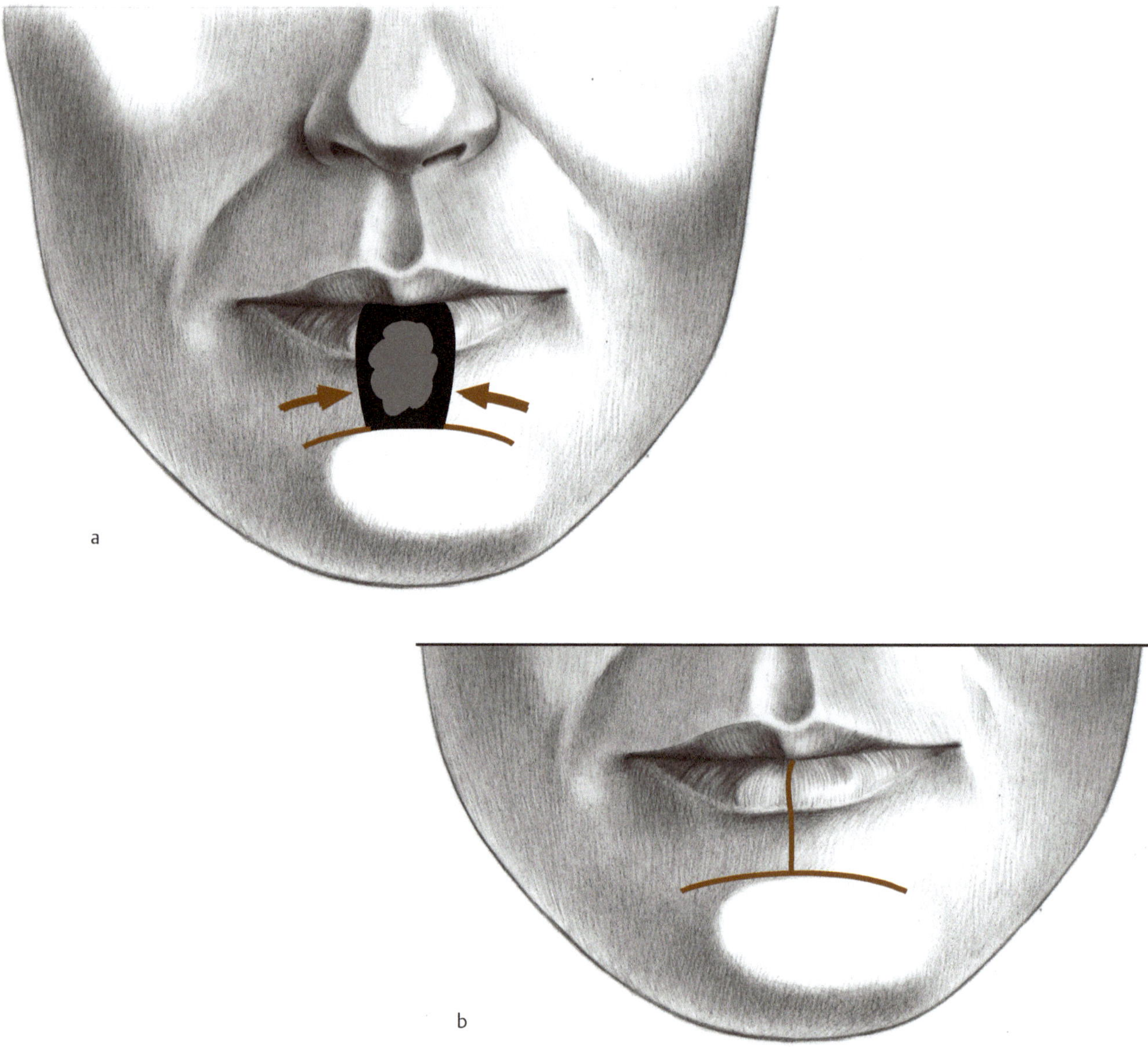

Fig. 9.11 (a, b) Bilateral advancement flap closure of the lower lip.

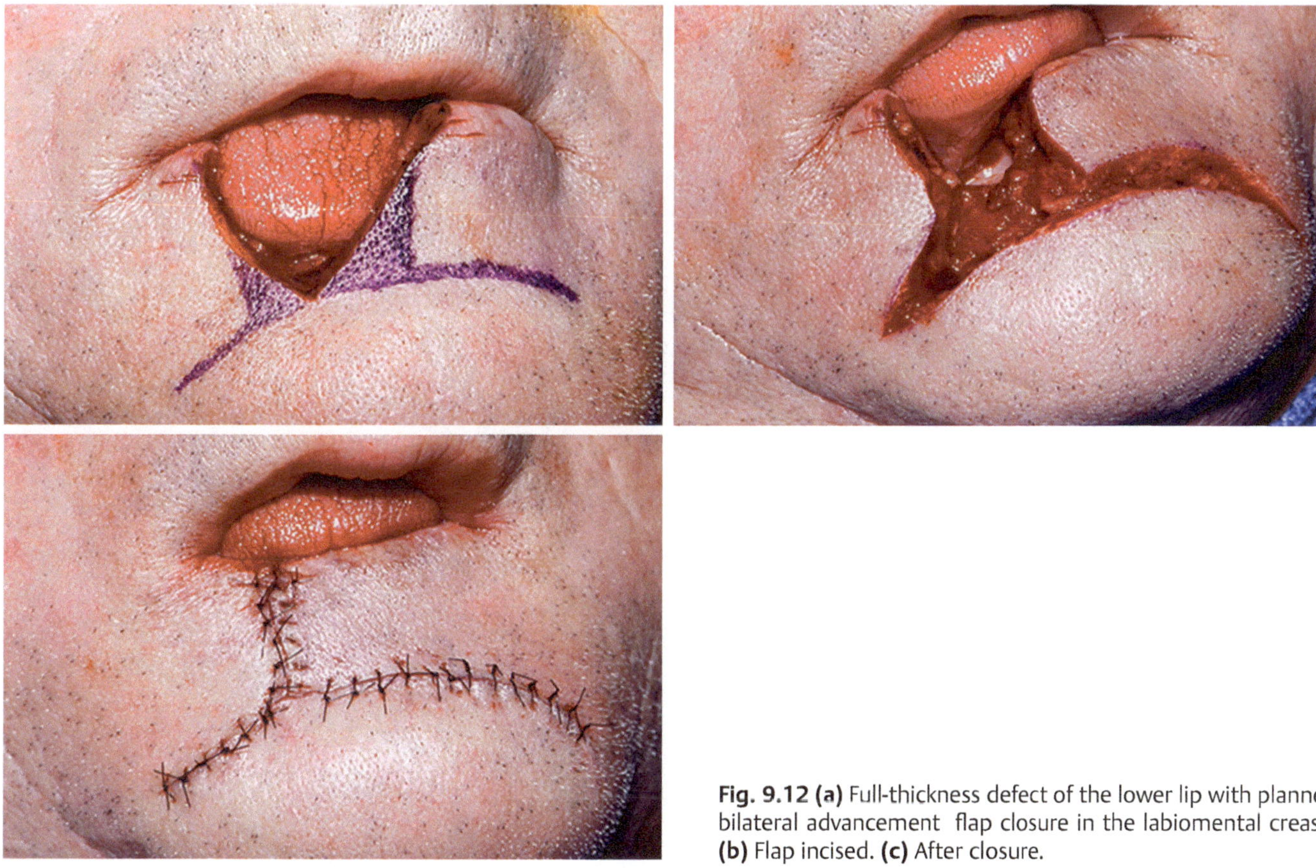

a b c

Fig. 9.12 (a) Full-thickness defect of the lower lip with planned bilateral advancement flap closure in the labiomental crease. **(b)** Flap incised. **(c)** After closure.

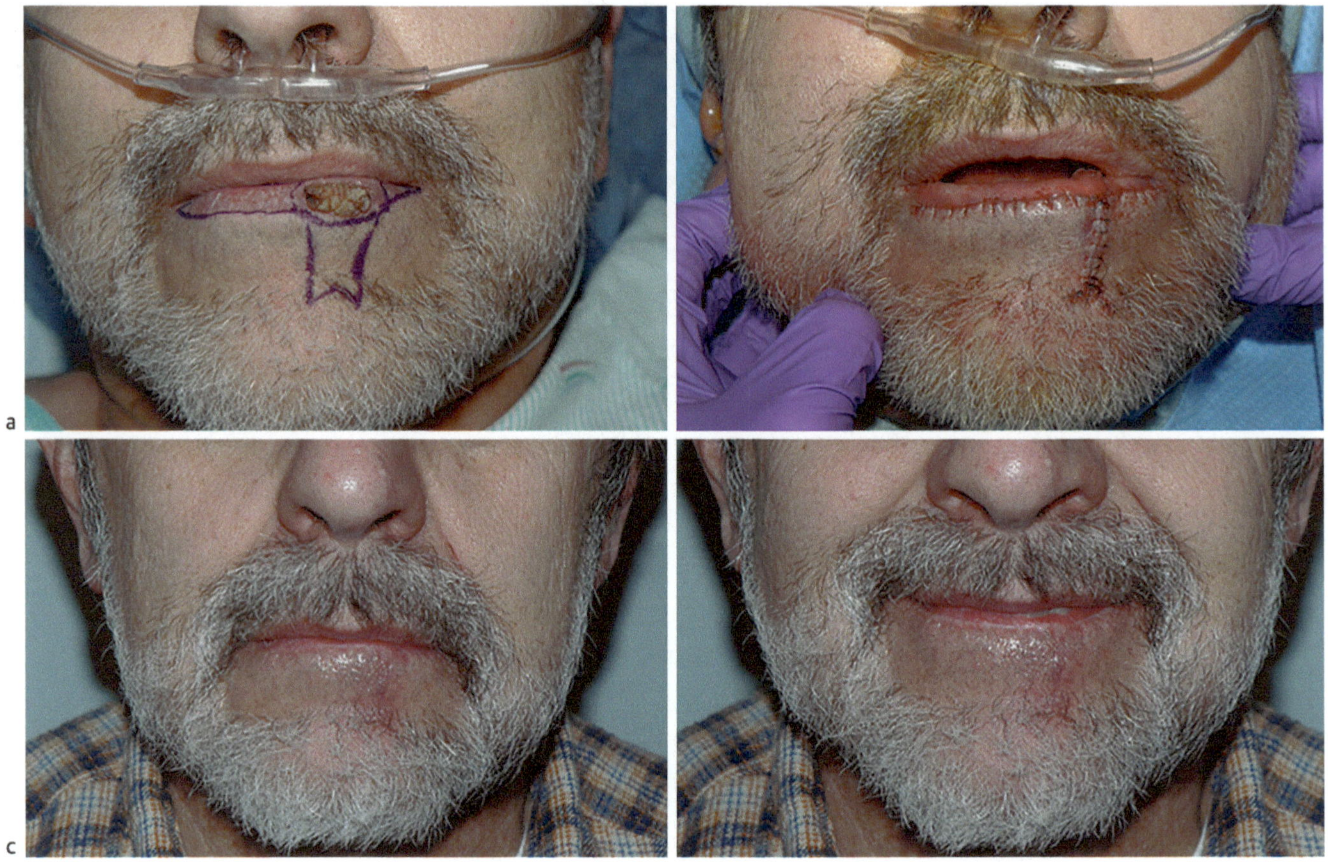

Fig. 9.13 (a) Lip lesion planned for vermilionectomy, full-thickness excision, and M-plasty excision at the labiomental sulcus to facilitate primary wedge closure. **(b)** After excision and three-layer closure. **(c)** Early postoperative appearance. **(d)** Oral competency and muscle function are intact with primary wedge closure.

Defects of the lateral one-third to one-half of the lower lip not involving the oral commissure can be reconstructed with the Abbe flap (**Fig. 9.14**). The white lines on both the upper and lower lips are marked with scratching or tattooing prior to local anesthetic injection. The flap is planned about one-half the size of the defect and is incised full-thickness down one side, along the inferiormost aspect, and three-fourths up the other side. Care is taken to dissect just across the vermilion border on the pedicled side of the flap. The flap is left pedicled on a small amount of mucosa and the labial artery. The flap is inset with a three-layer closure of skin, orbicularis oris, and mucosa. Care is taken to meticulously approximate the mucocutaneous junction on both sides of the flap and at the donor site. The donor site is also closed in three layers. The vascular pedicle is divided at 3 weeks, and mucosa is trimmed and inset as needed.

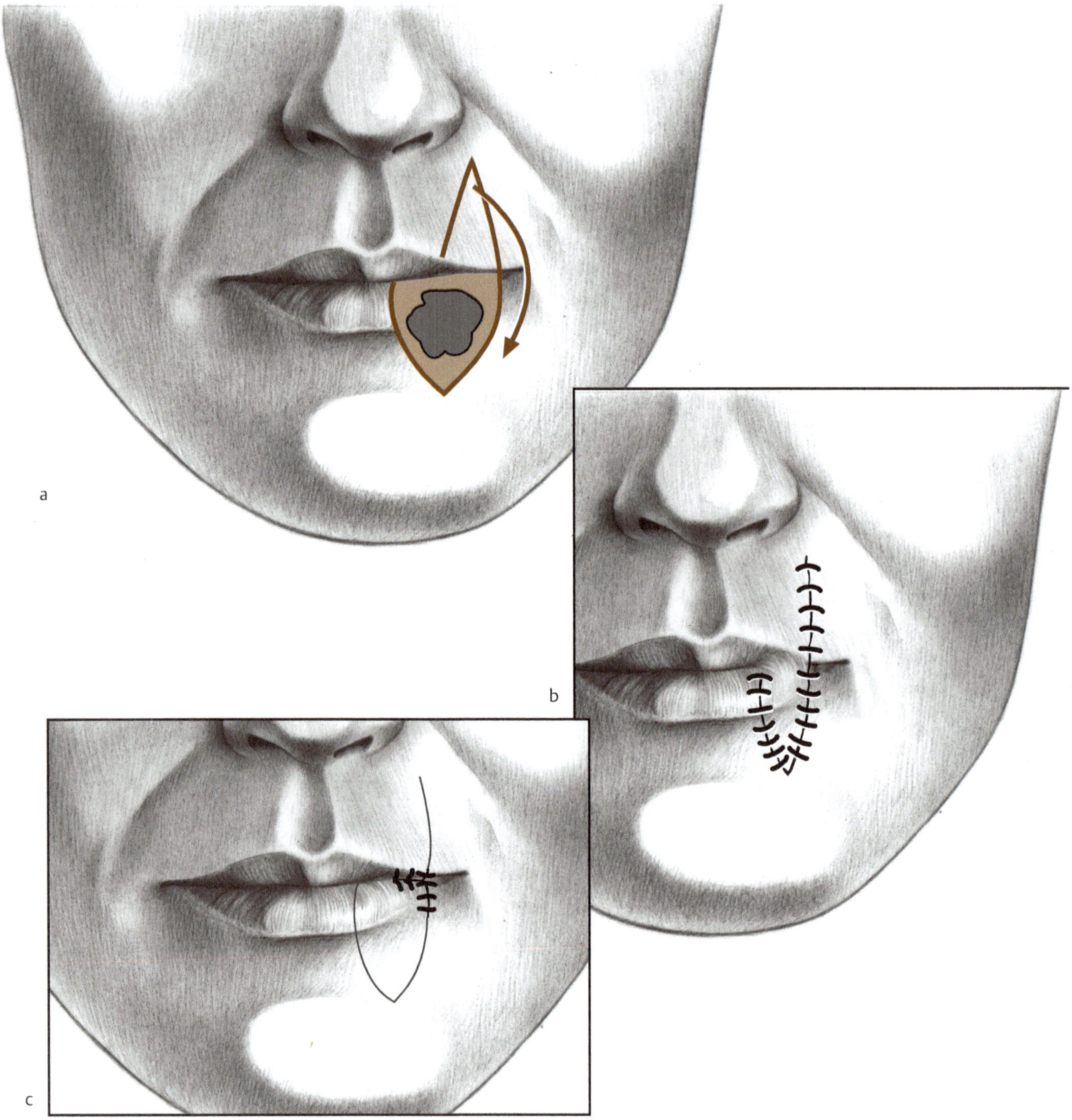

a

b

c

Fig. 9.14 (a–c) Abbe flap to a lower lip defect.

Lateral defects involving one oral commissure are best treated with an Estlander flap (**Fig. 9.15**). The repair not only fills the lip defect but is the first stage in commissure reconstruction. The incision is placed in the melolabial crease and, unlike the Abbe flap, is designed with a height 1 to 2 mm higher than that of the defect. While suturing the flap into place, some advancement of mucosa may be required to align the mucosa of the two lip segments.

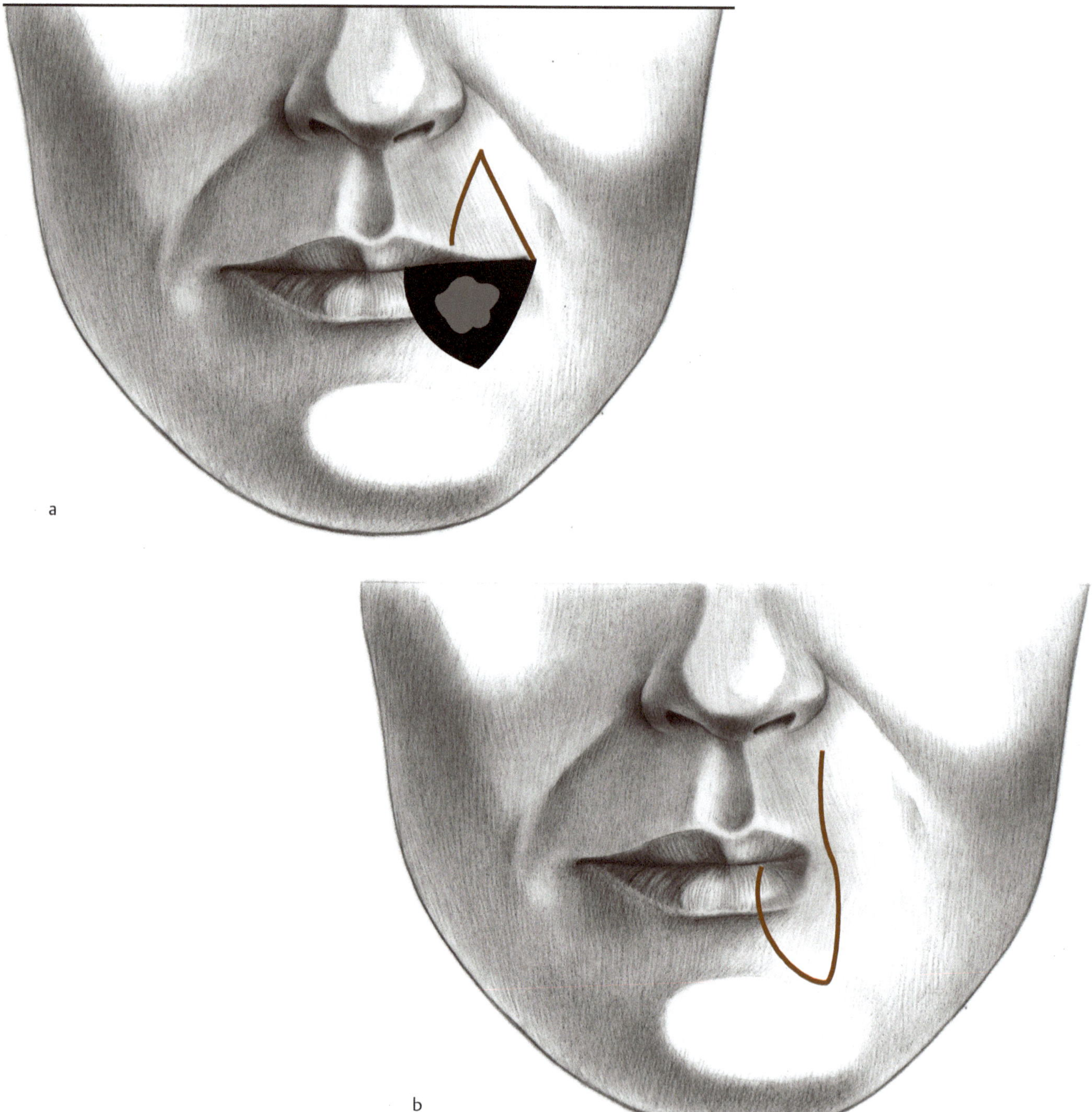

Fig. 9.15 (a, b) Estlander flap to the lower lip.

A commissuroplasty is performed at 3 months using the technique of Converse (**Fig. 9.16**). A triangle of skin, lateral to the planned commissure, is excised to the depth of the orbicularis oris muscle. The muscle is split at the area of the oral commissure. The mucosa from the lower lip segment is then incised, elevated in the plane superficial to the orbicularis oris muscle, and transferred to the new upper lip commissure. The mucosa of the intraoral lower lip is advanced outward to reconstruct the lower lip oral commissure mucosa.

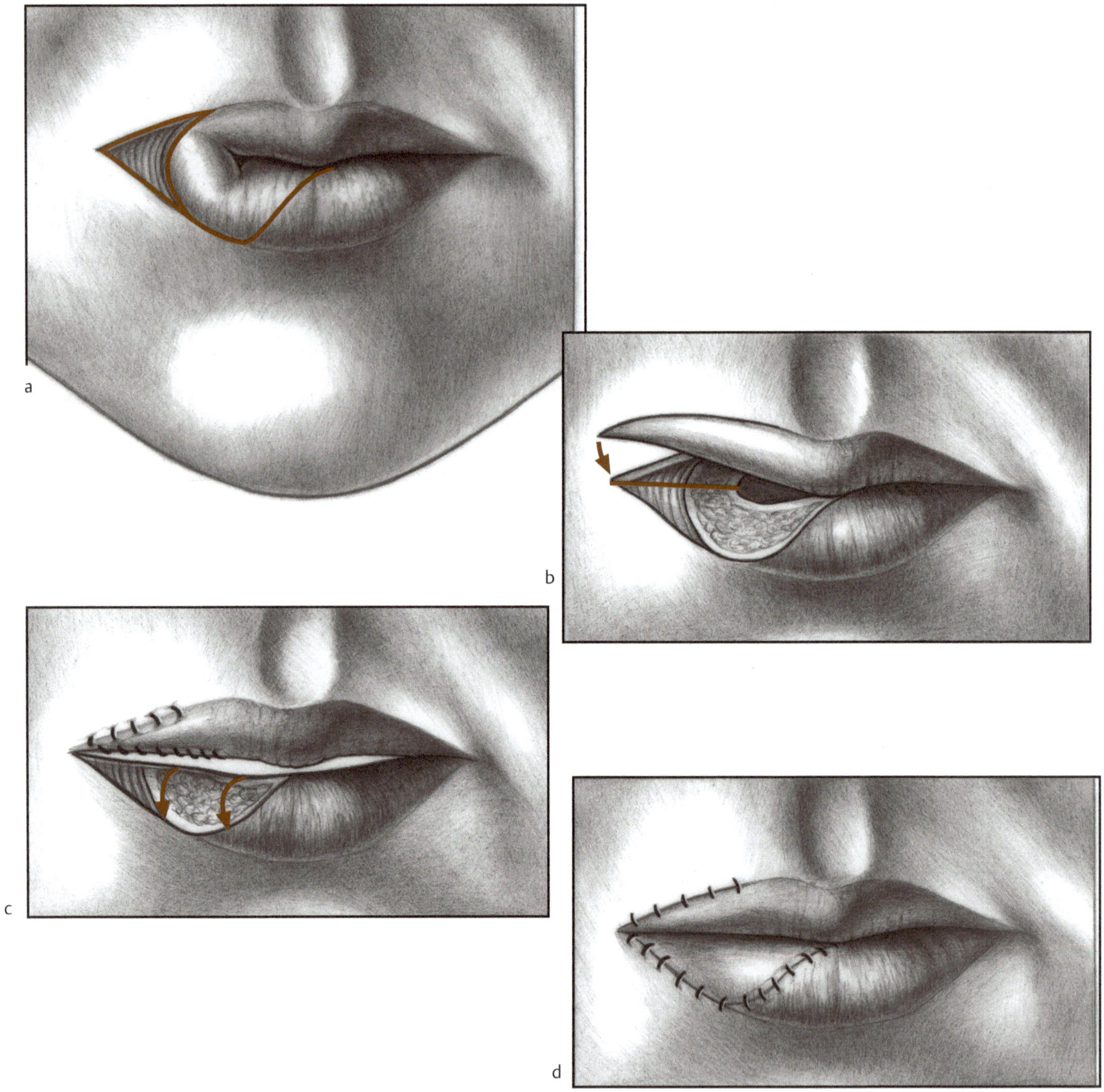

Fig. 9.16 (a–d) Commissuroplasty (after Converse).

The Karapandzic flap is especially useful for defects of one-half to two-thirds of the lower lip, but it can be used for total lower lip defects (**Fig. 9.17** and **Fig. 9.18**). This flap is easiest to apply in more central defects, where a complete lip is formed by rotating the bilateral flap of the upper lip and perioral tissue, both inferiorly and medially. The skin is marked and incised. Next, blunt dissection is used to identify and preserve the neurovascular supply to the orbicularis oris muscle. Muscle fibers may be separated carefully, but mucosa need not be incised. When sufficient mobilization has been accomplished to allow closure, a standard three-layer repair is accomplished in the midline. In contrast to the cross lip flaps, nerve preservation enables immediate muscular function. Preservation of the labial artery branches provides robust blood supply to these flaps in cases of preoperative irradiation. Use of the Karapandzic flap for defects larger than two-thirds of the lower lip is limited by the resultant severe microstomia.

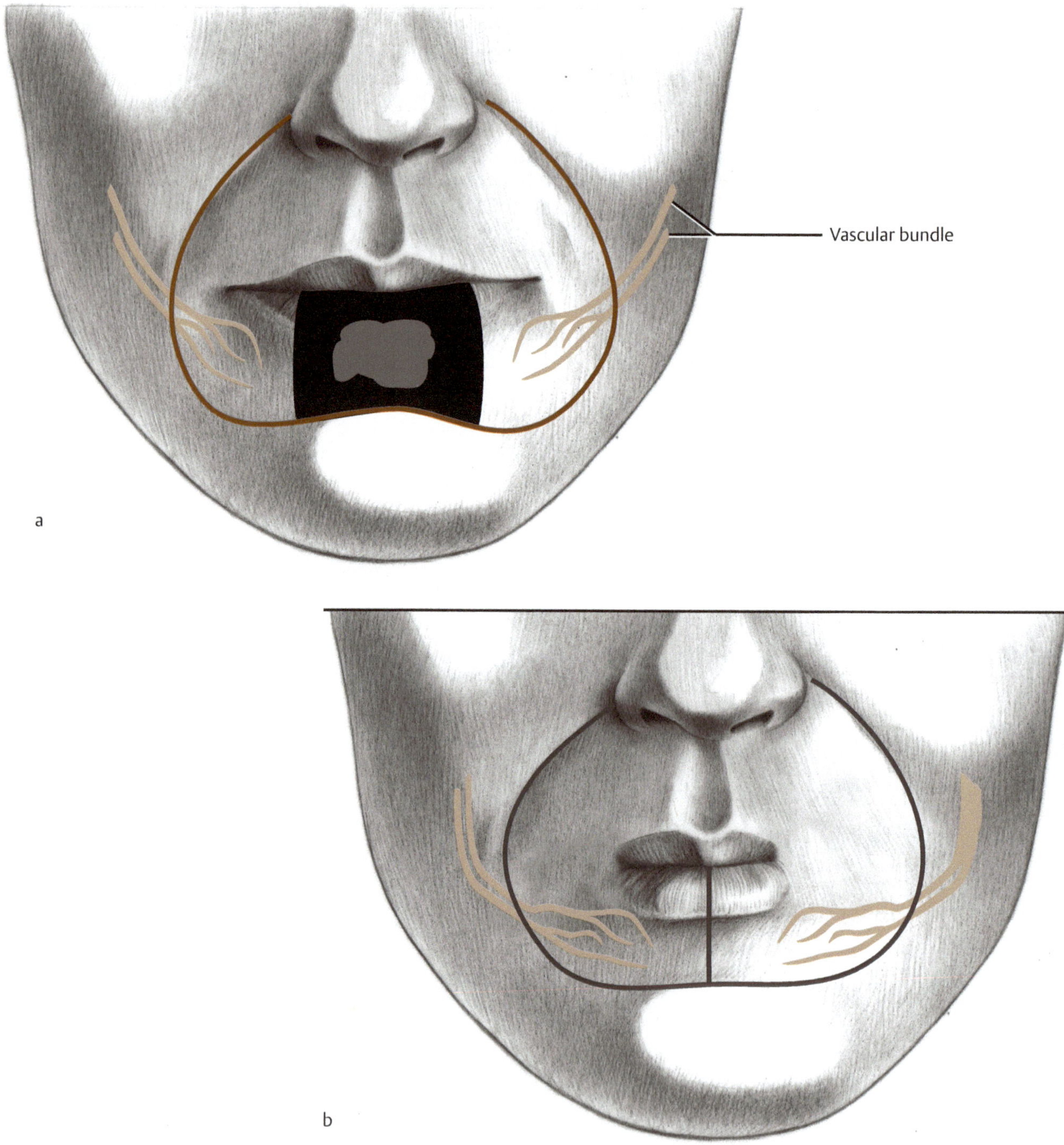

Fig. 9.17 (a, b) Karapandzic repair of the lower lip.

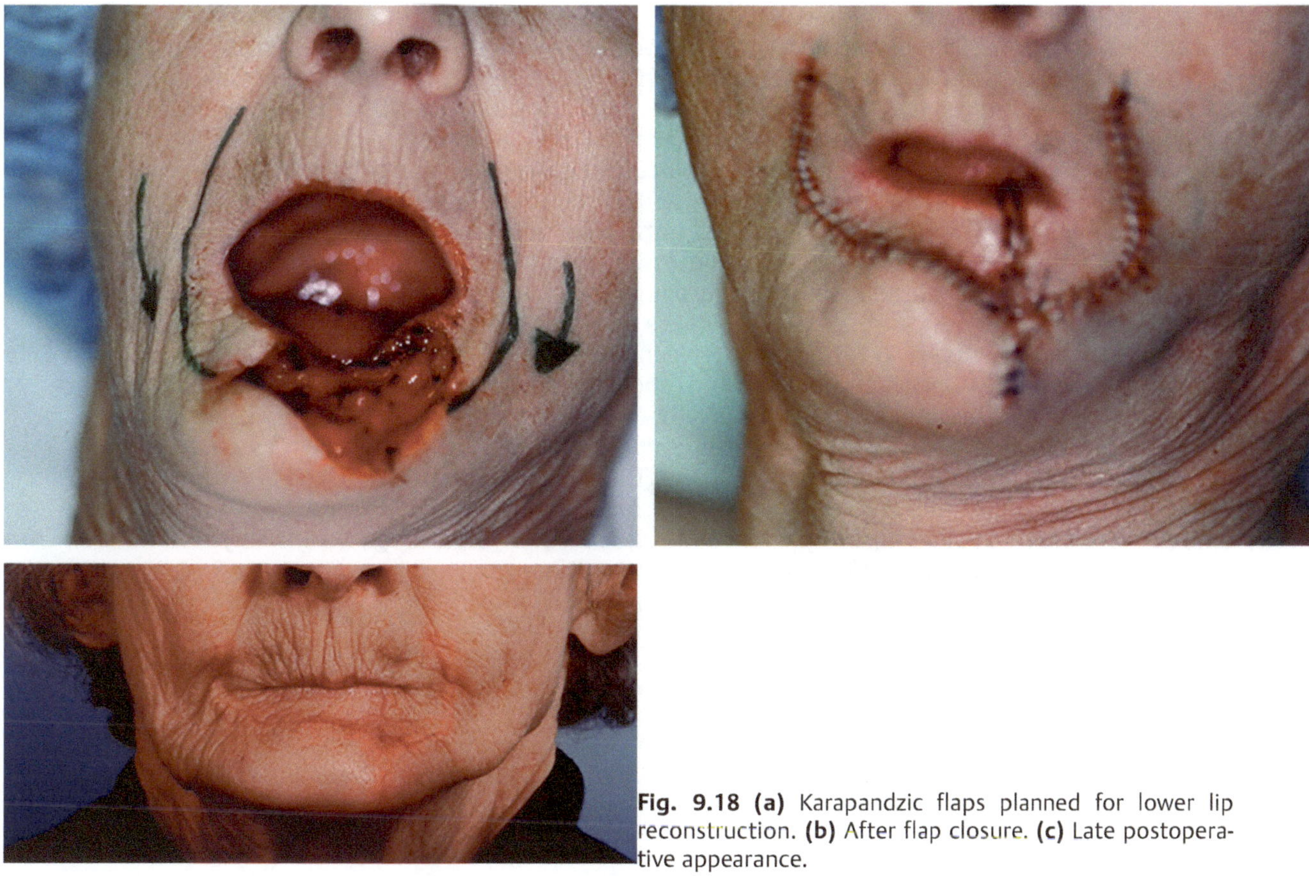

a b c

Fig. 9.18 **(a)** Karapandzic flaps planned for lower lip reconstruction. **(b)** After flap closure. **(c)** Late postoperative appearance.

Defects encompassing the entire lower lip can also be reconstructed using adjacent cheek tissue. Large, centrally located defects are closed with the Webster modification of the Bernard–Burow flap (**Fig. 9.19**). Large, horizontal cheek advancement flaps are designed with the upper border slightly superior to the oral commissure. The superior Burow triangle is designed with its apex in the melolabial fold, the medial side at the melolabial fold, and the lateral side connecting the apex with the horizontal line drawn from and slightly superior to the commissure. The triangle is modified somewhat to a half-crescent to assist closure; when closed, it will lie within the melolabial fold. The crescents of skin and subcutaneous tissue need not be excised until the flap has been mobilized and brought into position. The muscle is incised as far laterally as necessary to allow sufficient advancement for midline closure. A permanent suture at the base of the muscle incision helps re-create a modiolus at the commissure. Burow triangles of skin are excised along the inferior base of the flap as needed. The closure of the Burow triangle should lie in the crease between the mentum and the cheek. Intraoral mucosal flaps are created with the upper incision 4 or 5 mm above the level of the skin incision. The additional mucosa is used as an advancement flap to create a new vermilion, similar to the way a lip vermilionectomy is done. The labial sulcus is more easily preserved if a cuff of labial mucosa is left attached to the labial-alveolar groove at the time of tumor resection. The standard three-layer closure is undertaken. The major disadvantage of this technique is that the resultant lip is devoid of muscle function. The typical tightness of the neolip helps to provide oral continence while eating, but initially it does not provide movement during facial expression.

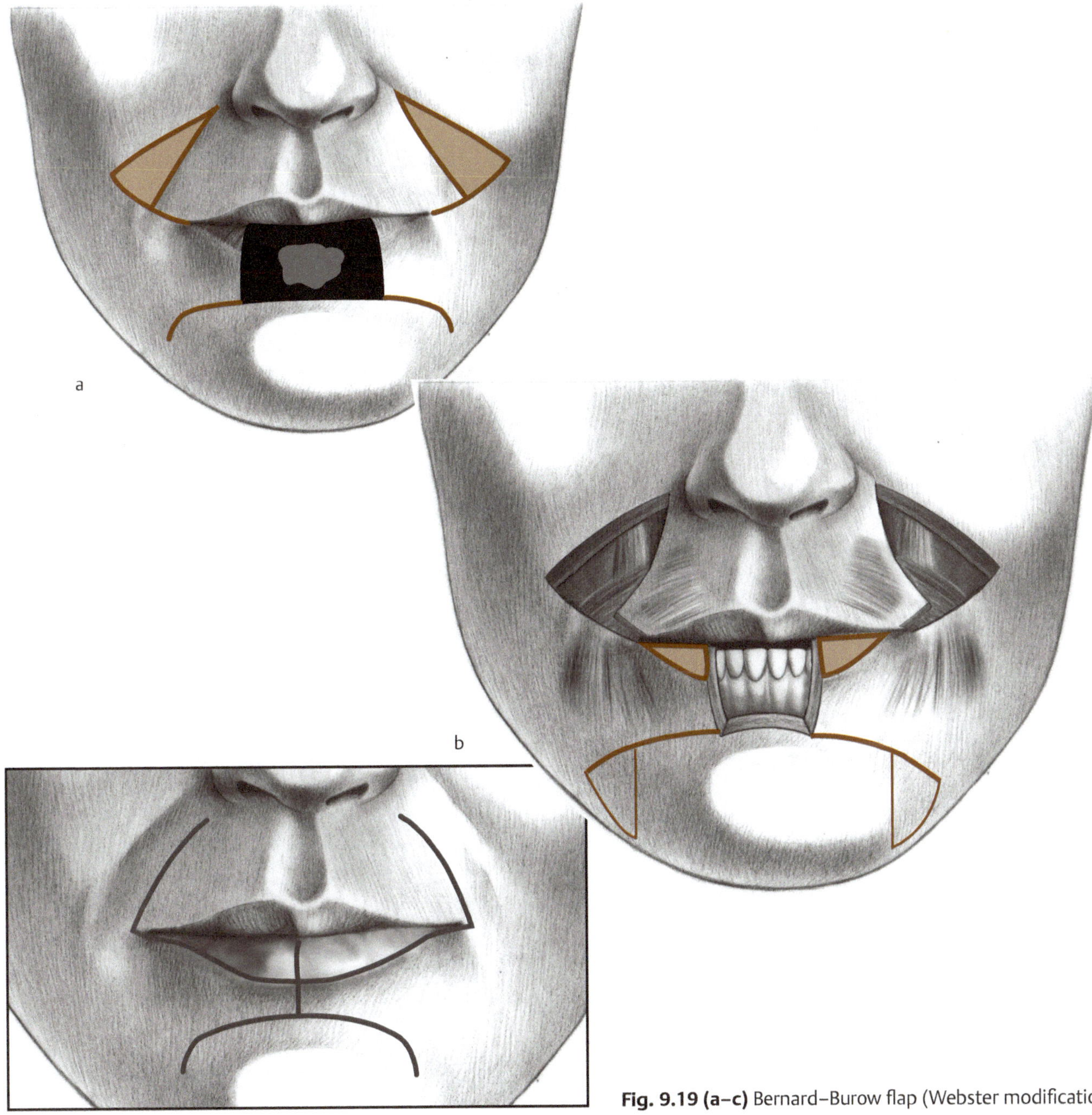

a b c

Fig. 9.19 (a–c) Bernard–Burow flap (Webster modification).

Other flaps of use in total lower lip reconstruction are the Gilles fan flap and the Gate flap (**Fig. 9.20**). Each can be done unilaterally or bilaterally. Depending on the situation, each has its advantage. The fan flap has a superiorly based pedicle, whereas the gate flap has an inferiorly based pedicle. Both provide additional tissue to the lip, so that microstomia is avoided. Yet each is limited because of the resultant lack of motor function and minimal return of sensation. The best answer for total lower lip reconstruction remains to be delivered.

Larger defects involving the lower lip, chin, and adjacent regions may be closed with a variety of regional flaps or free flaps that are beyond the scope of this book.

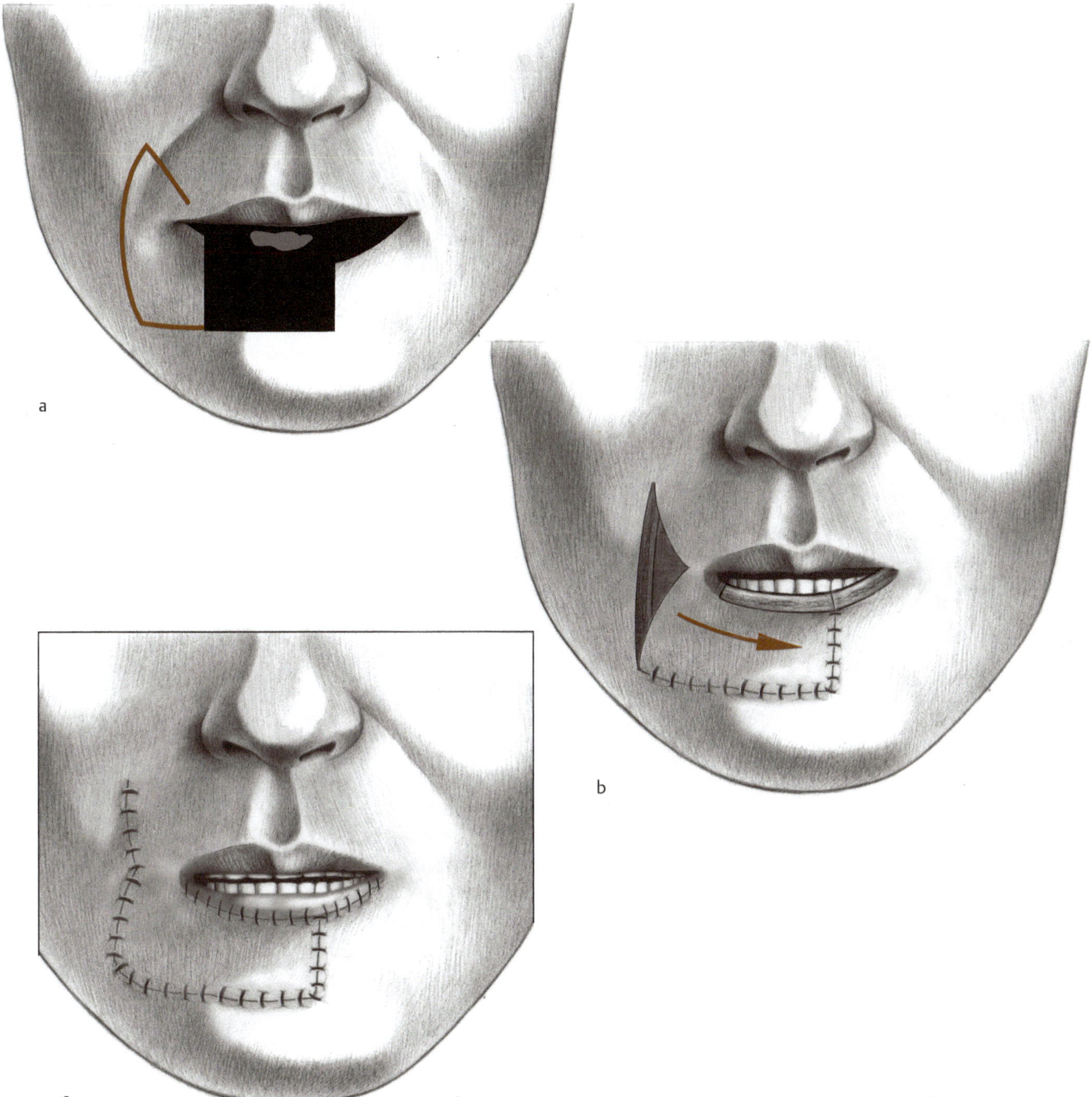

Fig. 9.20 (a–c) Unilateral Gilles fan flap.

♦ Upper Lip

Partial Thickness

Upper lip malignancies are almost always basal cell carcinomas and are usually located on perioral skin rather than the mucosa or vermilion. Repair of perioral skin defects is complicated by the near proximity of the vermilion and nose. Because the lip and nose lack excess skin, local flaps are usually transposed or advanced from the medial cheek.

Small superficial defects involving only the philtral subunit may be allowed to heal by secondary intention (**Fig. 9.21**). Another option is to excise the entire subunit and place a full-thickness skin graft (FTSG) either immediately or at a later time. The typical skin donor site is the preauricular or retroauricular area. Superficial defects of the vermilion are treated with mucosal advancement flaps from the infraoral lip or buccal mucosa.

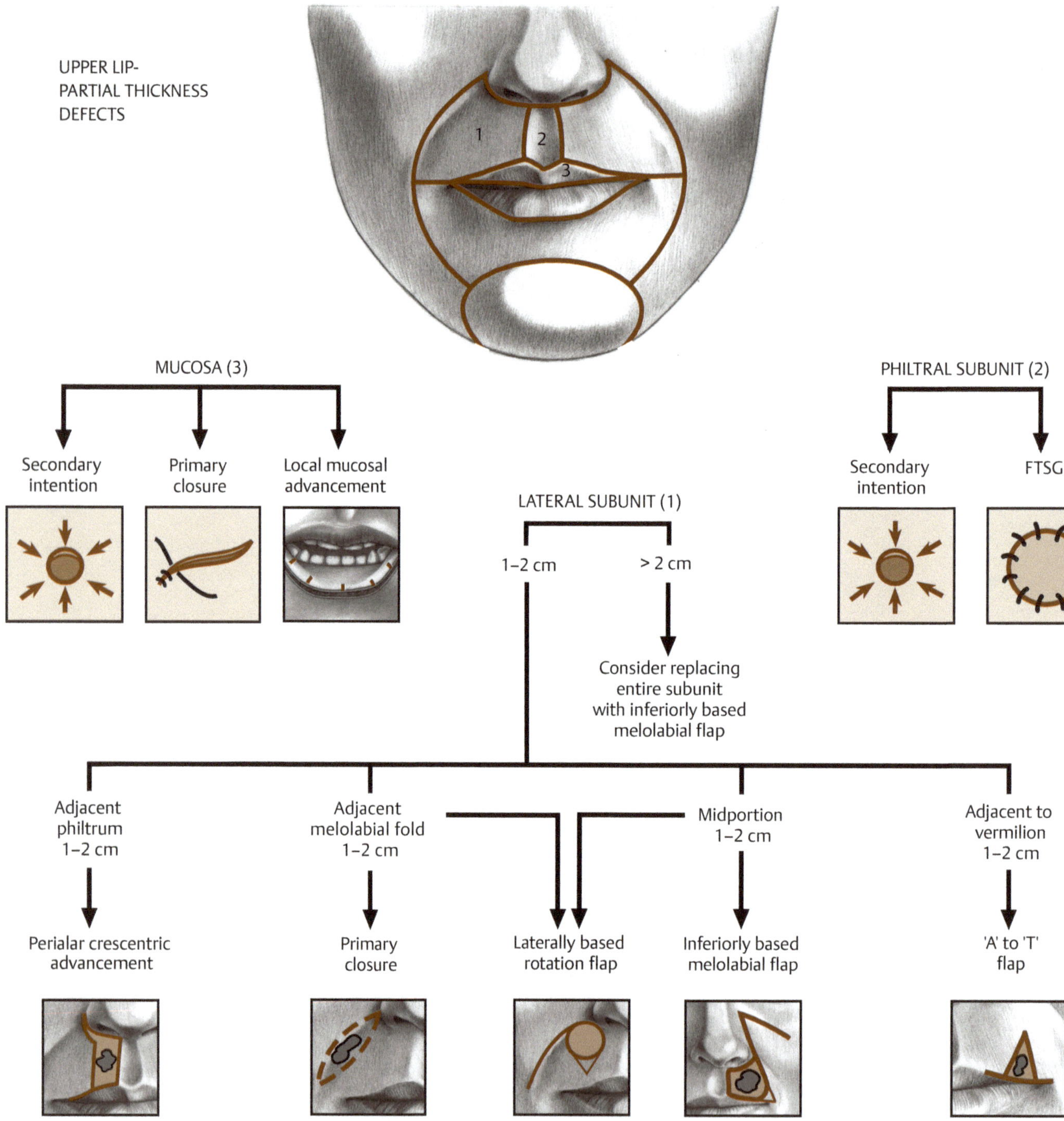

Fig. 9.21 Upper lip: partial-thickness defects.

Small to moderate-sized skin-only defects of the lateral upper lip subunit are closed primarily in the RSTLs. Defects overlying the melolabial fold are repaired with primary closure in the fold (**Fig. 9.22**). Small defects in the perialar melolabial crease can be allowed to heal by secondary intention with good results.

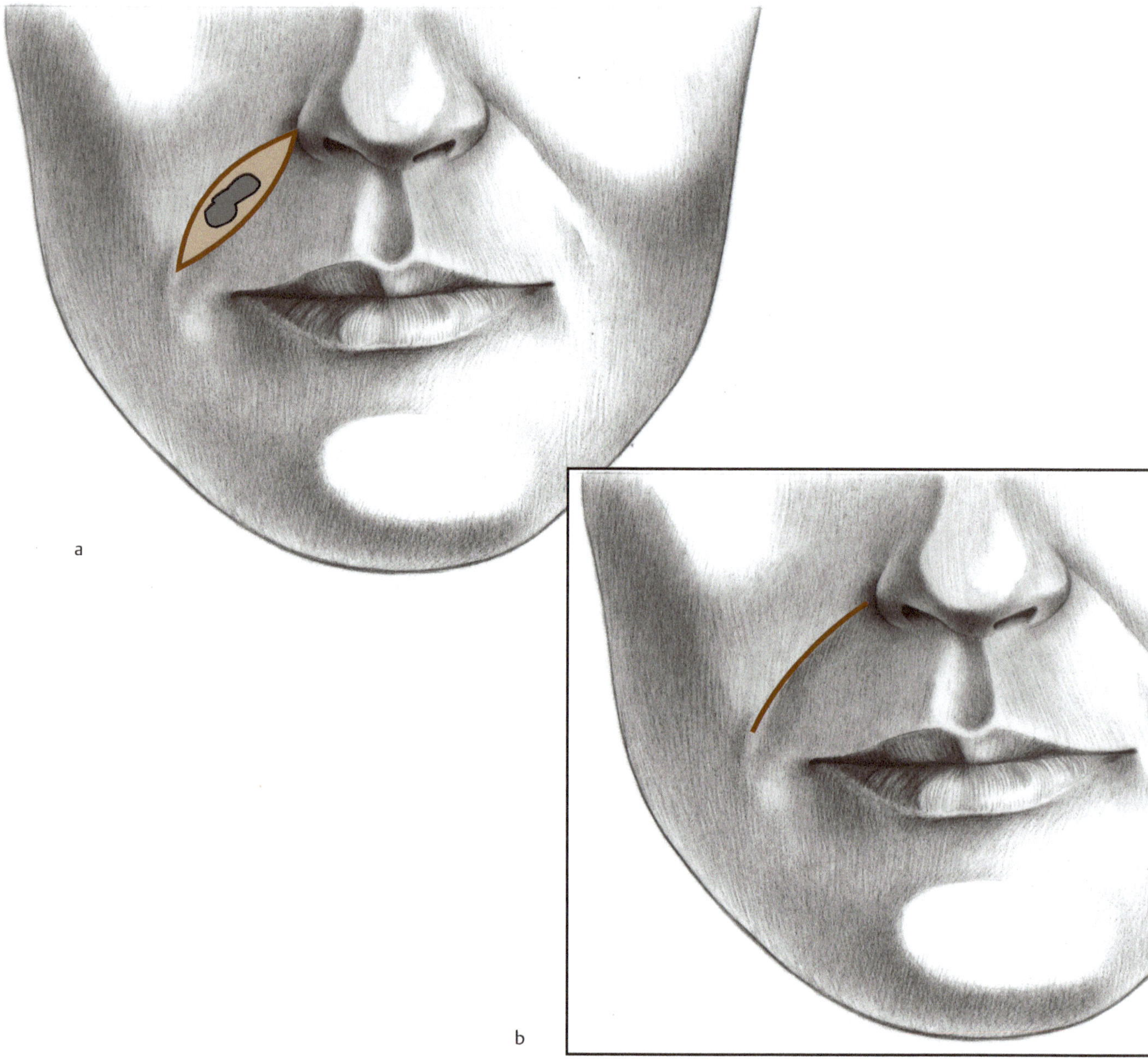

Fig. 9.22 (a, b) Primary closure in the melolabial fold.

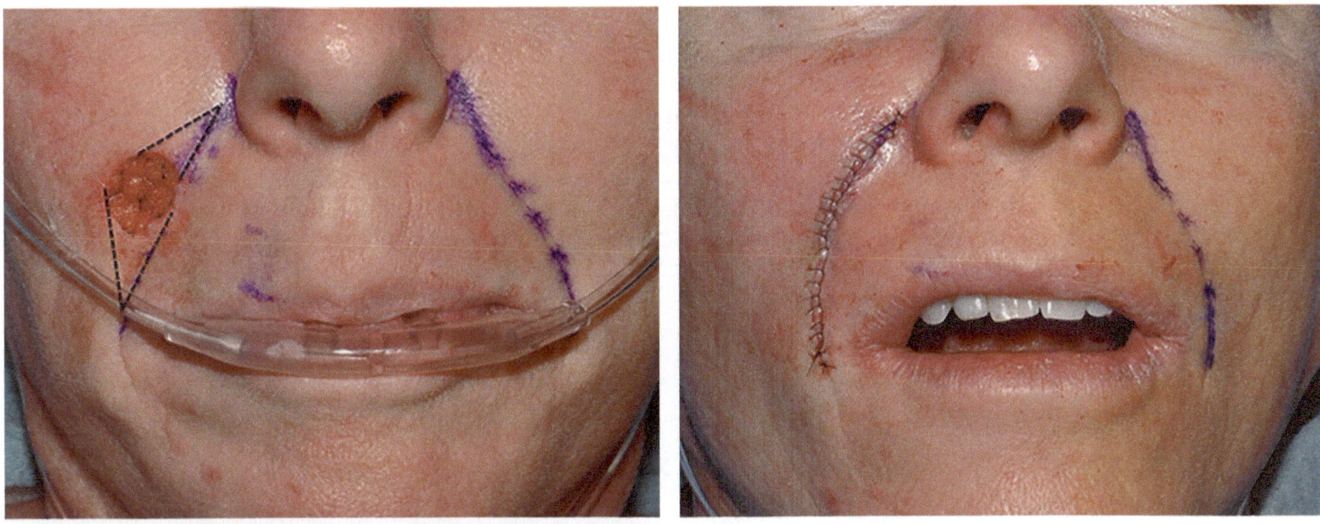

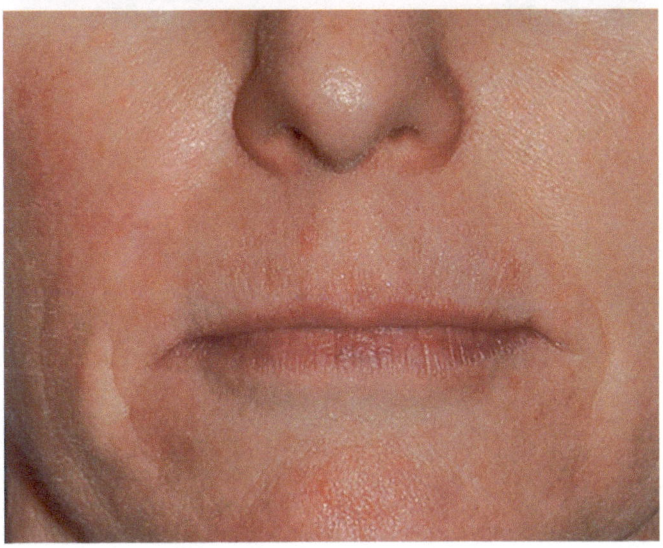

Fig. 9.22 (c) Melolabial lesion with template for excision, natural melolabial crease marked on contralateral side. **(d)** Melolabial primary closure. **(e)** Wound healed.

Larger defects adjacent to the melolabial fold but extending in an inferior direction can be repaired with an inferiorly based melolabial flap or a lateral rotation flap (**Fig. 9.23**). The lateral rotation flap is especially useful in men, as hair-bearing skin is used to reconstruct the mustache area. The lateral rotation flap is drawn initially within the melolabial crease but tapers out from the oral commissure to keep an approximate equidistance from this region to allow for greater tissue recruitment. The commissure may appear slightly elevated at the end of this procedure, but it usually returns to normal prior to the need for any secondary revision. If a dog ear is present at the vermilion border, extension of the incision into the upper vermilion border into the red lip can be accomplished to allow flattening and better contour to vermilion border (**Fig. 9.23f-g**).

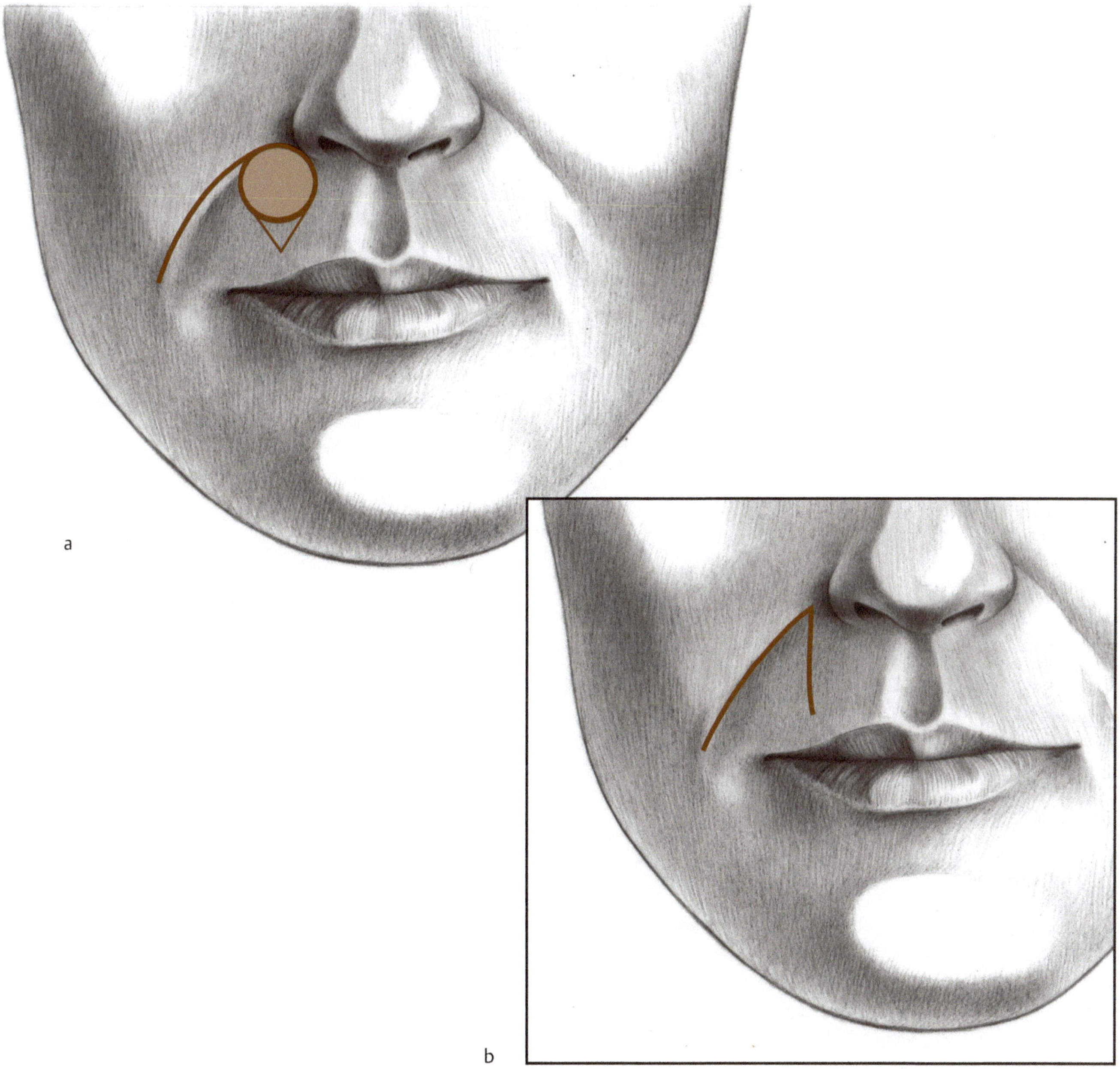

a

b

Fig. 9.23 (a, b) Laterally based rotation flap closure of the upper lip.

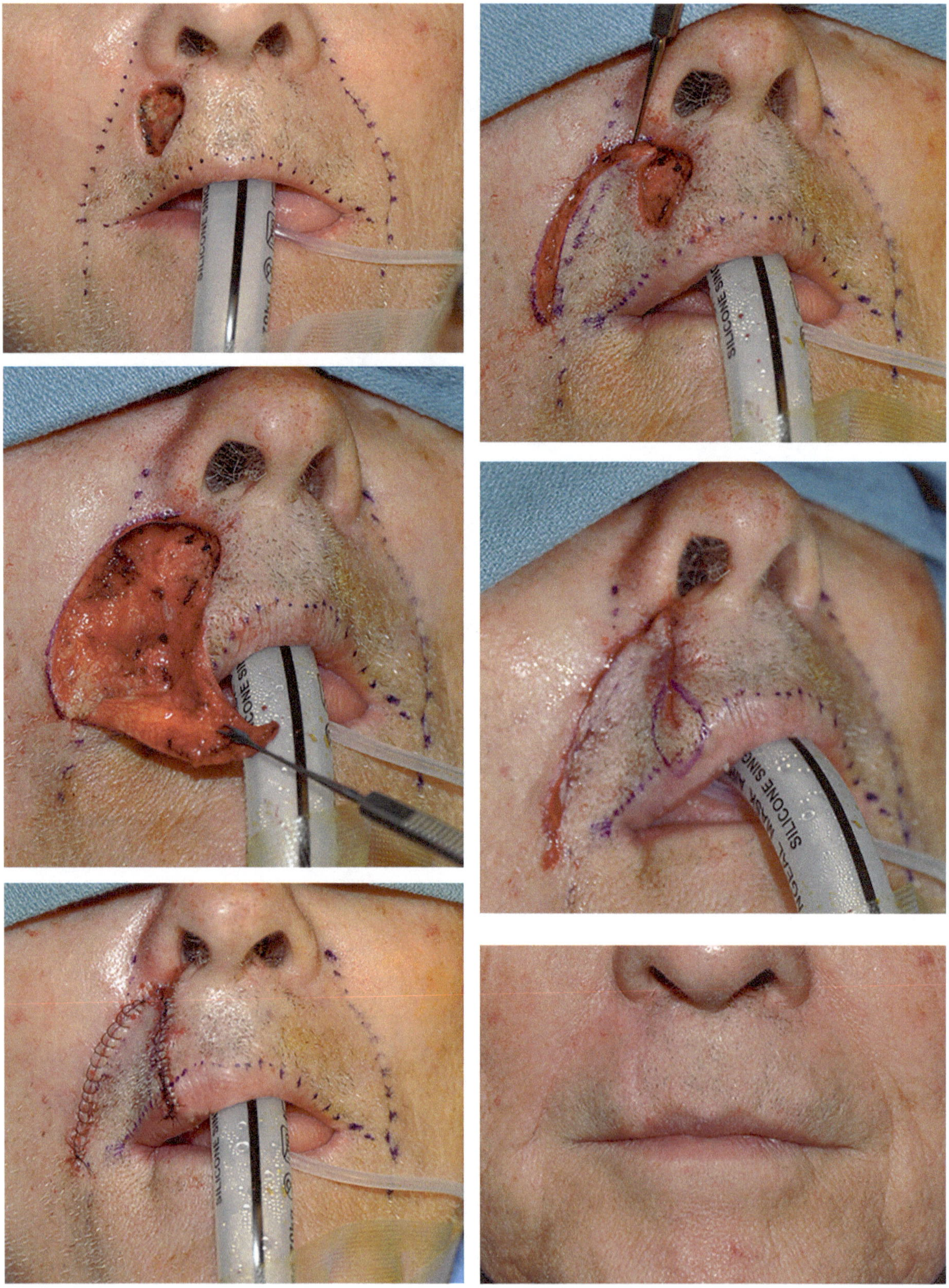

c d e f g h

Fig. 9.23 (c) Upper lip defect. **(d)** Melolabial rotation flap. **(e)** Melolabial rotation flap with demonstrated undermining. **(f)** Closure with dog ear at vermilion border. **(g)** Extension of incision into upper vermilion lip for excision of dog ear. **(h)** Wound healed.

Those defects close to the mucosa can be repaired with an A-to-T flap to avoid crossing the vermilion (**Fig. 9.24**). The releasing incision for the A-to-T flap is made at the anterior vermilion border for scar camouflage.

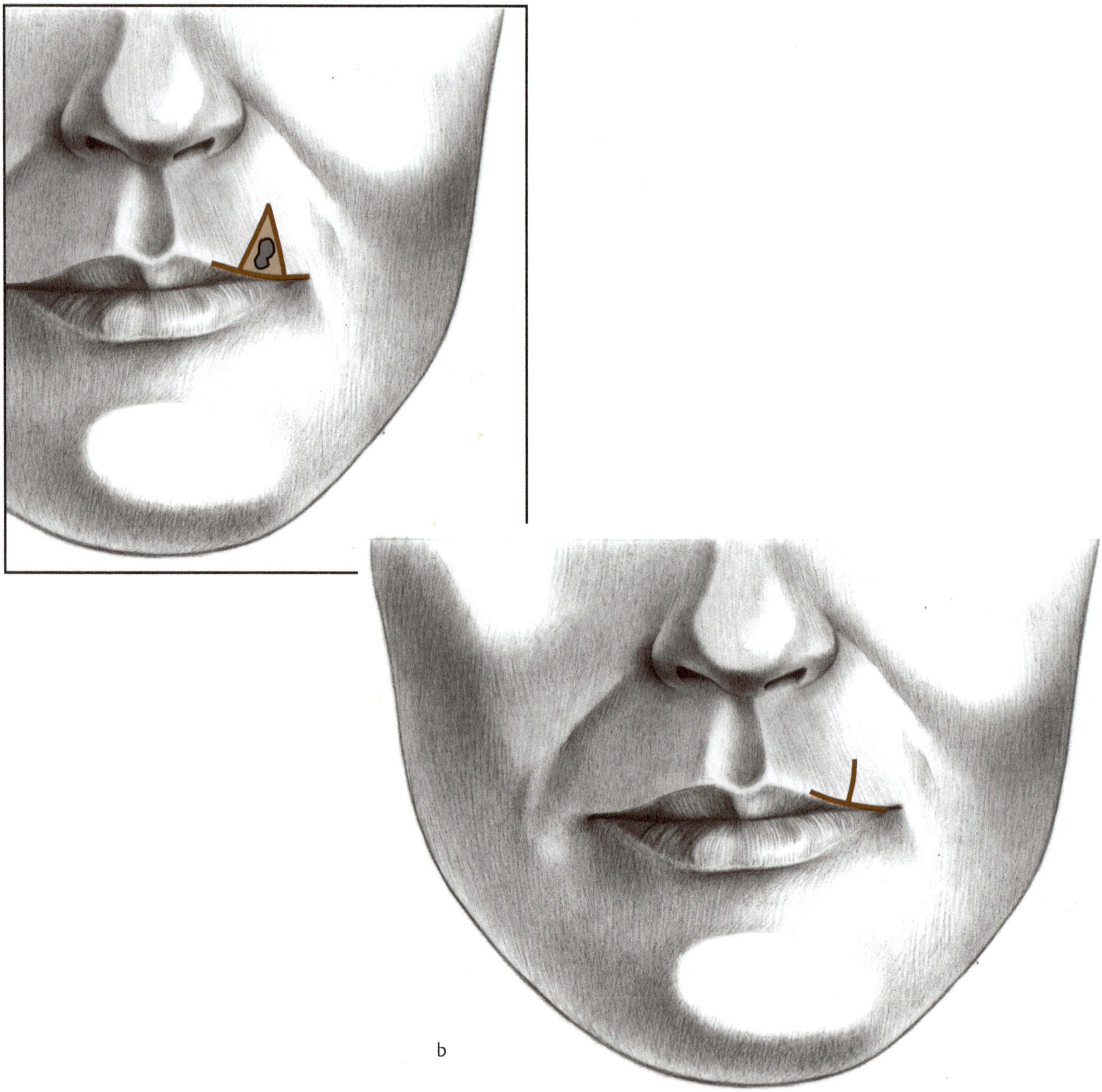

a

b

Fig. 9.24 (a, b) A-to-T flap at the vermilion border.

Small defects adjacent to the philtral ridge can be closed with an advancement flap with crescenteric skin excision around the alar base (**Fig. 9.25** and **Fig. 9.26**). If possible, the vertical scar is placed precisely at the philtral ridge. An inferior releasing incision at the vermilion can be added for larger defects.

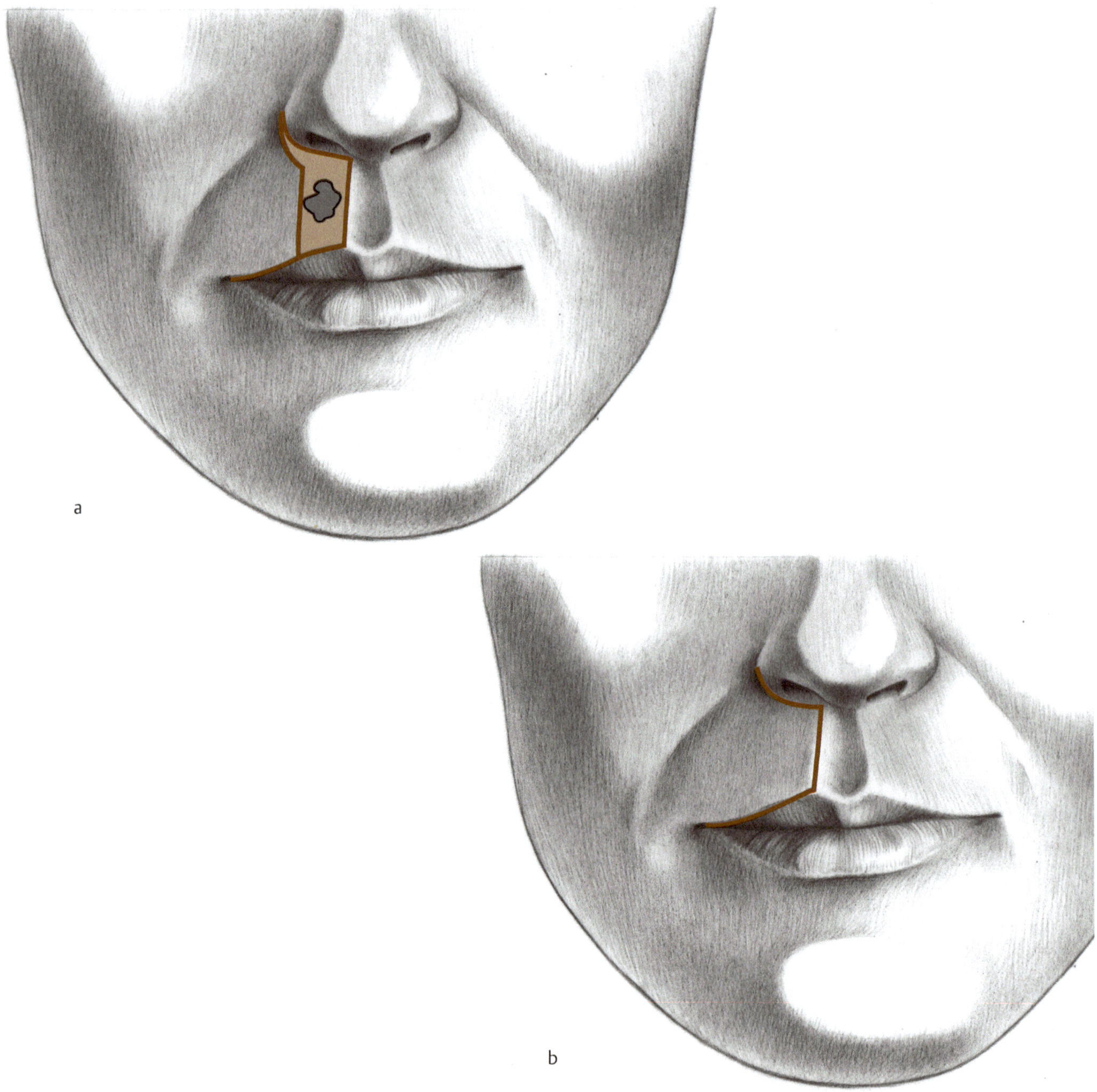

Fig. 9.25 (a, b) Perialar crescenteric advancement flap of upper lip skin.

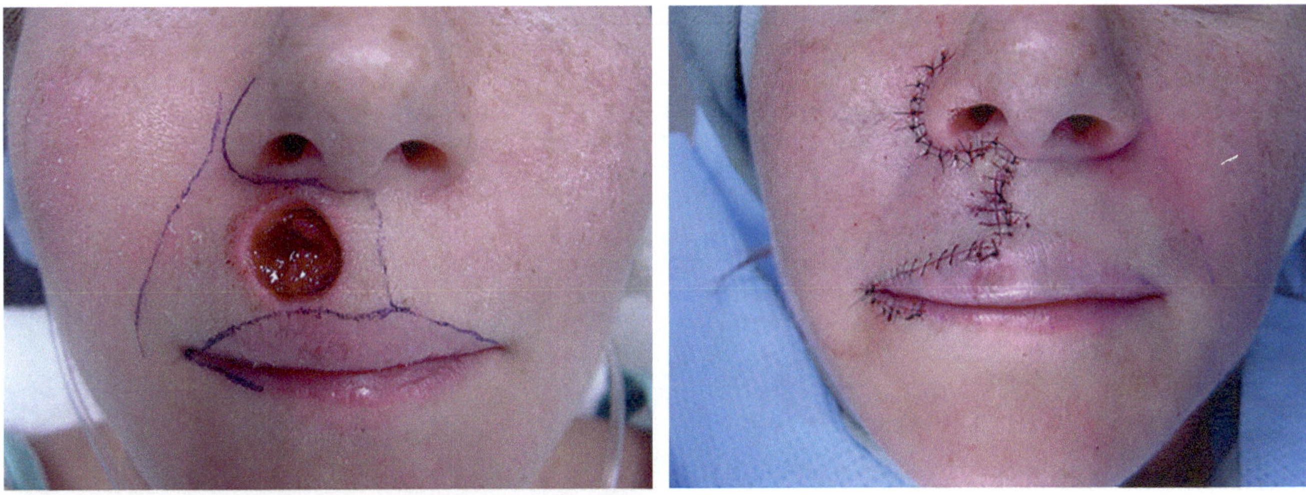

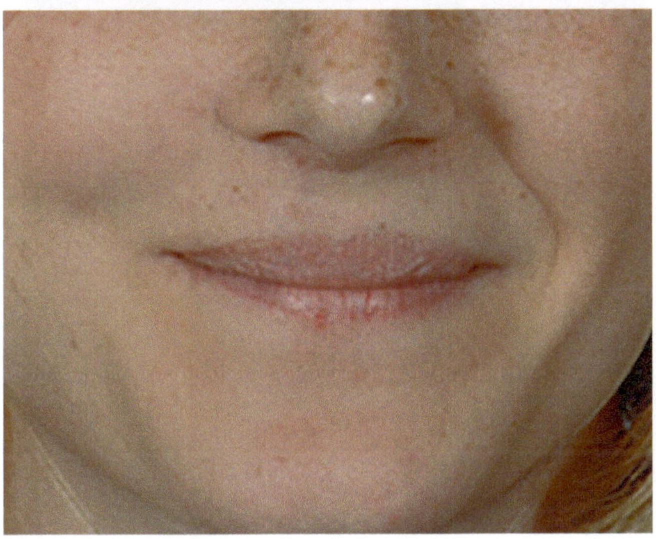

Fig. 9.26 (a) Important boundaries marked prior to right perialar crescenteric advancement flap reconstruction. **(b)** After flap inset. **(c)** Appearance late postoperatively.

In repairing superficial defects >2 cm of the lateral upper lip subunit, one should consider replacing the entire subunit. An inferiorly based transposition flap can be used to cover the entire lateral aesthetic unit in patients with adequate cheek laxity (**Fig. 9.27** and **Fig. 9.28**). The donor site closure is planned within the melolabial fold. This flap should be 1 to 2 mm wider than the defect to avoid retracting the lip upward as the wound contracts. The tip of the flap overlaps the philtral ridge and is trimmed to match the boundary of the medial aesthetic unit. The normal tissue of the subunit that is planned to be discarded is not removed until the melolabial fold has been elevated and is demonstrated to be of adequate size to cover the planned defect. The flap and cheek are elevated in the plane, just deep to the subdermal plexus. A deep, subcutaneous absorbable suture, located 1 or 2 cm from the flap edge, is anchored to the nasal spine to reduce closing tension without displacing the philtrum laterally. Similarly, the base of the donor site closure is approximated by using deep, permanent sutures to approximate the cheek flap to the piriform aperture periosteum.

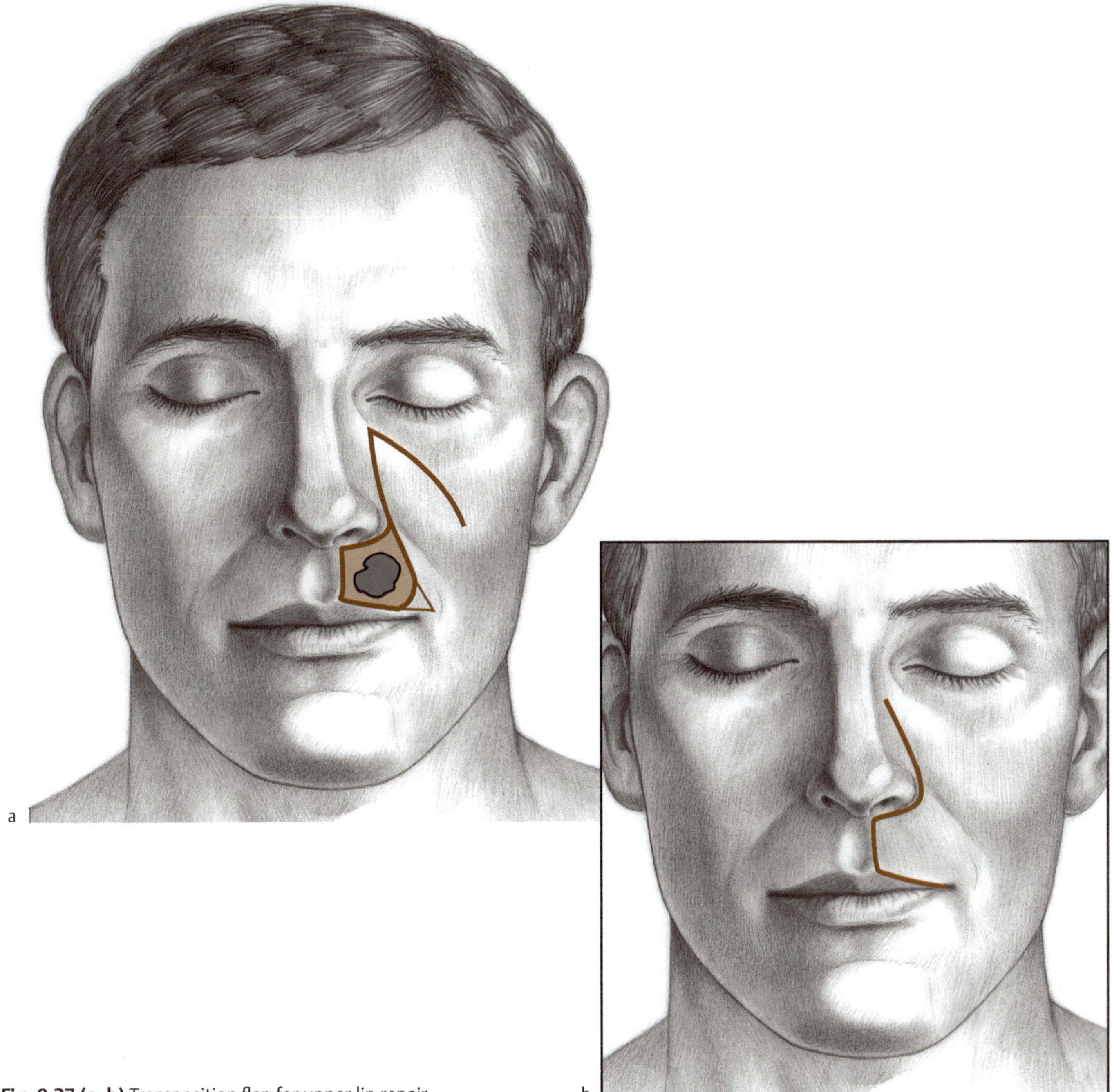

Fig. 9.27 (a, b) Transposition flap for upper lip repair.

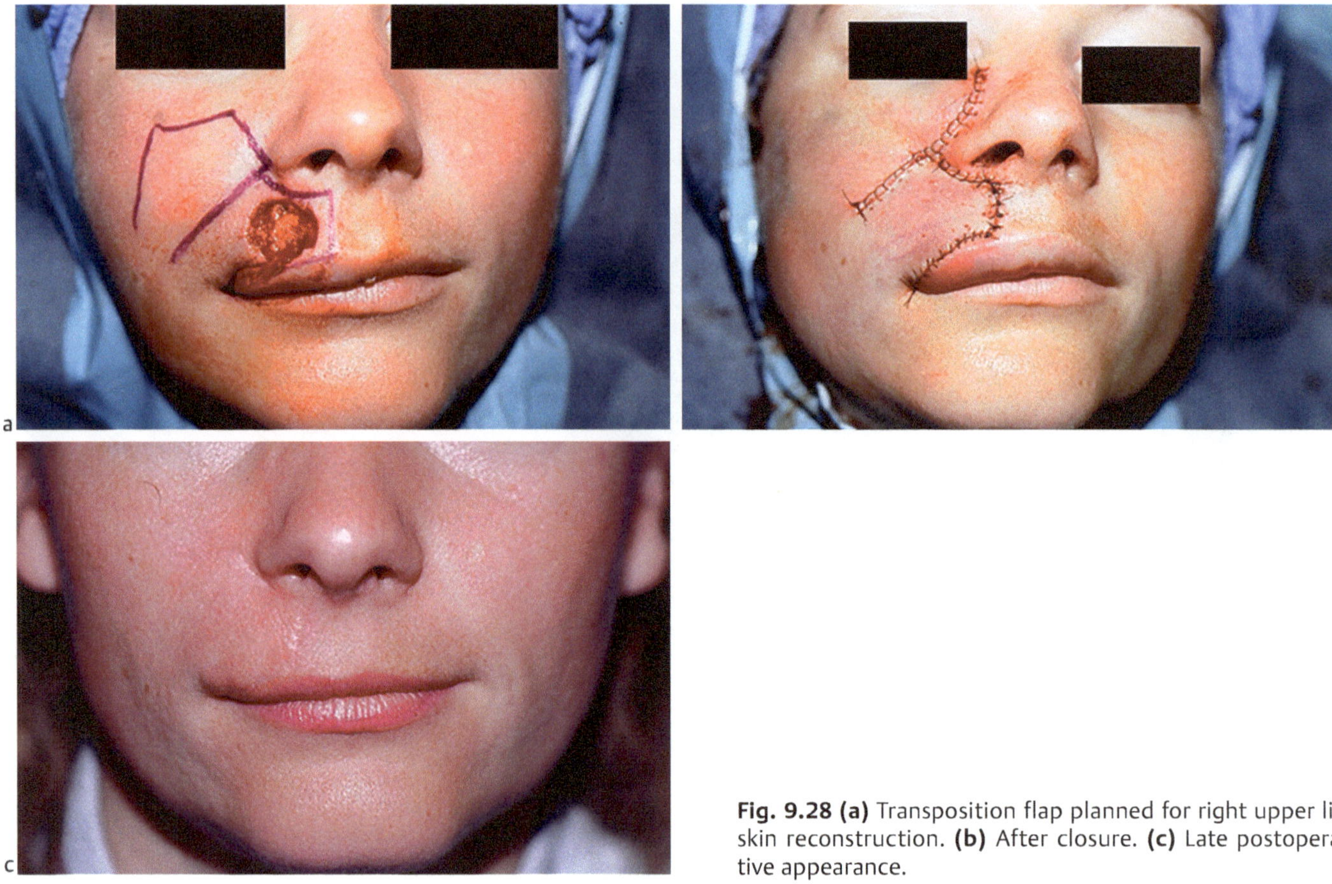

Fig. 9.28 (a) Transposition flap planned for right upper lip skin reconstruction. **(b)** After closure. **(c)** Late postoperative appearance.

Full Thickness

Full-thickness defects of the philtral subunit alone or in combination with lateral subunit defects are best treated with entire philtral subunit replacement (**Fig. 9.29**). This is done with an Abbe flap from the lower lip combined with a separate procedure for the other subunit defect (**Fig. 9.30** and **Fig. 9.31**). The Abbe flap is planned in the midline of the lower lip, with care not to cross the labiomental sulcus. As in the case of an Abbe flap for lower lip reconstruction, the flap is left pedicled on a small amount of mucosa and the labial artery. Both the flap and the donor sites are closed in three layers. Relaxing incisions in the labiomental sulcus may facilitate closure of the donor site. The vascular pedicle is divided at 3 weeks, and the mucosa is trimmed and inset as needed.

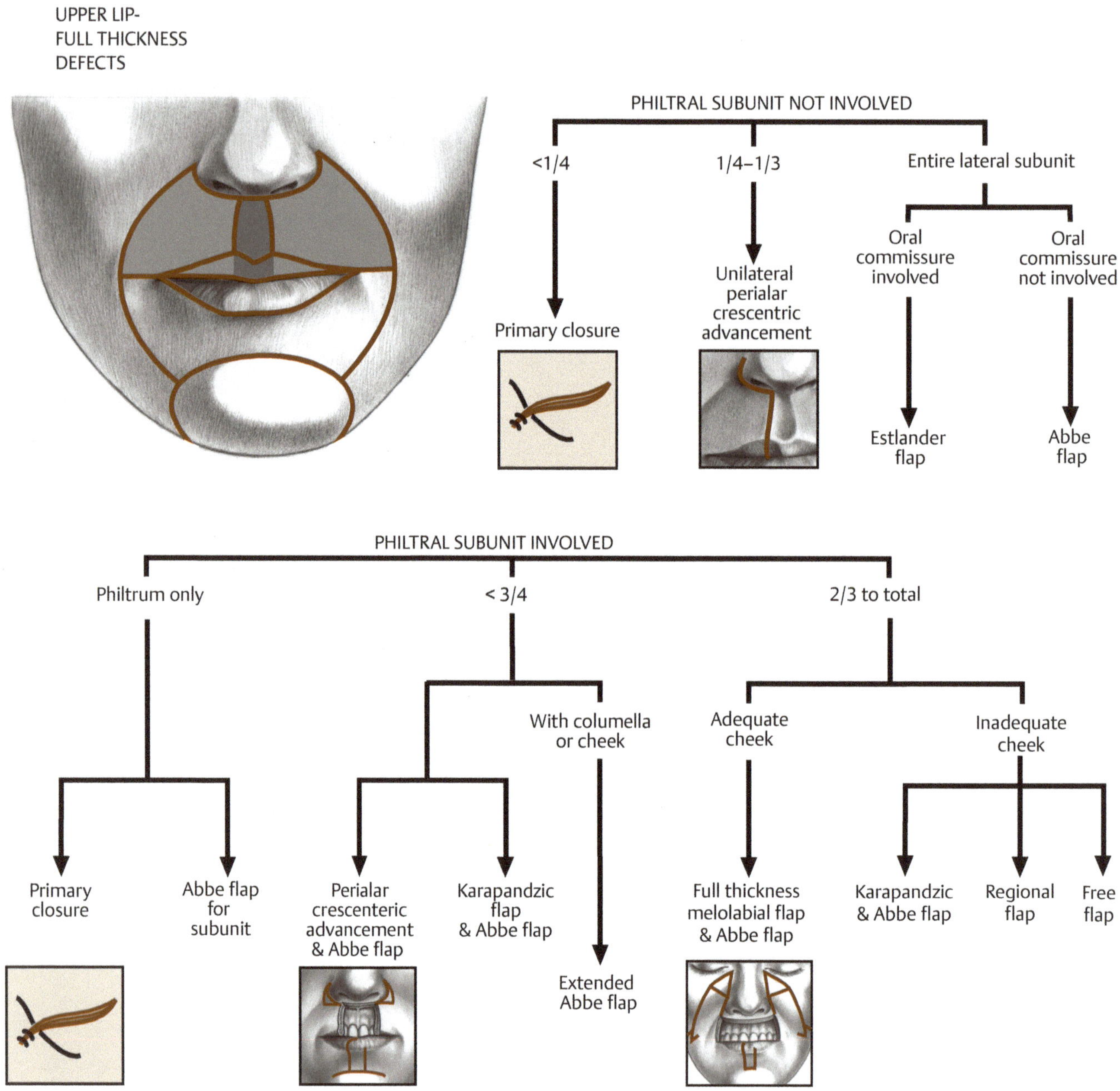

Fig. 9.29 Upper lip: full-thickness defects.

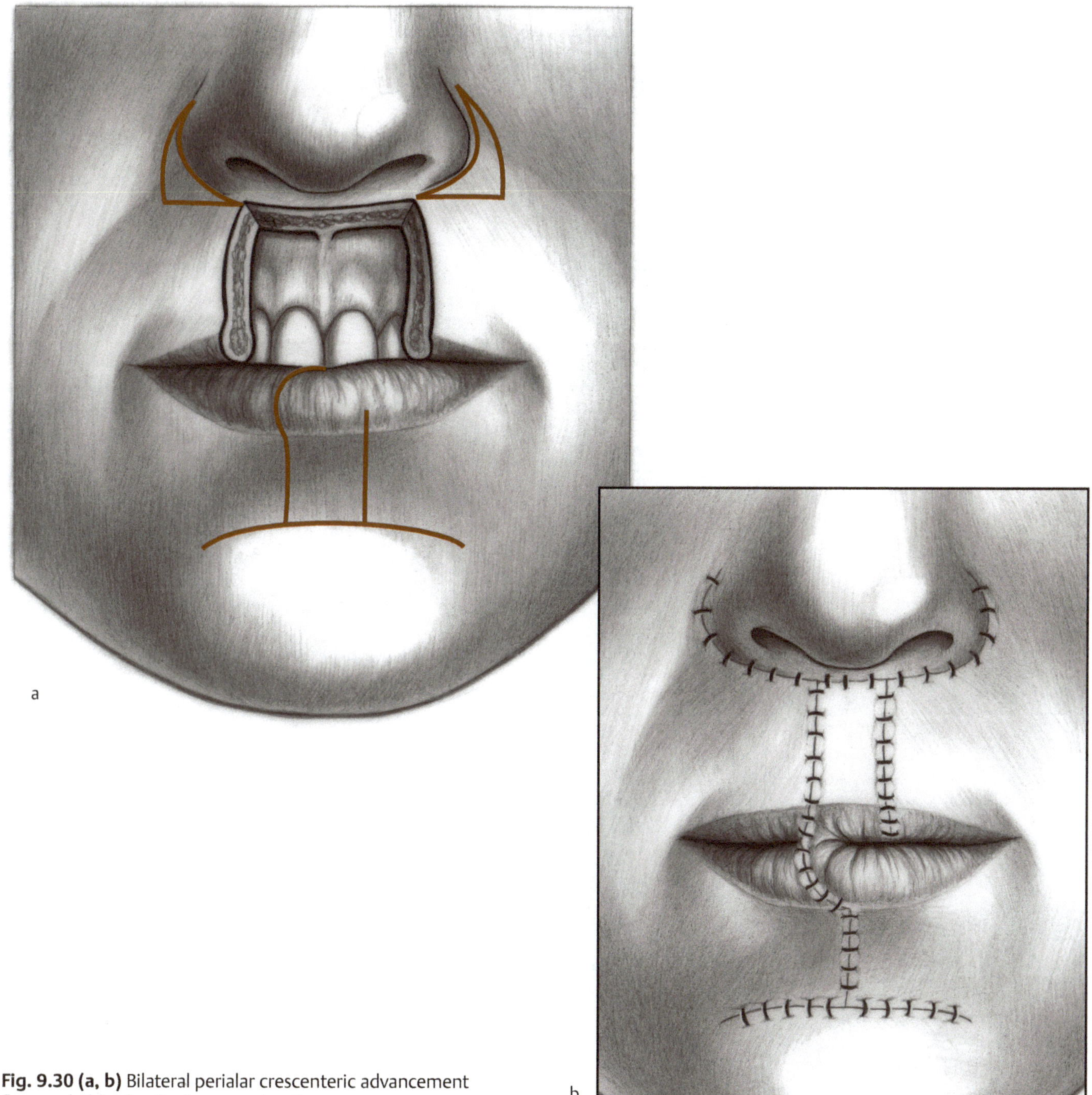

a

b

Fig. 9.30 (a, b) Bilateral perialar crescenteric advancement flaps and Abbe flap for lip reconstruction.

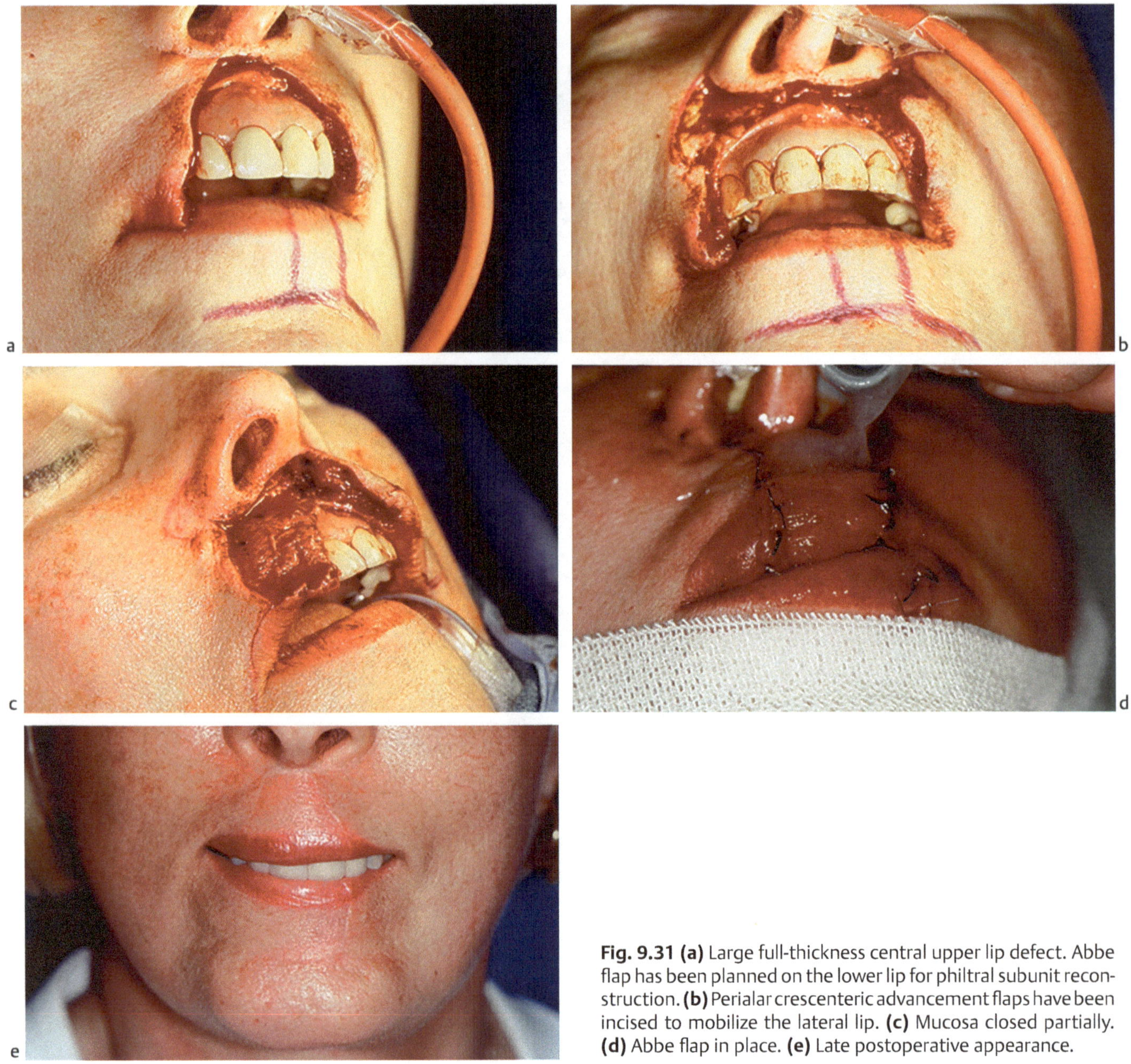

Fig. 9.31 (a) Large full-thickness central upper lip defect. Abbe flap has been planned on the lower lip for philtral subunit reconstruction. **(b)** Perialar crescenteric advancement flaps have been incised to mobilize the lateral lip. **(c)** Mucosa closed partially. **(d)** Abbe flap in place. **(e)** Late postoperative appearance.

Defects of one-fourth to one-third of the upper lip not involving the entire philtral unit can be closed primarily. This is done by standard wedge excision or rectangular excision with a perialar crescenteric advancement and three-layer closure of skin, orbicularis oris, and mucosa (**Fig. 9.32**). Prior to wedge excision, the mucocutaneous junction should be tattooed or scratched so that it can be meticulously reapproximated at closure.

Defects of one-half of the upper lip can be closed using unilateral or bilateral advancement flaps with perialar crescenteric pedicle excision. Tension on the lip itself should be minimized by deep sutures to the periosteum of the piriform aperture and nasal spine. The perialar crescenteric advancement can be done on both sides simultaneously and in combination with an Abbe flap to the philtrum to reconstruct defects up to three-fourths of the upper lip. In patients with minimal cheek laxity, most of the lateral subunits can be replaced with an Abbe flap from the lower lip. The subunit shape can be approximated by drawing a foil template from the intact corresponding subunit.

Defects involving the upper lip, cheek, and columella of the nose can be repaired with the extended Abbe flap (**Fig. 9.33**). This flap is designed the same as a standard Abbe flap but extends further into the chin and submental region to recruit more tissue.

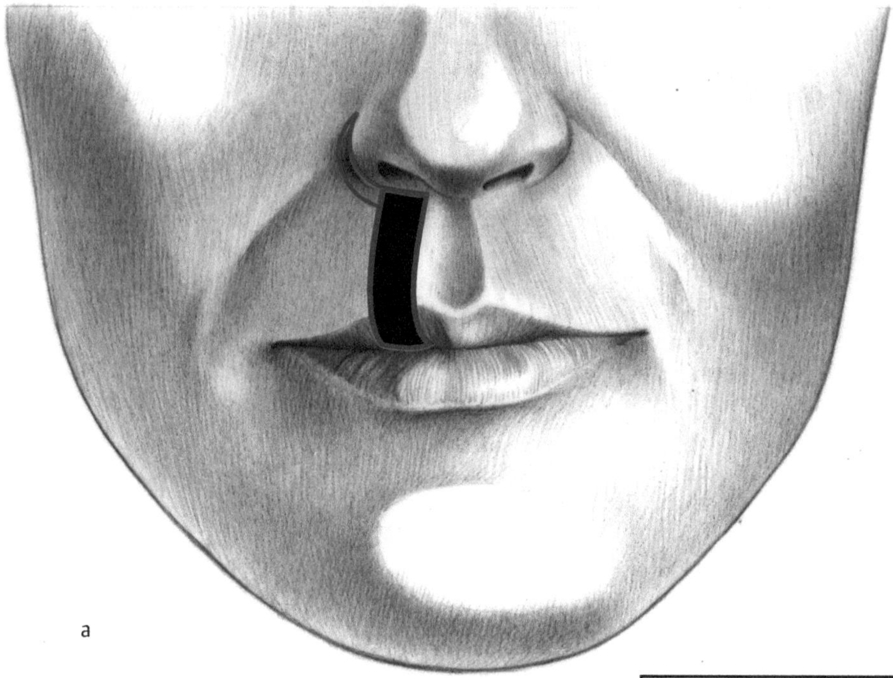

a

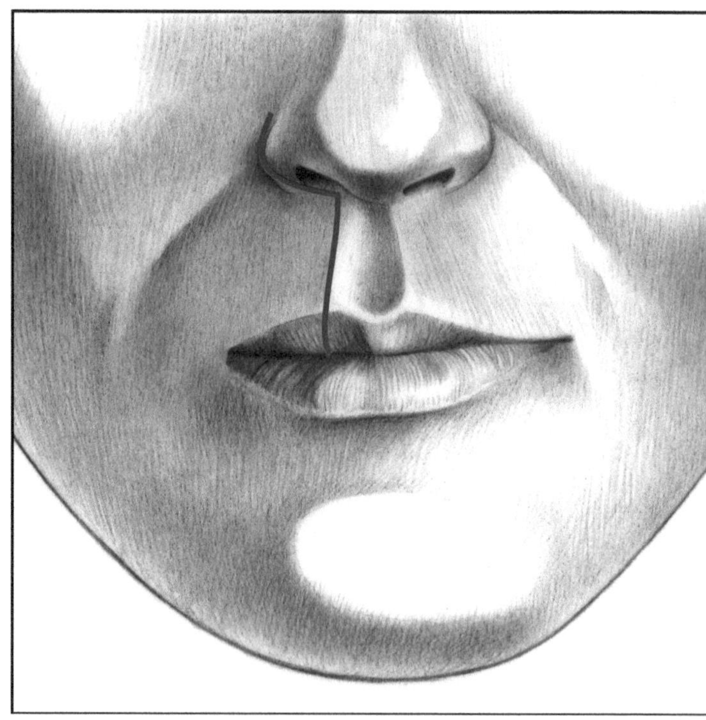

b

Fig. 9.32 (a, b) Primary wedge closure facilitated by unilateral perialar crescenteric flap advancement.

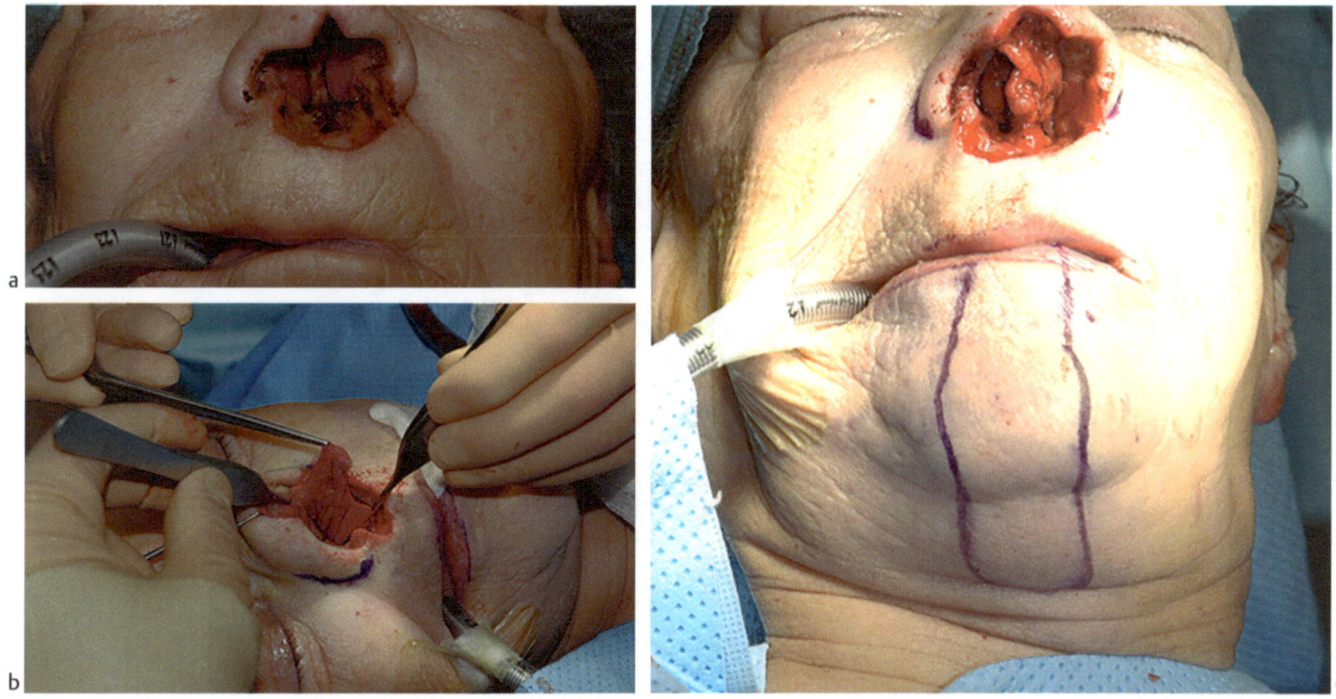

Fig. 9.33 (a) Defect of the columella, upper lip, and caudal septum. **(b)** Mucosal flap from the inferior turbinate to envelope cartilage grafts for tip support. **(c)** An extended Abbe flap is drawn on the lower lip and submental area.

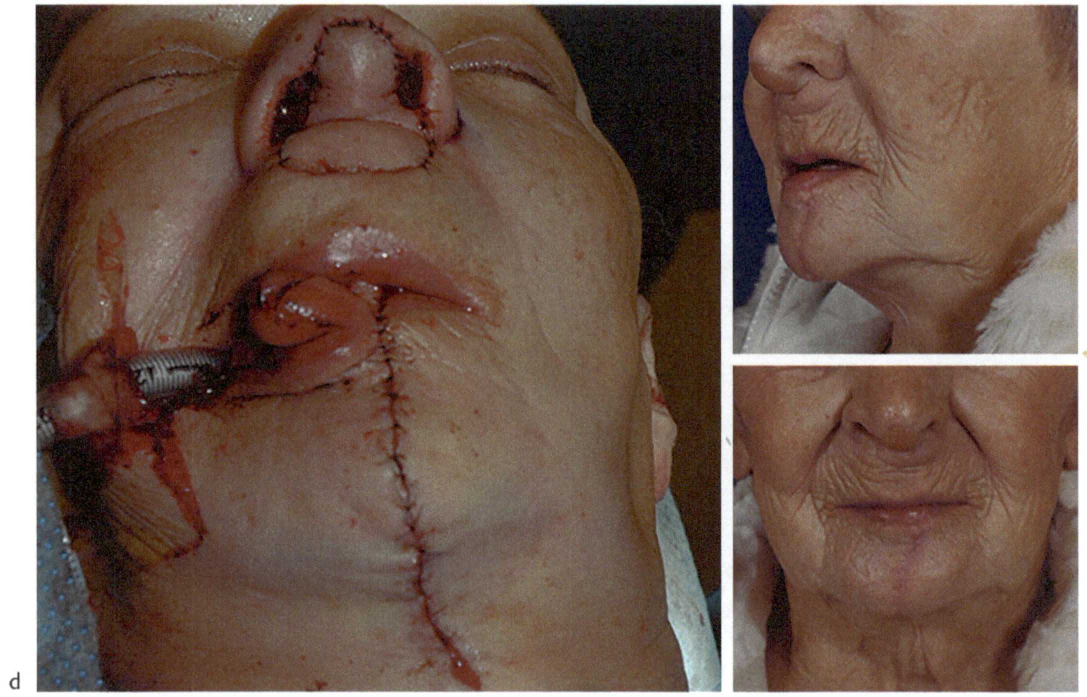

Fig. 9.33 (d) An extended Abbe flap shown in place with a pedicle from the lower lip and placed in under the upper lip. **(e)** Oblique view early postoperative after pedicle division. **(f)** Frontal view early postoperative with intact lip function.

Total upper lip defects are both uncommon and very difficult to reconstruct adequately. In patients with significant cheek laxity, the entire upper lip can be replaced by transposing full-thickness flaps from the cheeks and using an Abbe flap for the philtral subunit (**Fig. 9.34**). The melolabial flaps are incised full thickness, and the subcutaneous tissue near the pedicle, at the oral commissure, is left intact. The cheek tissue is rotated into place. The Abbe flap is performed as previously described, and a standard three-layer closure is done. The mucosa is advanced over the melolabial flaps to re-create the lip mucosa. Standing cones are excised to allow donor site closure within the melolabial and nasofacial creases.

In patients with insufficient cheek tissue, the reverse Karapandzic flap is an option (see discussion under Lower Lip and Chin: Full Thickness). The major drawback of this flap is the resultant microstomia. This can be especially problematic for patients who wear dentures and who may have trouble placing them. In some cases, regional flaps or free flaps may be used, but such procedures are beyond the scope of this book.

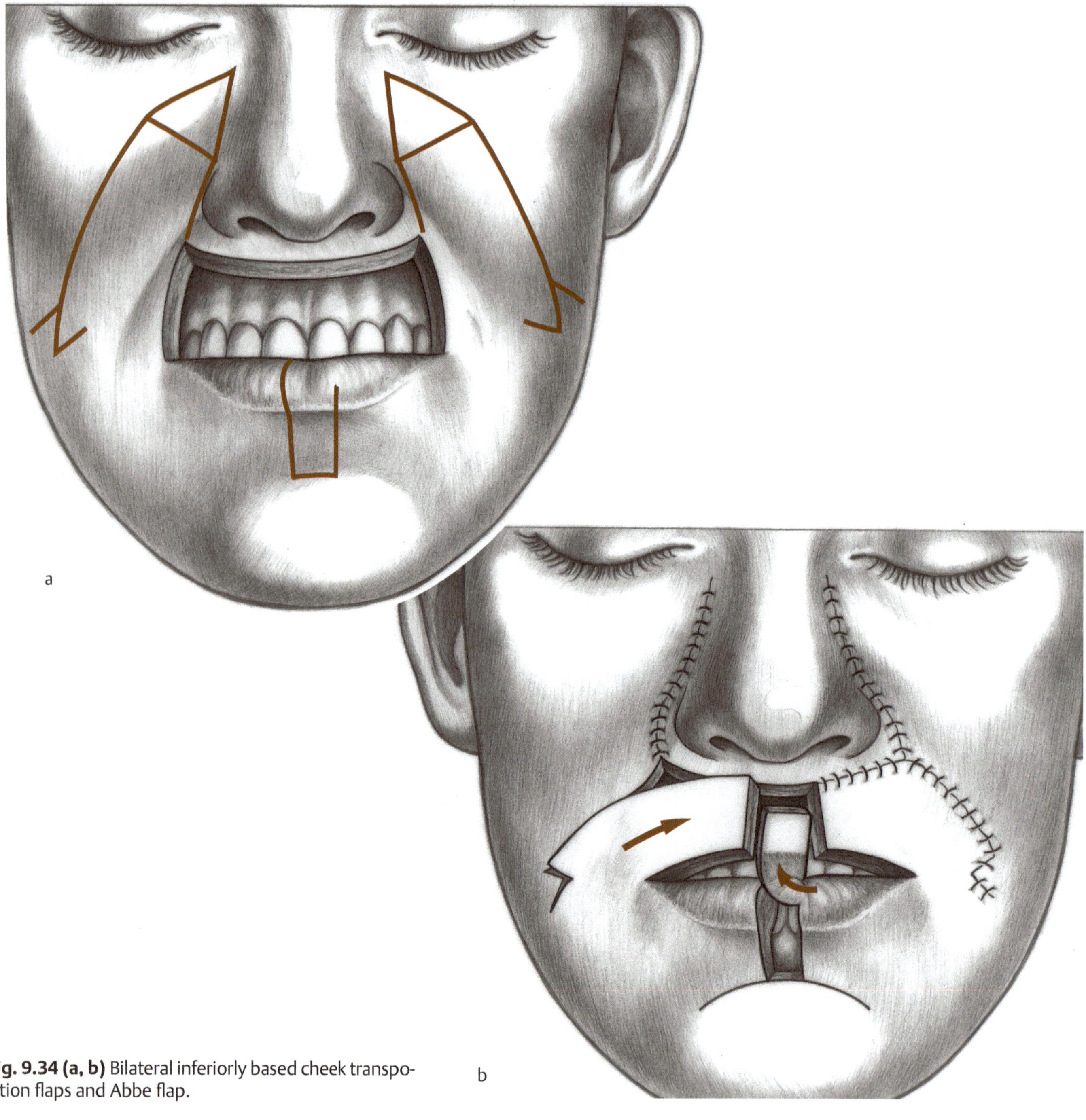

a

b

Fig. 9.34 (a, b) Bilateral inferiorly based cheek transposition flaps and Abbe flap.

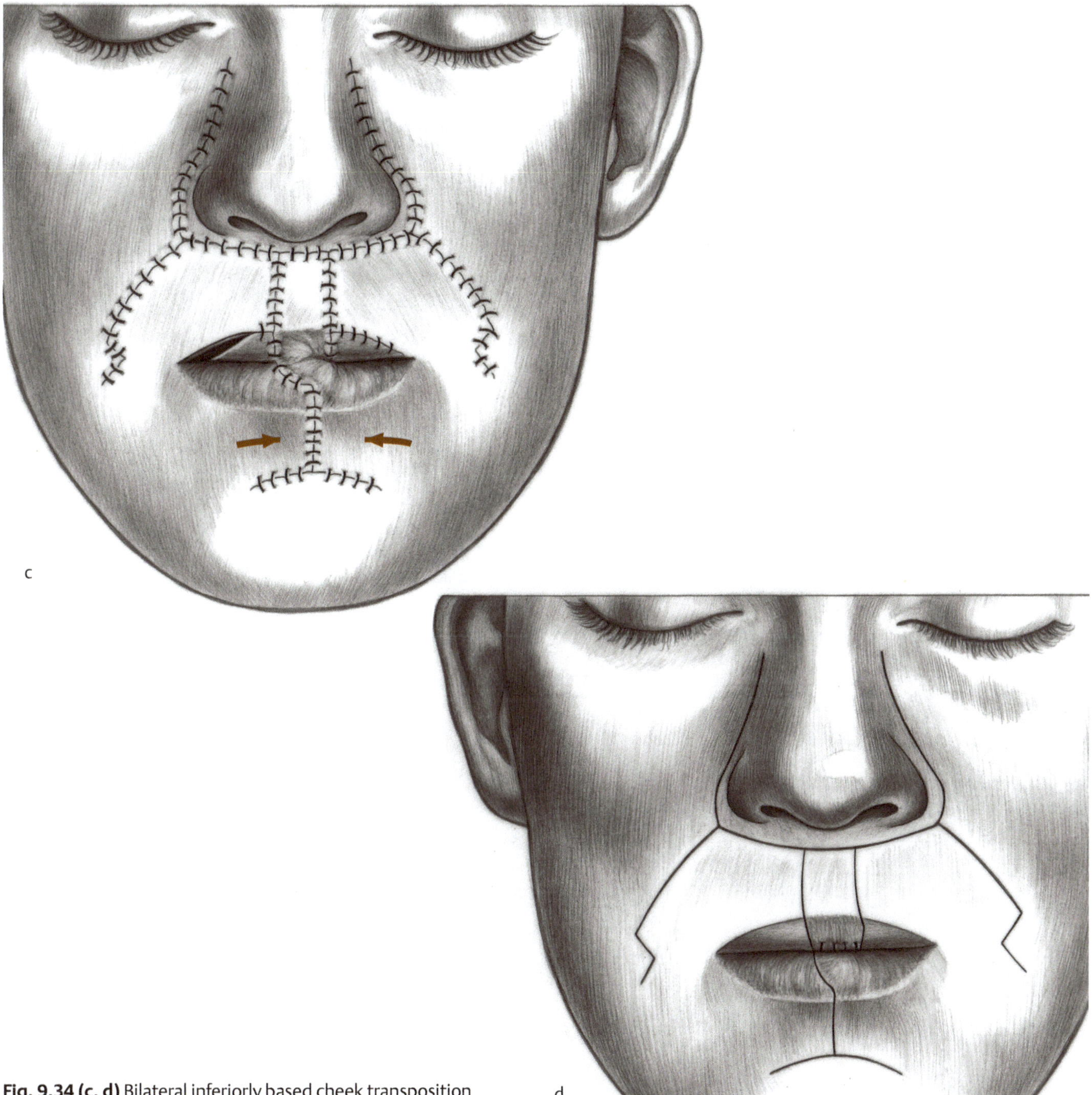
c

d

Fig. 9.34 (c, d) Bilateral inferiorly based cheek transposition flaps and Abbe flap.

Suggested Reading

Antia NH , Buch VI. Chondrocutaneous advancement flap for marginal defect of the ear. Plast Reconstr Surg 1967;39:472–477

Brent B. Reconstruction of traumatic ear deformities. Clin Plast Surg 1978;5:437–445

Brent B, Byrd HS. Secondary ear reconstruction with cartilage grafts covered by axial, random, and free flaps of temporoparietal fascia. Plast Reconstr Surg 1983;72:141–152

Bumsted RM. Methods of therapy and reconstruction of malignant auricular neoplasms. Facial Plast Surg 1987;5:19–27

Bumsted RM, Ceilley RI. Auricular malignant neoplasms: identifi cation of high-risk lesions and selection of method of reconstruction. Arch Otolaryngol 1982;108:225–231

Chen C, Chen ZJ. Reconstruction of the concha of the ear using a postauricular island fl ap. Plast Reconstr Surg 1990; 86:569–572

Converse JM. Traumatic deformities of the auricle. In: Surgical Treatment of Facial Injuries. Baltimore: Williams & Wilkins; 1974:11289–11334

Field LM. The single pedicle retroauricular advancement flap. J Dermatol Surg Oncol 1988;14:722–727

Krespi YP, Ries WP , Shugar JMA , et al . Auricular reconstruction with postauricular myocutaneous flap. Otolaryngol Head Neck Surg 1983;91:193–196

Mellette JR, Jr. Ear reconstruction with local flaps. J Dermatol Surg Oncol 1991;17:176–182

Millard DR, Jr. Reconstruction of one-third plus of the auricular circumference. Plast Reconstr Surg 1992;90:475–478

10 Graft Harvest Techniques

Summary

This chapter focuses on the surgical principles involved with harvest of grafting material for reconstruction principles discussed in previous chapters. We provide specific techniques for septal cartilage and perpendicular bone harvest for reconstruction of nasal defects. When such sources are deemed to be insufficient, the surgeon may consider auricular or costal cartilage harvesting. Lastly, we discuss techniques for harvesting split calvarial bone graft.

Keywords: costal cartilage, auricular cartilage, calvarial bone graft, septal cartilage, graft harvest, autologous

♦ Introduction

Certain autogenous grafts are commonly used in conjunction with the reconstructive techniques presented in this book (**Fig. 10.1**). The most common grafts harvested are septal cartilage and bone, conchal cartilage, costal cartilage and/or rib bone, and calvarial bone. The harvest techniques presented are not exhaustive, but they will provide reliable materials for the surgeon. The authors advocate the use of autogenous materials, in conjunction with maxillofacial plating where necessary, over the use of nonautogenous materials in most cases.

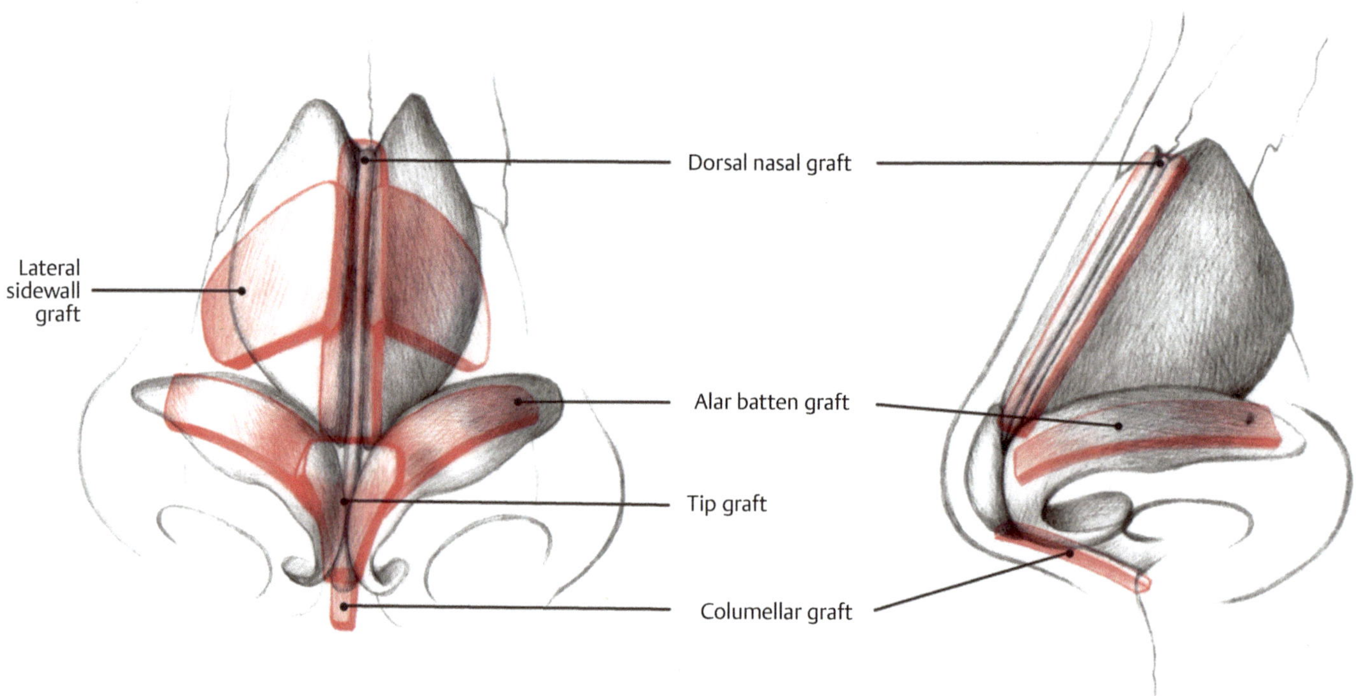

Fig. 10.1 Grafts commonly used in nasal reconstruction.

♦ Septal Cartilage and Bone

Septal cartilage grafts can be harvested from the quadrangular cartilage, with care to preserve the 1 cm caudal and dorsal strut that is necessary for nasal tip support (**Fig. 10.2**). Additionally, the perpendicular plate of the ethmoid bone and the vomer can also be used for grafting materials. These grafts are especially useful for nasal reconstruction where they are commonly used for nasal tip, nasal dorsum, nasal sidewall, and caudal septal reconstruction. The materials are very pliable, and holes can be drilled into the thin bone with an 18-gauge needle or septal auger for suture fixation. The grafts are harvested with standard septoplasty techniques.

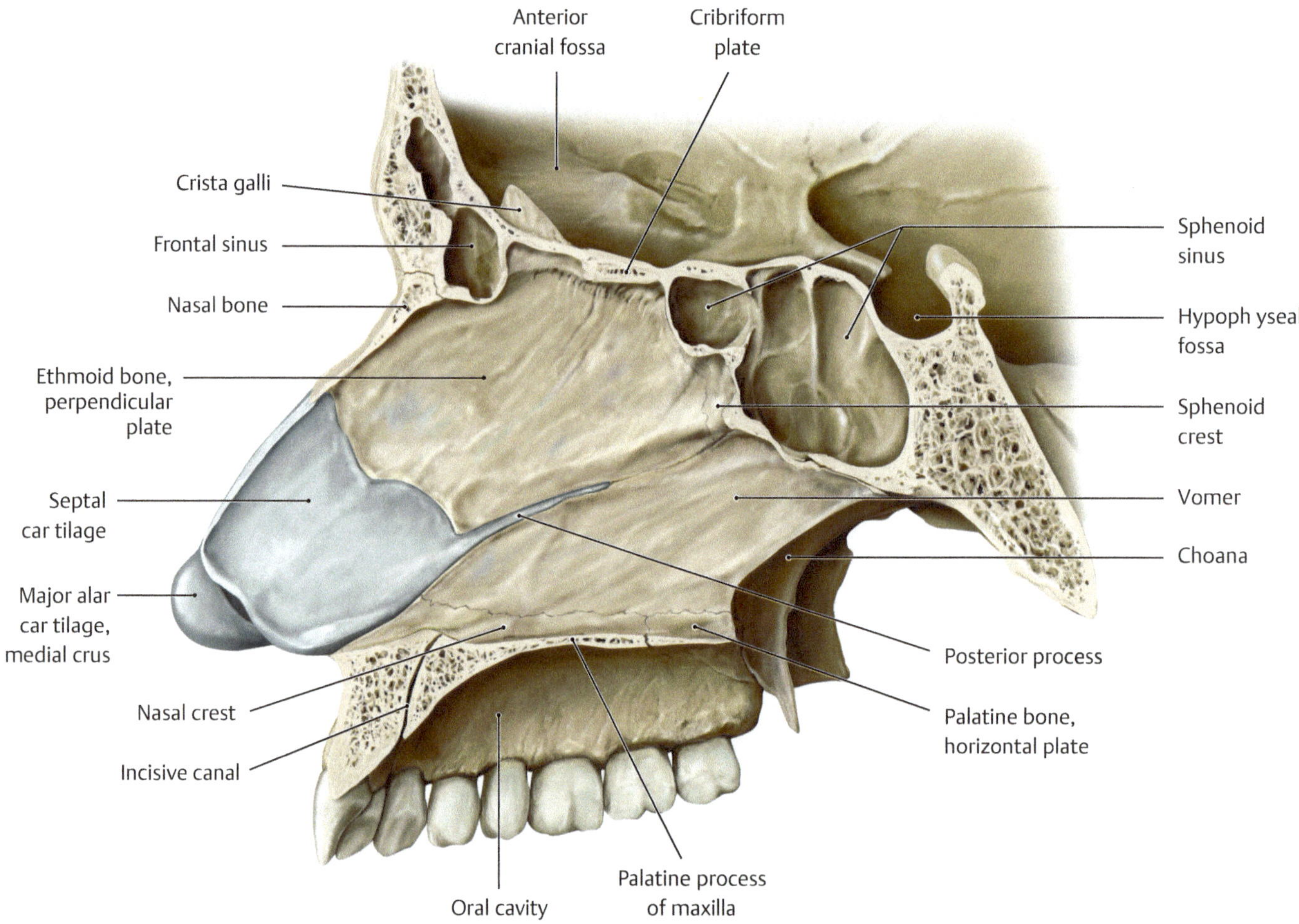

Fig. 10.2 Parasagittal section of the nasal septum viewed from the left side. The left lateral wall of the nasal cavity has been removed with the adjacent bones. The nasal septum consists of an anterior cartilaginous part, the septal cartilage, and a posterior bony part. The posterior process of the cartilaginous septum extends deep into the bony septum. Reproduced with permission from Schuenke M, et al. Thieme Atlas of Anatomy: Head and Neuroanatomy. New York: Thieme; 2007. Illustration by Karl Wesker.

♦ Ear Cartilage

Cartilage grafts are usually harvested from the concha cymba and/or the concha cavum. These grafts are useful in nasal and eyelid reconstruction. By restricting the harvest to these sites, the shape of the ear will not be distorted. The cartilage can be harvested from either an anterior incision following the antihelical fold boundary with the conchal cartilage or a posterior incision over the site to be harvested (**Fig. 10.3** and **Fig. 10.4**). The perichondrium can be left intact on the cartilage or in situ. In older patients, it is best to harvest the perichondrium with the cartilage, as the cartilage tends to slightly ossify with age and become brittle. The wound can be closed with 5–0 fast-absorbing suture and a tie-over bolster to prevent hematoma formation. A simple bolster can be fashioned from dental rolls (one on the back and one on the front) affixed with a 3–0 suture on Keith needles that pass through the site of graft harvest. The bolster is usually left in place 3 to 5 days.

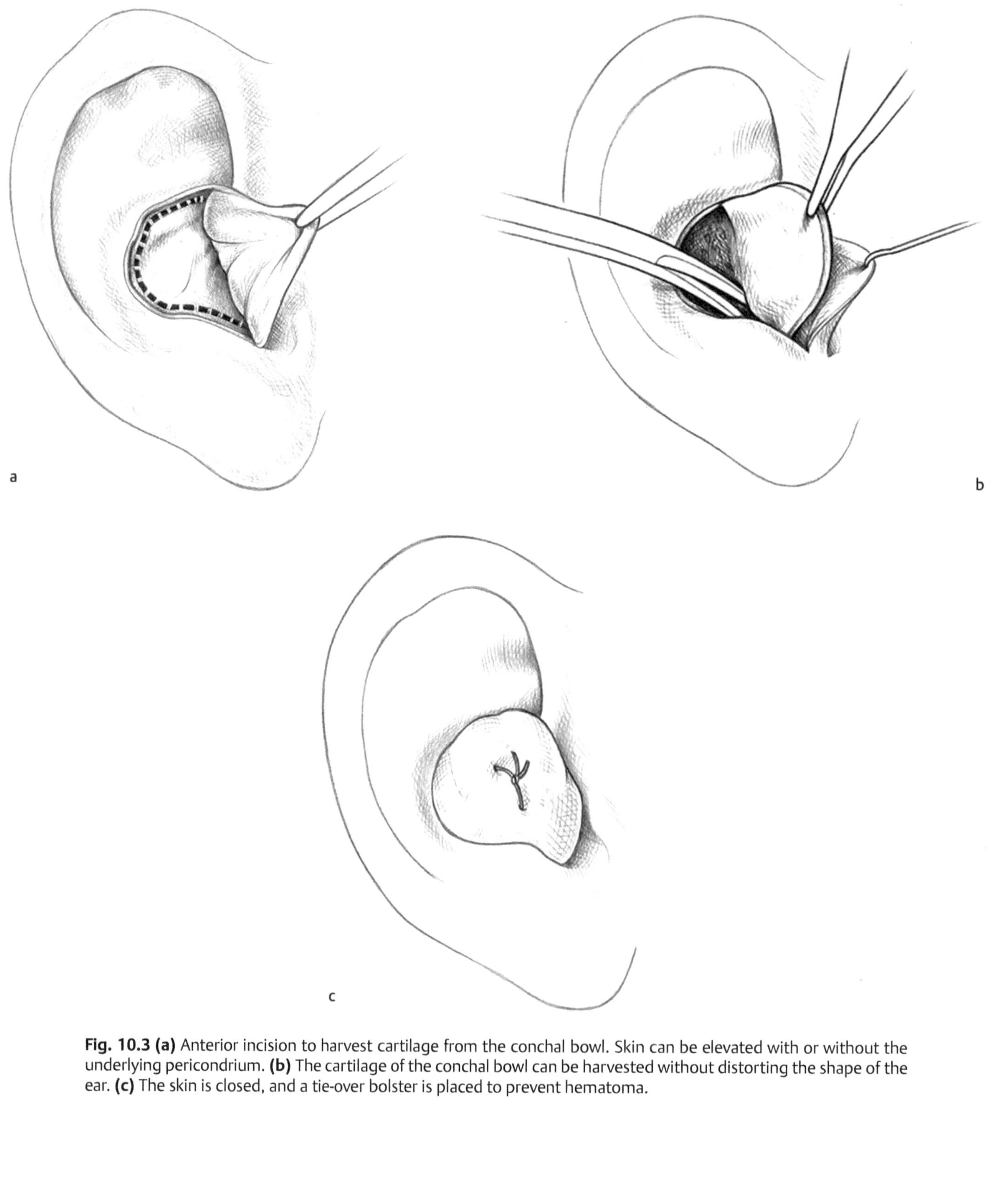

Fig. 10.3 **(a)** Anterior incision to harvest cartilage from the conchal bowl. Skin can be elevated with or without the underlying pericondrium. **(b)** The cartilage of the conchal bowl can be harvested without distorting the shape of the ear. **(c)** The skin is closed, and a tie-over bolster is placed to prevent hematoma.

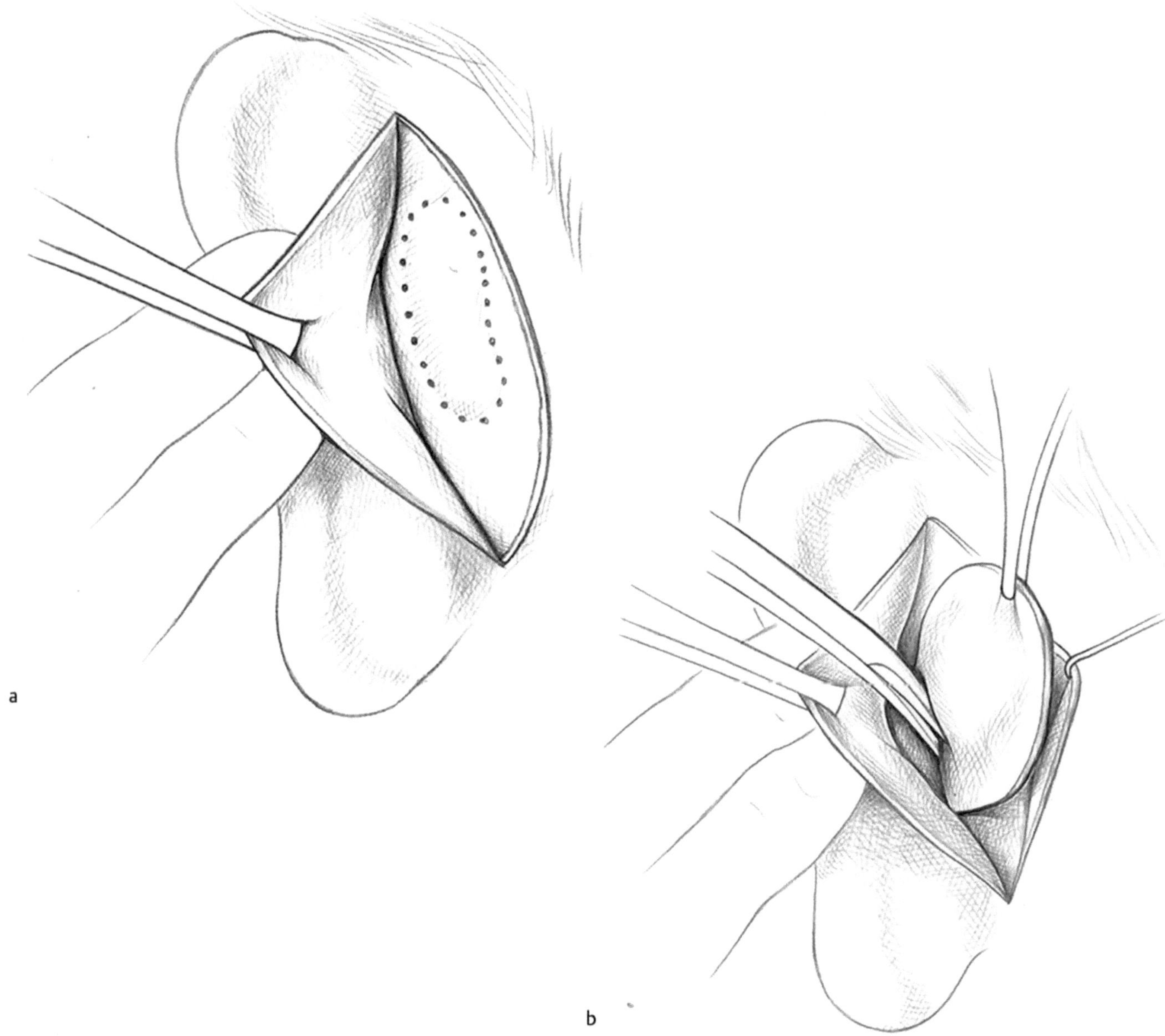

Fig. 10.4 (a) A postauricular incision may be used as well. (b) Same cartilage harvested from the postauricular excision.

♦ Costal Cartilage and Rib Bone

Costal cartilage is an excellent alternative to ear and septal cartilage when large cartilage grafts are needed. The 8th, 9th, and 10th ribs are the most common sites for harvest. They can be harvested as cartilage alone or include a portion of the rib bone to reconstruct the entire nasal dorsum.

The harvest starts by marking the appropriate rib for harvest (**Fig. 10.5**). Skin incision is made sharply for 3 to 5 cm over the chosen rib. Electrocautery or blunt dissection is performed through the underlying chest musculature until the perichondrium of the chosen rib is reached (**Fig. 10.6**). At that point, the perichondrium is incised with electrocautery, and the material to be harvested is circumferentially dissected at its medial extent with a septal elevator. Once the cartilage is elevated from the underlying tissue and pleura, a malleable retractor is placed under the medial margin of the graft site, and the cartilage is cut with a no. 10 blade. Then, by pulling the graft away from the chest wall, the rest of the posterior perichondrial dissection can be executed with little risk of pleural injury. The posterior graft is cut.

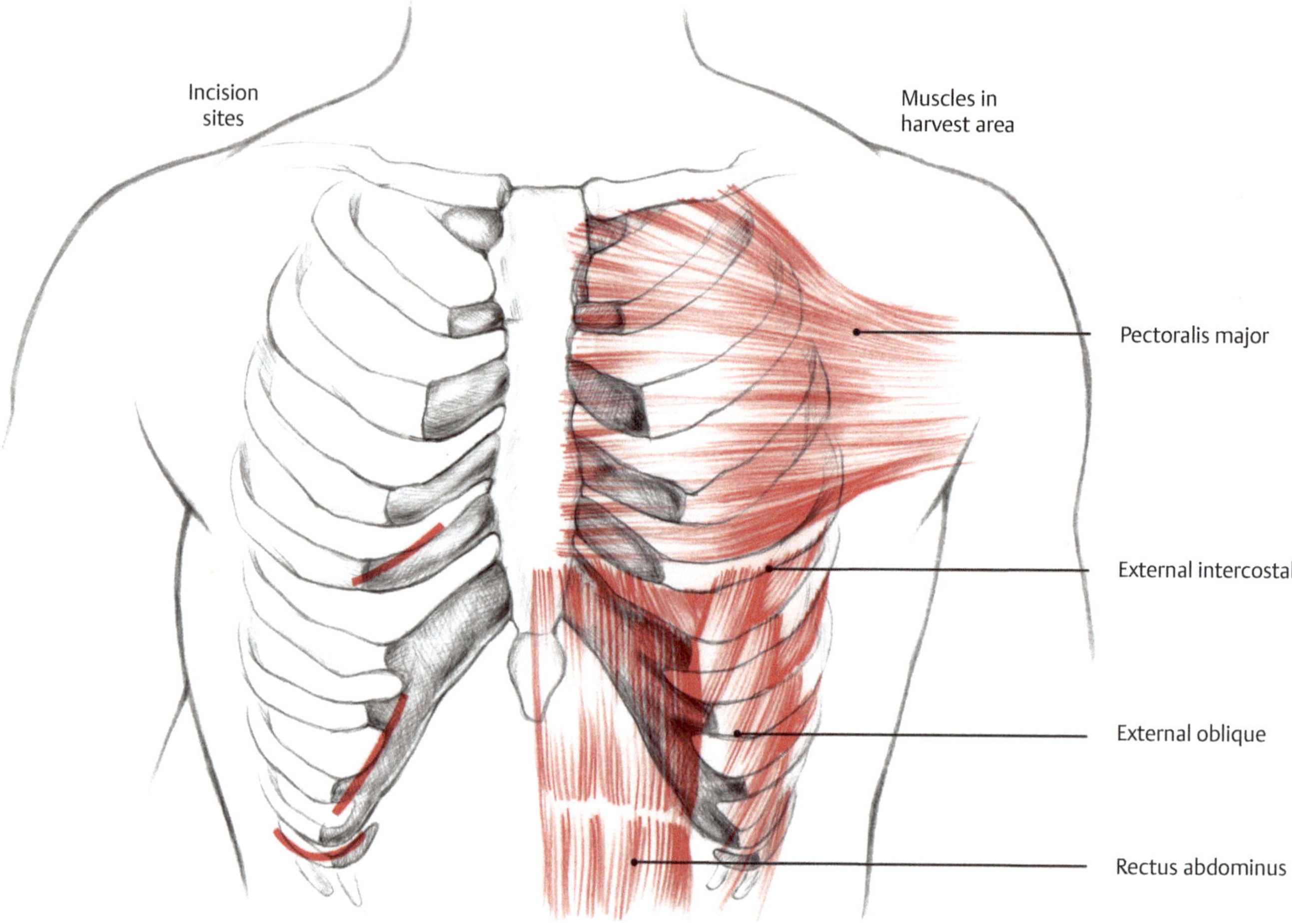

Fig. 10.5 Common incision sites to harvest rib bone and/or costal cartilage grafts.

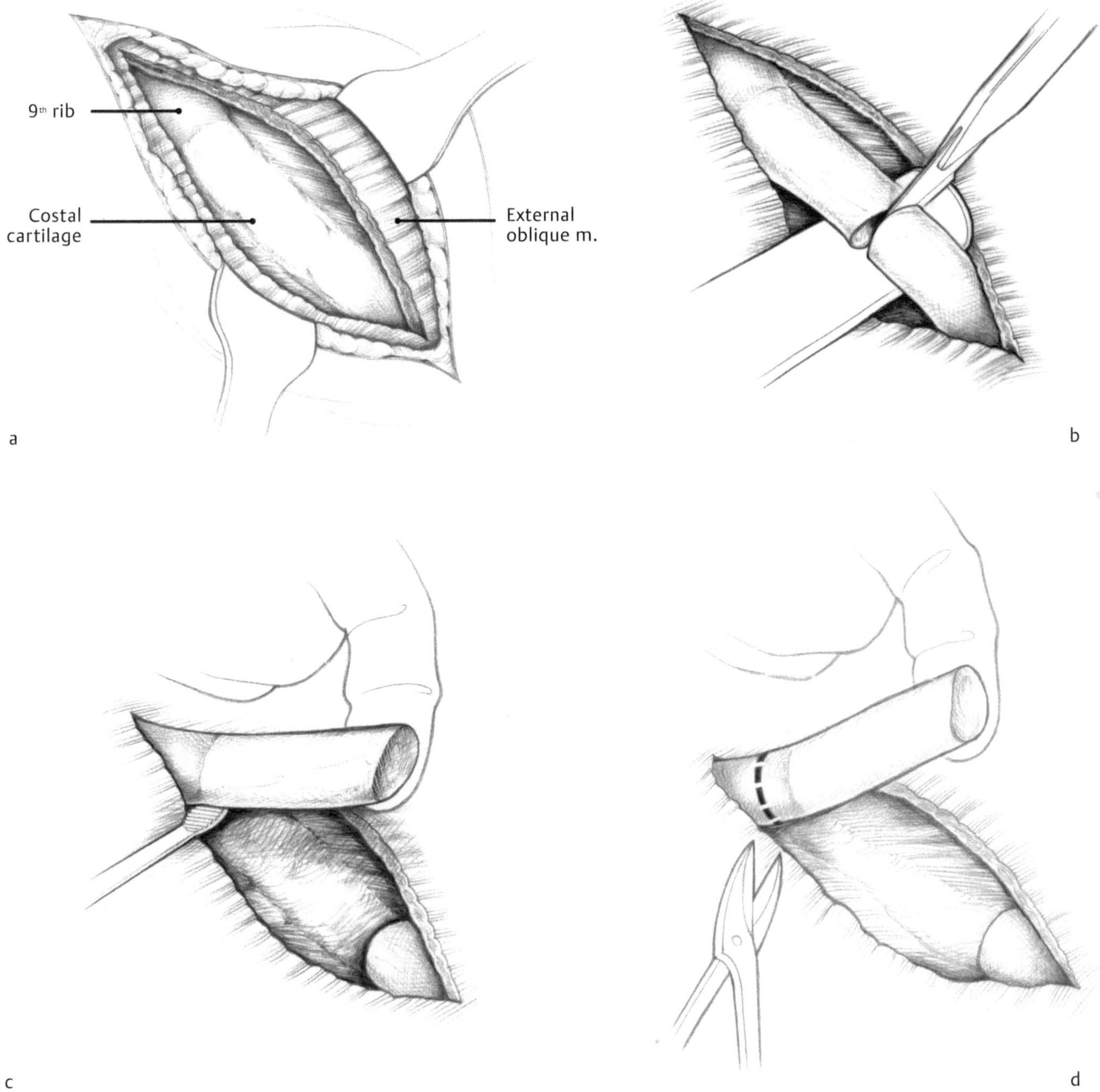

Fig. 10.6 (a) An incision is made over the rib to be harvested. **(b)** After subperichondrial elevation on the medial rib, an elevator is placed under the rib, and the rib is cut. **(c)** Subperichondrial and subperiosteal elevation is then done laterally under direct vision. **(d)** The rib is cut laterally.

Prior to closure, the cavity is filled with saline, and the anesthesiologist applies positive pressure ventilation. If there are bubbles present, a pleural defect is searched out. If a pleural tear is evident, it is treated by passing a soft rubber catheter into the defect (**Fig. 10.7**). Any air accumulated in the pleural space is evacuated. A "purse-string" suture of resorbable material is sewn around the catheter. The purse string is pulled tight and tied down as an assistant removes the catheter from the intrapleural space while applying suction to the catheter on the way out. The process is repeated until there are no longer air bubbles present. The intercostal space is injected with long-lasting local anesthetic, and the wound is closed in layers, including the perichondrium, the muscle and fascia, the subcutaneous tissue, and the skin. A suction drain in the subcutaneous layer is usually used to prevent hematoma formation.

Costal cartilage is quite thick. It can be split into thinner sheets by using a dermatome blade to split the material. Care must be taken to split the material equally on either side to prevent warping. The cartilage is then placed in an antibiotic solution for at least 15 minutes prior to use to assess for any warping. If the cartilage has not warped in that time frame, it does not tend to warp long term.

Rib bone can be split with a power saw. If it is split, the raw split surface should be put into contact with a raw bone surface and fixed with screws to stimulate osteoinduction and thereby prevent resorption.

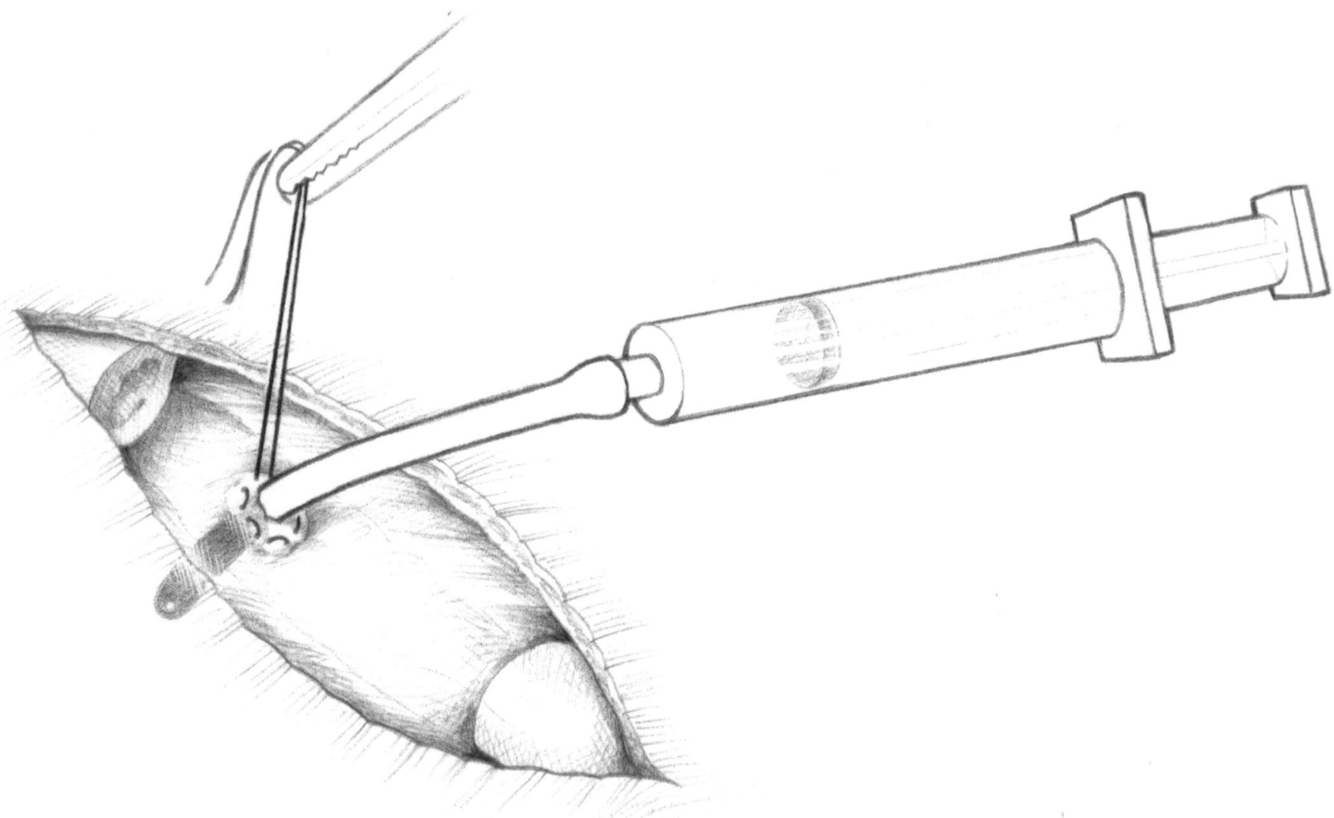

Fig. 10.7 Pleural defects are repaired with a purse-string suture.

♦ Split Calvarial Bone Graft

The outer table of calvarium is an excellent bone graft harvest site. The bone is thin but very rigid. The material is excellent for reconstruction of the anterior maxilla, nasal dorsum, orbital walls, and skull. The outer table is usually harvested from the parietal skull, at least 1 cm above the attachment of the temporalis muscle, and at least 2 cm from any suture lines, or the midline, where the bone becomes monocortical (**Fig. 10.8**). A coronal or hemicoronal incision is made, and the pericranium is elevated over the site for graft harvest. The bone to be harvested is outlined with a large cutting bur (**Fig. 10.9**). A trough is drilled with the cutting bur until the diploic space is encountered. This trough is usually ~5 to 10 mm wide, to accept an angled oscillating saw blade parallel to the inner table. The angled saw is then used to free the bone graft along all edges. It is best for the first graft to be harvested to be only 1.0 to 1.5 cm wide. Subsequent grafts are easier to harvest because of the large trough left by the removal of the first graft. Palpation under the graft for continued areas of adherence is done with a septal elevator. Usually, the last attachments can be freed by prying with the septal elevator. Hemostasis of the bone is achieved with bone wax. The wound is closed in layers with pericranial sutures and skin staples over a suction drain.

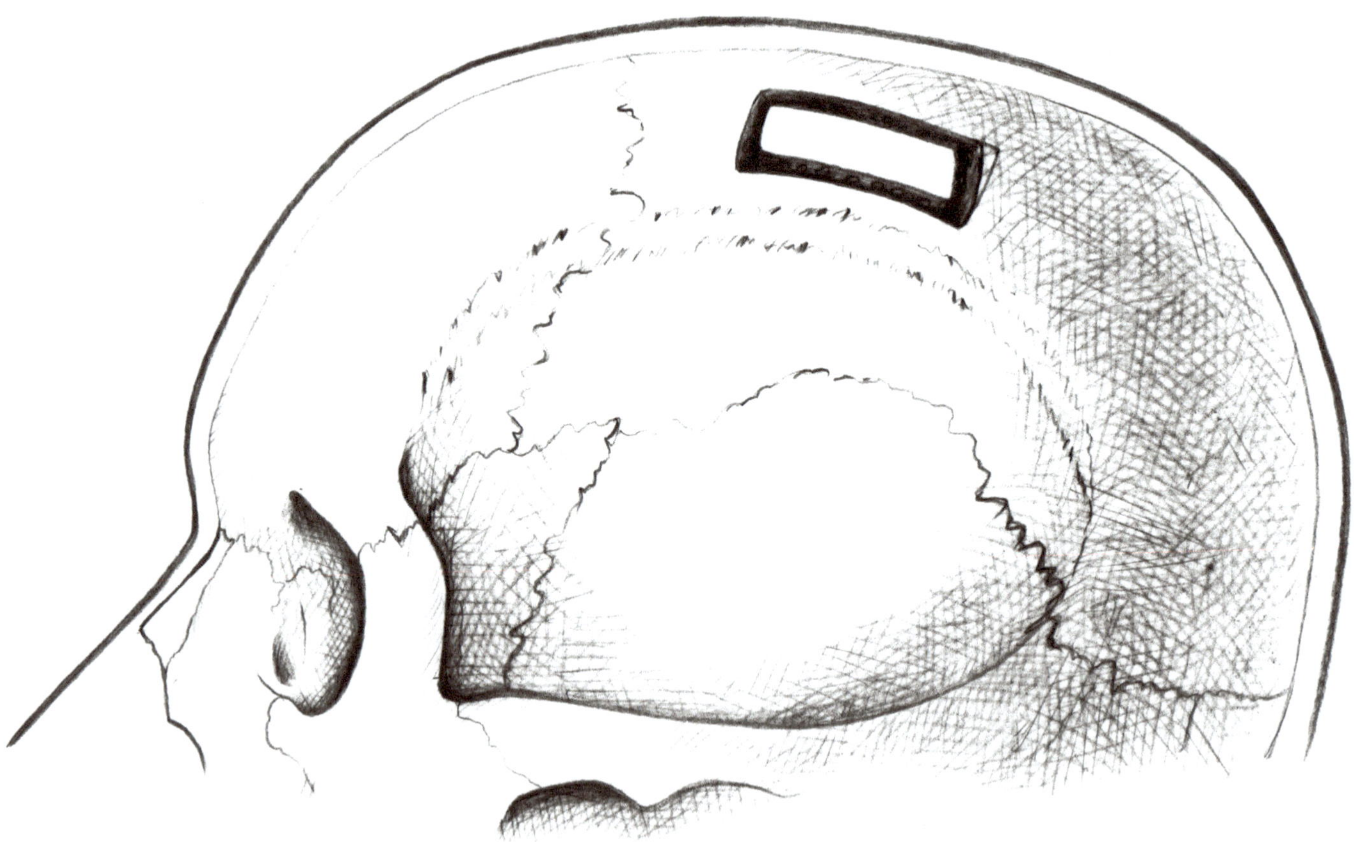

Fig. 10.8 Parietal skull is the usual site to harvest split calvarial bone grafts.

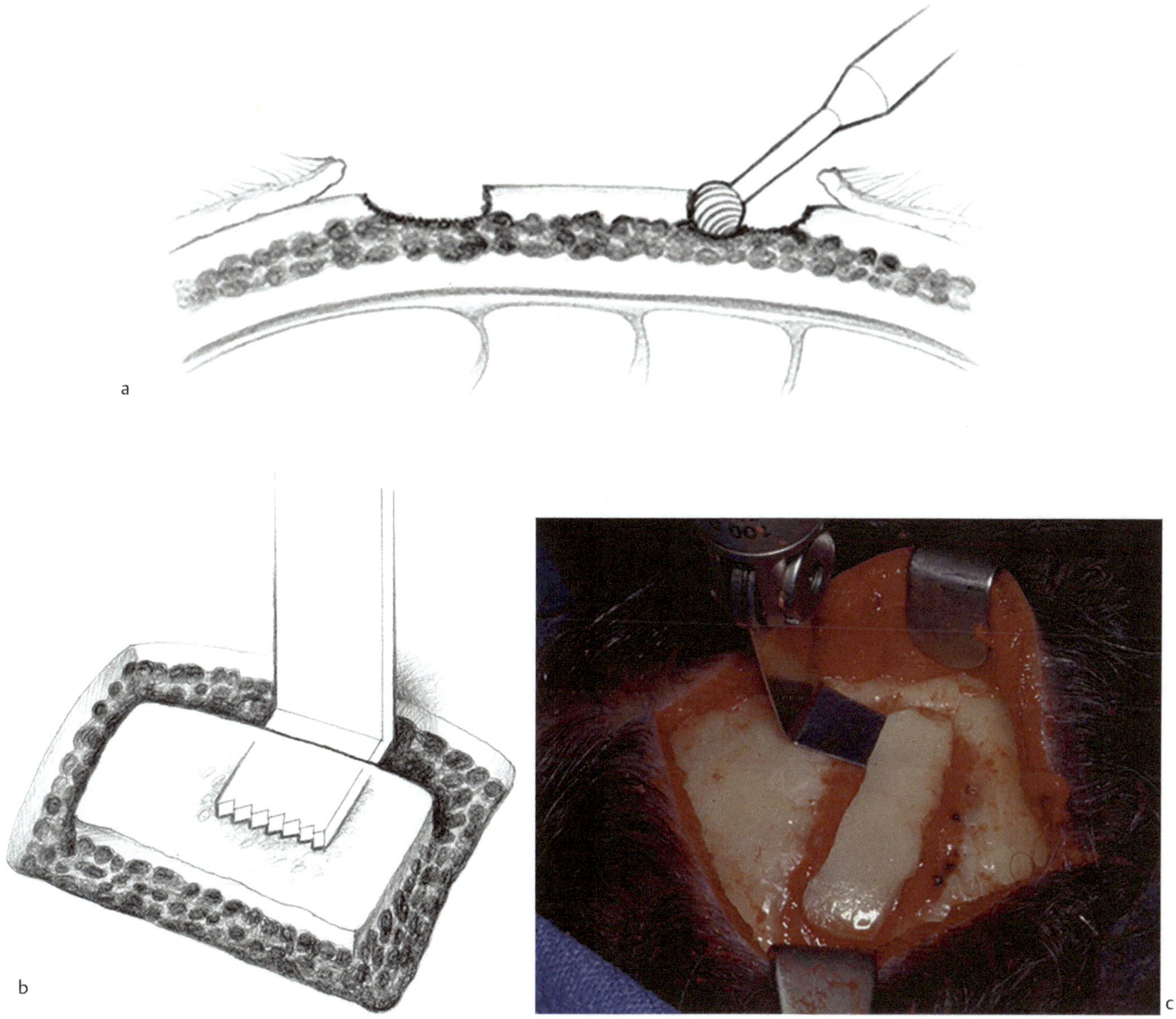

Fig. 10.9 (a) A trough is drilled around the planned graft and taken down to the diploic space of the skull. (b) The trough is tapered enough to facilitate a saw blade fitting into the diploic space parallel to the inner table. (c) Photograph of saw harvesting bone graft as described.

Suggested Reading

Khurana D, Sherris DA. Grafting materials for augmentation septorhinoplasty. Curr Opin Otolaryngol 1999;7:210–213

Otley CC, Sherris DA. Spectrum of cartilage grafting in cutaneous reconstructive surgery. J Am Acad Dermatol 1998;39(6):982–992

Sherris DA, Kern EB. The versatile autogenous rib graft in septorhinoplasty. Am J Rhinol 1998;12(3):221–227

Index

Note: Page numbers followed by *f* indicate figures.

F

G

H

T

U